Taste Versus Cancer

Taste Versus Cancer

David W Brown

Disclaimer

"I am not a doctor, but I have dedicated many years to researching the impact of a plant-based diet on cancer and exploring the harmful chemical processes that can affect our health. The information provided in this book is supported by scientific studies, all of which are available on thep53.com website for those who have purchased the book. While I do not offer personalized medical advice, I share insights from research studies and the conclusions drawn by scientists in the field. A plant-based diet has been shown to contribute to the reversal of certain cancers and other health conditions, and it may reduce the risk of developing certain cancers, as supported by the cited studies. To access the full list of references, please email proof of purchase to dave@thep53.com, and you will be given login credentials to view the sources used in this book." David W. Brown

This book is dedicated to my dad, who taught me to question everything and seek my own understanding. Throughout my life, I've embraced this challenge, knowing that truth will always prevail. Thanks for everything, Dad.

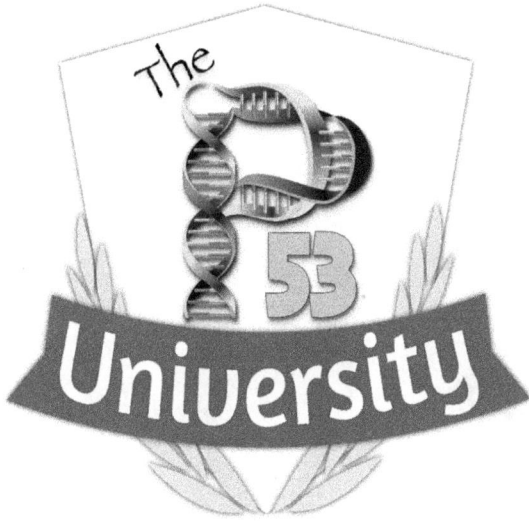

The P53 University

p53university.com

Introduction

In this book, *"Taste Versus Cancer,"* I will attempt to explain one of the most critical yet overlooked aspects of cancer treatment and prevention: diet. This book is born out of a deep concern for the increasing number of people who, despite being diagnosed with cancer, continue to make food choices that not only fuel their disease but also hinder their recovery. The relationship between taste and health is complex, often clouded by emotional, psychological, and environmental factors that drive individuals to prioritize short-term gratification over long-term well-being. In *"Taste Versus Cancer,"* I aim to unravel these complexities, providing readers with a comprehensive understanding of why certain dietary choices can either combat or exacerbate cancer.

This book is not just a critique of unhealthy eating habits but a call to action. Through real-life testimonials, scientific evidence, and a thorough exploration of the biochemical pathways involved in cancer growth, I hope to empower readers with the knowledge and motivation to make life-saving dietary changes. This is not merely a theoretical discussion; it is a deeply personal mission. I have witnessed firsthand the devastating consequences of poor dietary choices in loved ones who have lost their battles with cancer. This book is my attempt to prevent others from suffering the same fate. As I have stated before my job is to help people understand how to live a longer healthier life without the costly lies of Western medicine.

In this book, you'll notice that certain concepts, such as pathways, will be revisited multiple times. This repetition is intentional, as it's essential for providing a complete and thorough understanding of how these processes work together to impact health. This book will dive deep into the biochemistry processes involved, offering a thorough understanding, but don't worry—it's all presented in a way that's easy to follow and won't overwhelm you.

Eating Habits of People with Cancer

At the heart of *"Taste Versus Cancer"* lies the exploration of emotional eating disorders, which play a significant role in why many cancer patients struggle to adopt healthier diets. Emotional dysregulation, low self-esteem, body image issues, trauma, and stress are powerful drivers of unhealthy eating behaviors. These issues are often rooted in deep-seated psychological patterns and environmental influences, making them particularly challenging to address.

Emotional Dysregulation is a key factor in emotional eating. When individuals are unable to manage their emotions effectively, they may turn to food as a coping mechanism. This can lead to a vicious cycle where negative emotions trigger unhealthy eating, which in turn exacerbates emotional distress. Cancer patients, already burdened by the stress and anxiety of their diagnosis, are particularly vulnerable to this pattern.

Low self-esteem and body image issues further complicate the relationship between food and health. Many individuals with cancer struggle with feelings of inadequacy and self-loathing, which can lead them to make poor dietary choices as a form of self-punishment. The societal pressures to conform to certain body standards only exacerbate these feelings, making it difficult for individuals to prioritize their health.

Trauma and stress are also significant contributors to emotional eating. For many cancer patients, the trauma of their diagnosis and the stress of treatment can be overwhelming. Food becomes a source of comfort, a way to numb the pain and temporarily escape the harsh realities of their situation. However, this reliance on food for emotional comfort often leads to the consumption of unhealthy, cancer-promoting foods.

Learned behaviors and **environmental pathways** also play a role in emotional eating. Many unhealthy eating habits are passed down from generation to generation, becoming deeply ingrained in an individual's psyche. Additionally, the environment in which a person lives, including the availability of healthy food options and the influence of family and friends, can significantly impact their dietary choices.

In *"Taste Versus Cancer,"* I explore these emotional and psychological factors in-depth, providing readers with strategies to overcome them. By addressing the root causes of emotional eating, individuals can begin to make healthier choices that support their cancer treatment and improve their overall well-being.

Understanding Cancer: The Enemy Within

To effectively combat cancer, it is crucial to understand what it is and how it operates within the body. In *"Taste Versus Cancer,"* I provide a detailed explanation of the biological processes involved in cancer development, including oxidative stress and the production of •OH hydroxyl radicals. These highly reactive molecules are known to cause significant damage to cellular components, leading to mutations and the uncontrolled cell growth characteristic of cancer.

Oxidative stress, caused by an imbalance between free radicals and antioxidants in the body, is a major contributor to cancer development. When the body is unable to neutralize free radicals effectively, they can damage DNA, proteins, and lipids, leading to the initiation and progression of cancer. The •OH hydroxyl radical is particularly dangerous because it is highly reactive and can cause extensive damage to cellular structures. This radical is often generated through environmental factors such as radiation, pollution, and certain chemicals, as well as through unhealthy dietary choices.

Understanding these processes is essential for making informed dietary choices. By reducing oxidative stress through the consumption of antioxidant-rich foods, individuals can help prevent the initiation and progression of cancer. In *"Taste Versus Cancer,"* I explain how a plant-based diet, particularly the P53 Diet & Lifestyle, can help achieve this by providing the body with the nutrients it needs to combat oxidative stress effectively.

Cancer Growth: Pathways of Destruction

Cancer is a complex disease, driven by multiple biological pathways that promote the growth and spread of malignant cells. In *"Taste Versus Cancer,"* I explore some of the key pathways involved in cancer progression, including the Ras pathway, the PI3K/AKT/mTOR pathway, and angiogenesis.

The Ras pathway is one of the most commonly mutated pathways in cancer. Ras proteins are involved in transmitting signals from outside the cell to the cell's nucleus, promoting cell growth and division. When Ras proteins are mutated, they can become permanently activated, leading to uncontrolled cell proliferation and tumor growth. This pathway is particularly relevant in cancers such as pancreatic, lung, and colorectal cancer.

The PI3K/AKT/mTOR pathway is another critical pathway in cancer development. This pathway regulates various cellular processes, including growth, survival, and metabolism. In many cancers, mutations in the PI3K/AKT/mTOR pathway lead to its hyperactivation, promoting cancer cell survival and resistance to treatment. This pathway is a major target for cancer therapies, but it is also influenced by diet. Certain dietary factors, such as high levels of saturated fats and sugars, can activate this pathway, further promoting cancer growth.

Angiogenesis, the process by which new blood vessels form from existing ones, is essential for tumor growth. Without a blood supply, tumors cannot grow beyond a certain size. However, cancer cells can secrete factors that stimulate angiogenesis, allowing them to grow and spread. In *"Taste Versus Cancer,"* I discuss how certain plant-based foods, such as those rich in polyphenols, can inhibit angiogenesis and starve tumors of the nutrients they need to grow.

Tumor Suppressor Genes: The Body's Defense Mechanisms

While many pathways promote cancer growth, the body also has natural defense mechanisms in the form of tumor suppressor genes. These genes act as brakes on cell division, preventing the uncontrolled growth that leads to cancer. In *"Taste Versus Cancer,"* I explore two of the most important tumor suppressor pathways: the p53 pathway and the RB1 pathway.

The **p53 pathway** is often referred to as the "guardian of the genome" because of its crucial role in maintaining genomic stability. When DNA is damaged, p53 is activated and either halts cell division to allow for repair or triggers apoptosis (programmed cell death) if the damage is irreparable. However, in many cancers, the p53 gene is mutated, rendering it unable to perform its protective functions. This allows cancer cells to proliferate unchecked. I explain how certain dietary choices, such as those rich in antioxidants, can support the p53 pathway and help prevent cancer.

The **RB1 pathway** is another critical tumor suppressor pathway. The RB1 protein regulates the cell cycle, ensuring that cells only divide when they are supposed to. When the RB1 gene is mutated, cells can divide uncontrollably, leading to cancer. In *"Taste Versus Cancer,"* I discuss how a plant-based diet can support the RB1 pathway and help prevent cancer progression.

Types of Cancers: A Diverse Enemy

Cancer is not a single disease but a collection of related diseases, each with its own unique characteristics and challenges. In *"Taste Versus Cancer,"* I provide an overview of the most common types of cancer, including breast cancer, lung cancer, colorectal cancer, and prostate cancer. For each type, I discuss the specific pathways involved in its development and how diet can play a role in prevention and treatment.

For example, **breast cancer** is often driven by hormonal factors, particularly estrogen. Certain plant-based foods, such as flaxseeds and soy, contain phytoestrogens that can help modulate estrogen levels and reduce the risk of breast cancer. Similarly, **colorectal cancer** is strongly associated with diet, particularly the consumption of red and processed meats. I explain how a plant-based diet, rich in fiber and antioxidants, can help prevent colorectal cancer.

The Dark Side of Conventional Therapies: Chemotherapy, Radiation, and Antibiotics

While diet plays a crucial role in cancer prevention and treatment, it is also important to address the potential harms of conventional cancer therapies. In *"Taste Versus Cancer,"* I explore the dark side of chemotherapy, radiation, and antibiotics, which can cause significant damage to healthy cells and lead to secondary cancers.

Chemotherapy-induced secondary cancers are a serious concern, as the very treatments used to combat cancer can sometimes cause new cancers to develop. This occurs because chemotherapy drugs are highly toxic and can damage DNA, leading to mutations. In *"Taste Versus Cancer,"* I discuss the pathways involved in chemotherapy-induced mutations and how a plant-based diet can help mitigate some of the damage caused by these treatments.

Radiation therapy is another common cancer treatment that comes with significant risks. It has the potential to cause radiation-induced carcinogenesis, where the radiation itself induces the formation of new cancers. This occurs because radiation can cause DNA damage, leading to mutations that drive cancer development. In *"Taste Versus Cancer,"* I explore the cellular pathways affected by radiation and the biological pathways involved in radiation-induced cancer.

Similarly, antibiotics, which are often prescribed to cancer patients to prevent infections, may also contribute to cancer growth. Emerging research suggests that prolonged or excessive antibiotic use can disrupt the gut microbiome, weaken the immune system, and foster conditions that encourage tumor growth. In *"Taste Versus Cancer,"* I delve into the pathways through which antibiotics can potentially promote cancer and the role a plant-based diet plays in restoring balance and supporting immune health.

By understanding the risks associated with these conventional therapies, individuals can make more informed decisions about their treatment options and explore complementary approaches, such as adopting a plant-based diet, to support their overall health and well-being.

"Taste Versus Cancer" is more than just a book; it is a call to action. It challenges the conventional wisdom surrounding cancer treatment and prevention, offering a new paradigm that places diet at the forefront of the battle against this devastating disease. By exploring the emotional, psychological, and biological factors that drive unhealthy eating habits in cancer patients, and by providing practical strategies for making healthier choices, this book aims to empower individuals to take control of their health and their future.

I am filled with hope that this book will make a meaningful difference in the lives of those battling cancer. It is my sincere wish that through this book, readers will gain the knowledge, motivation, and inspiration they need to make dietary changes that could save their lives. The fight against cancer is not just about killing cancer cells; it is about nurturing the body, mind, and spirit to create an environment where cancer cannot thrive. This book is my contribution to that fight, and I believe it has the potential to be my best work yet.

David W. Brown - Author/Researcher

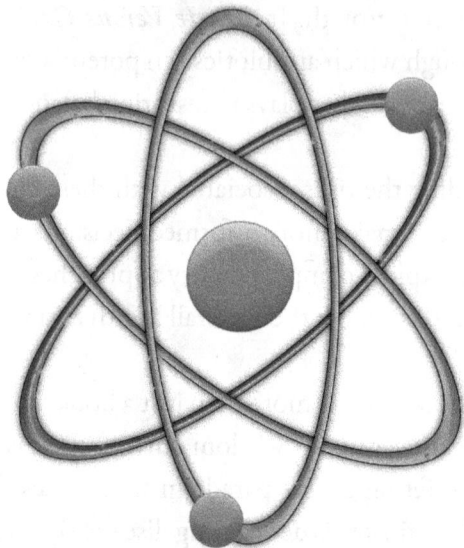

GIVE A FREE RADICAL A HOME!

EAT YOUR FRUIT!
thep53.com

Table of Contents

Chapter 1

Eating Habits of People with Cancer.....1
Emotional Eating Disorders.....9

Chapter 2

What is Cancer.....17
Oxidative Stress.....32
Hydroxyl Radicals (•OH).....35
P13K/AKT/mTOR Pathway.....41
RAS Pathway.....48

Chapter 3

Tumor Suppressor Genes.....57
TP53.....61
RB1.....69
BRCA1 and BRCA2......75
APC.....84
WT1......93
VHL.....101
NF1.....107
NF2.....113
CDKN2A.....117
PTEN.....124
SMAD4......131

TP73.....140
CDH1......145
DCC.....150
MEN1.....157
TSC1 and TSC2......164
STK11 (LKB1).....170
FHIT......176
MUTYH.....182
CHEK2.....187
BAP1......194

Chapter 4

Types of Cancer.....203
Bladder.....205
Brain.....211
Breast......220
Cervical.....237
Colon.....243
Endometrial.....251
Esophageal......261
Gallbladder.....270
Head and Neck.....278
Kidney.....289
Leukemia.....298
Liver.....309
Lung......317
Non-Hodgkin Lymphoma.....327
Ovarian.....337
Pancreatic......346
Parathyroid......354
Prostate.....364

Retinoblastoma.....373
Skin.....380
Stomach.....389
Testicular.....398
Thyroid.....407
Vaginal.....415

Chapter 5

Chemo/Radiation/Antibiotics.....425
Chemotherapy.....425
Radiation.....432
Antibiotics.....437

Chapter 6

Angiogenesis.....445

Chapter 7

Cancer Fuel: Sugar, Sodium & Saturated Fats.....453
Sugar.....453
Sodium.....457
Saturated Fats.....463

Chapter 8

Animal Products Linked to Cancer.....471
Dairy.....471

Meat.....480
Heme Iron Linked To Gene Mutations......486
Eggs......492
Fish & Seafood.....498

Chapter 9

Nutrient Deficiencies & Cancer.....507

Chapter 10

Plant-Based Diet Role in Cancer Reversal.....515
The Role of Vitamin C in Cancer Reversal.....522
Finding Testimonials.....529

Chapter 11

Call to Action.....533
Closing Statement.....539
P53 University.....543

Eating Habits of People with Cancer

C hanging dietary habits is one of the most powerful ways to impact health, prevent disease, and even reverse certain medical conditions. However, despite growing evidence that poor dietary choices significantly contribute to the development and progression of diseases like cancer, many individuals remain resistant to adopting healthier eating habits. This resistance persists even when confronted with a life-threatening diagnosis, such as cancer. The question then arises: why do people choose not to change their diet even if it means dying from cancer?

The reasons are multifaceted, deeply rooted in cultural, psychological, physiological, and societal factors. To understand the reluctance to change one's diet in the face of severe illness, it is essential to explore the complexity of human behavior, beliefs, habits, and how these aspects interplay with food choices. I will delve into the primary reasons why people resist dietary change, particularly when their life may depend on it, including emotional ties to food, the addictive nature of certain foods, cultural conditioning, lack of awareness or misinformation, fear of the unknown, and the role of medical advice in perpetuating unhealthy habits. This subject is very close to me after watching people choose bad food habits over staying alive. I just find this subject so hard to understand. I work with people each day to explain to them how to get control of their health by eating a plant-based diet and exercising.

Emotional Ties to Food

Food is more than sustenance. For many, it is deeply intertwined with emotional well-being, social experiences, and personal identity. From childhood, we are conditioned to associate food with comfort, celebration, family gatherings, and cultural traditions. Over time, these emotional connections become embedded in our psyches, making the idea of changing one's diet feel like an affront to personal identity and a loss of an emotional outlet. I will cover emotional eating disorders later in this chapter.

1. **Comfort Eating and Stress**: People often use food as a coping mechanism to deal with stress, anxiety, or depression. Studies have shown that comfort foods, typically high in fat, sugar, and salt, can temporarily reduce stress and make people feel better emotionally. In the case of cancer patients, who are often dealing with immense physical and emotional distress, the allure of comfort foods can be even stronger. The thought of giving up these foods, which have provided emotional solace throughout their lives, can feel overwhelming and undesirable, even in the face of a serious illness.

2. **Cultural and Familial Bonds**: For many individuals, food is a way to connect with their heritage and maintain cultural identity. Traditional dishes are often passed down through generations, symbolizing family, community, and continuity. Suggesting a drastic change in diet may feel like an abandonment of culture or familial connections, which can cause an emotional conflict. Many people see traditional foods as integral to their social lives and may resist dietary changes that could alienate them from family gatherings or cultural events, especially during such vulnerable times as battling cancer.

3. **Emotional Eating Patterns**: Some individuals develop emotional eating patterns early in life, where food is used to self-

soothe during difficult times. When faced with the physical and emotional toll of cancer, giving up comforting and familiar foods can feel like one more loss to endure, making the transition to a healthier diet harder. This emotional attachment to food can be a powerful barrier to dietary change, even when the person is aware of the negative health implications of their choices.

The Addictive Nature of Certain Foods

Certain foods, especially those high in sugar, fat, and salt, have been shown to have addictive properties. These foods can trigger the release of dopamine, a neurotransmitter associated with pleasure and reward, in the brain. Over time, people can become reliant on the temporary high provided by these foods, similar to how individuals develop addictions to substances like drugs or alcohol.

1. **Food Addiction**: Research suggests that processed foods, particularly those high in sugar and fat, can lead to addictive behaviors in some individuals. The combination of sugar, fat, and salt in highly processed foods activates the brain's reward system in much the same way as drugs of abuse, leading to cravings and overeating. Once addicted, it becomes extremely difficult to stop consuming these foods, even when a person knows they are harmful to their health. The biochemical dependence on these foods can be so strong that cancer patients may continue to eat them despite the knowledge that these foods can fuel cancer growth and contribute to poor health outcomes.

2. **Dopamine and Reward Systems**: Dopamine is a neurotransmitter in the brain that plays a key role in motivation and reward. When we eat something pleasurable, dopamine is released, reinforcing the behavior and making us want to repeat it. The food industry has mastered the science of combining ingredients like sugar, fat, and salt to create hyper-palatable foods that trigger

massive dopamine release. Over time, the brain becomes desensitized to normal levels of dopamine, and individuals need more of the "pleasurable" food to achieve the same reward, similar to how addictions to drugs develop. This cycle makes it extremely difficult for people to break free from unhealthy eating habits, even when faced with a life-threatening illness like cancer.

3. **Withdrawal Symptoms**: When people try to cut out addictive foods, they may experience withdrawal symptoms, including irritability, fatigue, depression, and intense cravings. These symptoms can make it difficult to maintain the dietary changes, particularly for cancer patients who are already dealing with physical pain and emotional distress. The fear of these withdrawal symptoms can prevent people from even attempting dietary change, as the short-term discomfort may seem too much to bear, especially when they are already struggling with a serious illness.

Cultural Conditioning

Cultural conditioning plays a significant role in shaping our dietary habits and food preferences. From a young age, we are exposed to societal norms and cultural messages about food, which can be difficult to break away from later in life, even when faced with a diagnosis of cancer.

1. **Societal Norms and Marketing**: The food industry spends billions of dollars on advertising to create and reinforce societal norms around food. From fast food to sugary snacks, advertisements often depict unhealthy foods as enjoyable, convenient, and even necessary for happiness. These marketing messages are ingrained in our culture, making it difficult to view food differently, even when we know the health risks involved. For someone with cancer, changing their diet means going against societal norms and the messages they have been bombarded with their entire lives, which can be intimidating and isolating.

2. **Family and Social Expectations**: In many cultures, food is an integral part of social life. Family gatherings, holidays, and celebrations often revolve around food, and the pressure to conform to family and social expectations can be overwhelming. When a cancer patient is told to change their diet, it often means giving up the foods that have been a part of their cultural or family traditions. This can create feelings of isolation or guilt, as they may feel they are letting down their loved ones or missing out on important social interactions.

3. **Resistance to Change**: Humans are creatures of habit, and changing long-standing habits, especially when it comes to food, can be particularly challenging. Many people grow up eating a certain way, and the idea of adopting a radically different diet feels daunting. For cancer patients, who are already dealing with significant changes in their health, energy levels, and daily routines, the idea of overhauling their diet can feel like one more insurmountable obstacle. The comfort and familiarity of their current eating habits often outweigh the perceived benefits of dietary change, even if it could improve their chances of survival.

Misinformation and Lack of Awareness

A significant barrier to dietary change, especially in the context of cancer, is misinformation and a lack of awareness about the impact of diet on health. Many people are simply unaware of how much their diet influences cancer development and progression, or they have been misled by inaccurate information.

1. **Conflicting Information**: The internet is filled with conflicting information about diet and cancer, making it difficult for individuals to know what to believe. Some sources claim that certain diets or foods can cure cancer, while others downplay the role of diet altogether. This flood of conflicting information can leave

cancer patients feeling confused and unsure of what changes to make. As a result, many people choose to stick with their current diet rather than risk making changes based on advice they do not fully trust or understand.

2. **Trust in Traditional Medical Advice**: Many cancer patients rely heavily on the advice of their doctors, but unfortunately, not all medical professionals emphasize the role of diet in cancer treatment. In some cases, patients may be told that dietary changes will not make a significant difference in their cancer prognosis, leading them to believe that changing their diet is unnecessary. This can perpetuate the belief that diet is not a crucial factor in cancer survival, even when mounting evidence suggests otherwise.

3. **Myths about "Healthy" Foods**: There are also widespread myths about what constitutes a healthy diet. For example, many people believe that as long as they are eating low-fat or low-calorie foods, they are eating healthily, even if those foods are highly processed and contain harmful additives. Others may believe that as long as they are eating "organic" or "natural" foods, they do not need to worry about the impact of their diet on their health. These misconceptions can prevent people from making the necessary dietary changes to improve their health and reduce their cancer risk.

Fear of the Unknown

For many people, the idea of changing their diet is daunting because it involves stepping into the unknown. They may not know how to prepare healthy meals, what foods to eat, or how to maintain a balanced diet. This fear of the unknown can be a significant barrier to dietary change, particularly for cancer patients who may already feel overwhelmed by their diagnosis and treatment.

1. **Lack of Knowledge**: Many people simply do not know how to eat a healthy diet, especially if they have spent most of their lives eating processed or fast food. The thought of learning how to cook new meals, read nutrition labels, or plan balanced meals can feel overwhelming, particularly for cancer patients who may be dealing with fatigue, nausea, or other side effects of treatment. This is where the P53 Diet can come into play with all the plant-based recipes and easy meal planning it takes fear away. Visit thep53.com for more details.

2. **Fear of Failure**: Some people fear that they will not be able to stick to a new diet and will end up failing in their attempt to change their eating habits. This fear of failure can prevent people from even trying, as they may believe it is better to continue with their current diet than to risk failing at a new one. For cancer patients, who may already be feeling a loss of control over their health, the idea of failing at dietary change can feel like one more failure in a long list of struggles.

3. **Comfort in Familiarity**: The familiarity of one's current diet can provide a sense of comfort and stability in an otherwise chaotic and uncertain time. For cancer patients, who are dealing with significant physical and emotional changes, the idea of changing their diet can feel like losing one more piece of their normal life. The comfort and familiarity of their current eating habits may feel like one of the few things they can control, making it difficult to let go, even if it could improve their health.

The Role of Medical Advice

Finally, the role of medical advice cannot be underestimated when it comes to dietary change. Many cancer patients rely heavily on their doctors for guidance, but unfortunately, not all medical professionals emphasize the importance of diet in cancer treatment.

1. **Limited Nutritional Training**: Many doctors receive little to no training in nutrition during medical school, which can lead to a lack of emphasis on the role of diet in disease prevention and treatment. As a result, some cancer patients may not receive adequate guidance on how to change their diet to support their treatment and recovery. Without clear and consistent advice from their doctors, patients may be less likely to make dietary changes, especially if they are not aware of the potential benefits.

2. **Focus on Medication and Treatment**: In many cases, the focus of cancer treatment is on medication, surgery, and other medical interventions, with little attention given to the role of diet. This can create the perception that diet is not an important factor in cancer treatment, leading patients to believe that changing their eating habits will not make a significant difference in their prognosis. When patients are told that diet is not a priority, they are less likely to make the effort to change their eating habits, even if it could improve their health and survival outcomes.

3. **Inconsistent Messaging**: Even when doctors do recommend dietary changes, the messaging can be inconsistent or vague, making it difficult for patients to know exactly what changes to make. For example, some patients may be told to "eat a healthy diet" without clear guidance on what that means in practice. This lack of clarity can leave patients feeling confused and unsure of how to proceed, leading them to stick with their current diet rather than making changes they do not fully understand.

The reasons why people resist changing their diet, even in the face of a cancer diagnosis, are complex and multifaceted. Emotional attachments to food, the addictive nature of certain foods, cultural conditioning, misinformation, fear of the unknown, and the role of medical advice all play a significant role in shaping people's dietary choices. For cancer patients, the prospect of changing their diet can feel overwhelming, particularly when they are already dealing with the physical and emotional toll of their illness. However, understanding the underlying reasons for this resistance can help to develop more effective strategies for encouraging dietary change, ultimately improving health outcomes for those facing serious illness.

Emotional Eating Disorders

Emotional eating disorders are a subset of eating disorders characterized by the consumption of food in response to emotions rather than physical hunger. These disorders can be complex, involving psychological, physiological, and environmental factors. The pathways leading to emotional eating disorders often include biological mechanisms, psychological triggers, and social influences. Understanding these pathways is crucial for developing effective prevention and treatment strategies.

Biological Pathways

1. **Genetic Predisposition**
   Research suggests that genetic factors play a significant role in the development of emotional eating disorders. Individuals with a family history of eating disorders or other mental health conditions may be more susceptible to emotional eating. Genetic predisposition can influence neurotransmitter systems, hormones, and brain structures involved in emotion regulation and appetite control.
2. **Neurotransmitter Imbalance**
   Neurotransmitters, such as serotonin, dopamine, and norepinephrine, are chemicals in the brain that regulate mood, appetite, and reward pathways. Imbalances in these neurotransmitters can lead to emotional dysregulation and cravings for certain foods.

For instance, low levels of serotonin are associated with depression and anxiety, which can trigger emotional eating as a coping mechanism.

3. **Hormonal Influences**

Hormones such as cortisol, insulin, and ghrelin play a critical role in regulating appetite and stress responses. Chronic stress can lead to elevated cortisol levels, which increase cravings for high-fat and high-sugar foods. Insulin resistance, commonly associated with metabolic disorders, can also influence hunger signals and food intake. Ghrelin, known as the "hunger hormone," stimulates appetite and is often elevated in individuals with emotional eating tendencies.

4. **Brain Structure and Function**

Brain imaging studies have shown that individuals with emotional eating disorders often have altered brain activity in regions associated with reward processing, impulse control, and emotion regulation. The prefrontal cortex, responsible for decision-making and self-control, may be less active, while the amygdala, involved in emotional responses, may be overactive. These brain changes can make it difficult for individuals to resist emotional eating urges.

Psychological Pathways

1. **Emotional Dysregulation**

Emotional dysregulation, or the inability to manage and respond to emotions appropriately, is a key psychological pathway in emotional eating disorders. Individuals may turn to food as a way to soothe negative emotions such as sadness, anxiety, boredom, or loneliness. This coping mechanism can provide temporary relief but often leads to feelings of guilt and shame, perpetuating the cycle of emotional eating.

2. Low Self-Esteem and Body Image Issues

Many individuals with emotional eating disorders struggle with low self-esteem and negative body image. Societal pressures to achieve a certain body type can exacerbate these feelings, leading to disordered eating behaviors. Emotional eating may serve as a way to numb or distract from these negative self-perceptions, but it ultimately reinforces the underlying issues.

3. Trauma and Stress

Trauma, including physical, emotional, or sexual abuse, is a significant risk factor for emotional eating disorders. Traumatic experiences can disrupt normal emotional processing and lead to maladaptive coping strategies such as emotional eating. Chronic stress, whether from personal relationships, work, or other sources, can also contribute to the development of emotional eating patterns.

4. Learned Behaviors

Emotional eating can be a learned behavior, often modeled by family members or peers. If an individual grows up in an environment where food is used as a reward or comfort, they may internalize these behaviors and turn to food in times of emotional distress. Additionally, cultural norms and media messages promoting food as a source of comfort can reinforce emotional eating tendencies.

Environmental Pathways

1. Food Environment

The availability and accessibility of highly palatable, energy-dense foods play a crucial role in emotional eating. Modern food environments are often characterized by an abundance of convenient, unhealthy food options that are marketed as quick fixes for emotional distress. The easy access to these foods can make it challenging for individuals to make healthier choices, especially during times of stress or emotional upheaval.

2. **Social Influences**

   Social relationships and dynamics can impact emotional eating behaviors. For example, social gatherings and celebrations often revolve around food, reinforcing the association between eating and emotional experiences. Peer pressure and social norms can also influence eating behaviors, with individuals feeling compelled to eat in certain ways to fit in or gain approval.

3. **Cultural Factors**

   Cultural attitudes towards food, body image, and emotions can shape an individual's relationship with eating. In some cultures, emotional expression is discouraged, leading individuals to find alternative ways to cope with their feelings, such as through food. Additionally, cultural beliefs about ideal body types and dieting can contribute to disordered eating patterns and emotional eating.

4. **Economic Stress**

   Economic factors, such as financial insecurity or poverty, can contribute to emotional eating disorders. Limited financial resources can restrict access to healthy food options, leading individuals to rely on cheaper, less nutritious foods. Economic stress can also increase overall stress levels, prompting individuals to turn to food as a coping mechanism.

Pathways of Intervention and Treatment

1. **Cognitive-Behavioral Therapy (CBT)**

   CBT is a widely used therapeutic approach for treating emotional eating disorders. This therapy focuses on identifying and changing negative thought patterns and behaviors related to food and emotions. Techniques such as cognitive restructuring, behavioral experiments, and mindfulness practices can help individuals develop healthier coping strategies and improve emotional regulation.

2. **Dialectical Behavior Therapy (DBT)**

   DBT, originally developed for borderline personality disorder, has been adapted for treating emotional eating disorders. DBT emphasizes skills training in areas such as emotion regulation, distress tolerance, interpersonal effectiveness, and mindfulness. These skills can help individuals manage their emotions more effectively and reduce reliance on food for emotional comfort.

3. **Nutritional Counseling**

   Working with a P53 Certified Plant-Based Nutrition Specialist can provide individuals with the knowledge and tools to develop healthier eating habits. Nutritional counseling can help individuals understand the impact of food on their mood and energy levels, as well as provide guidance on balanced meal planning and mindful eating practices.

4. **Mindfulness and Meditation**

   Mindfulness-based interventions, such as Mindfulness-Based Stress Reduction (MBSR) and Mindful Eating, can help individuals develop a more conscious and balanced relationship with food. These practices encourage individuals to pay attention to their physical hunger and fullness cues, as well as their emotional triggers for eating, promoting greater self-awareness and control.

5. **Support Groups and Peer Support**

   Support groups and peer support can provide a sense of community and understanding for individuals struggling with emotional eating disorders. Sharing experiences and challenges with others who have similar struggles can reduce feelings of isolation and provide practical tips and encouragement for managing emotional eating.

Preventative Strategies

1. **Early Intervention and Education**
   Educating individuals about healthy coping strategies and the risks of emotional eating from an early age can help prevent the development of disordered eating behaviors. Schools, families, and community programs can play a vital role in promoting emotional literacy, healthy eating habits, and positive body image.

2. **Promoting Emotional Resilience**
   Building emotional resilience through practices such as stress management, problem-solving, and emotional expression can reduce the likelihood of turning to food for comfort. Encouraging activities that promote mental well-being, such as exercise, hobbies, and social connections, can also support emotional health.

3. **Creating Supportive Environments**
   Creating environments that support healthy eating and emotional well-being can reduce the risk of emotional eating disorders. This includes promoting access to nutritious food options, reducing the availability of unhealthy food choices, and fostering supportive social networks that encourage positive emotional expression and coping strategies.

4. **Addressing Societal and Cultural Pressures**
   Challenging societal and cultural pressures related to body image, dieting, and emotional expression can help reduce the prevalence of emotional eating disorders. This involves promoting diverse body representations in media, encouraging body positivity, and advocating for policies that support mental health and well-being.

Emotional eating disorders are complex conditions influenced by a combination of biological, psychological, and environmental factors. Understanding the pathways that contribute to emotional eating is essential for developing effective prevention and treatment strategies. By addressing genetic predispositions, neurotransmitter imbalances, emotional dysregulation, social influences, and other contributing factors, we can help individuals develop healthier relationships with food and emotions. Comprehensive approaches that include therapy, nutritional counseling, mindfulness practices, and support networks are key to managing and overcoming emotional eating disorders. Preventative measures, such as early education, promoting emotional resilience, and creating supportive environments, are also crucial in reducing the incidence of these disorders. Through a multifaceted approach, we can better support individuals in achieving emotional and physical well-being.

2

What is Cancer?

C ancer is a broad term that encompasses a group of diseases characterized by the uncontrolled growth and spread of abnormal cells
in the body. These cells can invade and destroy normal tissue, and they
have the ability to spread to other parts of the body, a process known as
metastasis. Understanding cancer involves exploring its underlying biological mechanisms, the factors that contribute to its development, and
the various types of cancers that can affect the human body. It's
thought-provoking to consider how, despite the vast amounts of money
funneled into cancer research in the United States over the years, the
prevalence of cancer has actually increased—from 5% in 1950 to 5.4% in
2022. Similarly, the percentage of people who died from cancer has also
risen, from 17% in 1950 to 18% in 2022.

The Biology of Cancer

At its core, cancer is a disease of the cells, the basic units of life. The
human body is made up of trillions of cells that grow, divide, and eventually die in a regulated manner. This process is controlled by a complex
system of signals that ensure cells function correctly, reproduce at the
right time, and die when they are no longer needed. Cancer arises when
this regulatory system breaks down, leading to the uncontrolled proliferation of cells.

Cells become cancerous due to mutations in their DNA, the genetic
material that contains the instructions for cell behavior. These mutations can be inherited from parents or acquired during a person's

lifetime due to environmental factors such as exposure to carcinogens (substances that can cause cancer), radiation, or hypoxia. Some of the key genes involved in cancer development include oncogenes, which promote cell growth and division, and tumor suppressor genes, which inhibit cell division and promote cell death. When mutations occur in these genes, they can lead to the development of cancer. According to cancer studies about 92% of all cancers are somatic mutations (environment) with roughly 8% germline mutations (hereditary).

Types of Cancer

Cancer is not a single disease but rather a collection of related diseases. There are over 100 different types of cancer, each classified based on the type of cell or tissue from which it originates. I will only cover the top cancers in this book due to page limitations. The most common types of cancer include:

- **Carcinomas**: These are cancers that originate in the epithelial cells, which line the inside and outside surfaces of the body. Carcinomas account for the majority of cancer cases and include cancers of the skin, lungs, breast, prostate, and colon.
- **Sarcomas**: These cancers arise from connective tissues such as bone, cartilage, fat, muscle, or blood vessels. Sarcomas are less common than carcinomas.
- **Leukemias**: Leukemia is a type of cancer that originates in the blood-forming tissues of the bone marrow and leads to the production of large numbers of abnormal white blood cells. These abnormal cells crowd out normal blood cells, leading to symptoms like anemia, infections, and bleeding.
- **Lymphomas**: Lymphomas are cancers that develop in the lymphatic system, a part of the immune system that includes the lymph nodes, spleen, and thymus. Lymphomas can be classified into Hodgkin lymphoma and non-Hodgkin lymphoma, depending on the type of cell involved.

- **Central nervous system cancers**: These cancers begin in the tissues of the brain and spinal cord. Examples include gliomas, which arise from glial cells, and meningiomas, which develop in the meninges, the protective membranes around the brain and spinal cord.

The Process of Cancer Development

The development of cancer is a multistep process that involves the accumulation of genetic mutations over time. This process can be divided into three main stages: initiation, promotion, and progression.

- **Initiation**: The initiation stage occurs when a normal cell undergoes a genetic mutation that affects its ability to regulate its growth and division. These mutations can be caused by exposure to carcinogens, errors during DNA replication, or inherited genetic factors.
- **Promotion**: During the promotion stage, the initiated cell begins to proliferate abnormally, forming a mass of cells known as a tumor. This stage is often influenced by factors that stimulate cell growth, such as hormones or chronic inflammation. The tumor may remain benign (non-cancerous) at this stage, meaning it does not invade nearby tissues or spread to other parts of the body.
- **Progression**: In the progression stage, the tumor becomes malignant (cancerous). The cells within the tumor acquire additional mutations that enable them to invade surrounding tissues and spread to distant sites in the body through the bloodstream or lymphatic system. This process is known as metastasis and is responsible for the majority of cancer-related deaths.

Hallmarks of Cancer

Cancer cells exhibit a number of distinctive characteristics that differentiate them from normal cells. These characteristics, known as the "hallmarks of cancer," were first described by researchers Douglas Hanahan and Robert Weinberg in 2000 and have since become a framework for understanding cancer biology. The hallmarks of cancer include:

- **Sustaining proliferative signaling**: Cancer cells have the ability to continuously signal themselves to grow and divide, bypassing the normal regulatory mechanisms that control cell proliferation.
- **Evading growth suppressors**: Cancer cells are able to evade the signals that normally inhibit cell growth, allowing them to continue dividing uncontrollably.
- **Resisting cell death**: Normal cells undergo a process called apoptosis, or programmed cell death when they are damaged or no longer needed. Cancer cells, however, are able to resist these death signals and survive even when they should not.
- **Enabling replicative immortality**: Most normal cells can only divide a limited number of times before they stop growing and enter a state called senescence. Cancer cells, however, can maintain their ability to divide indefinitely, making them "immortal."
- **Inducing angiogenesis**: Tumors need a blood supply to grow and survive. Cancer cells can induce the formation of new blood vessels (angiogenesis) to supply the tumor with oxygen and nutrients.
- **Activating invasion and metastasis**: Cancer cells have the ability to invade surrounding tissues and spread to other parts of the body, forming secondary tumors.

In addition to these original hallmarks, two emerging characteristics have been added to the framework:

- **Deregulating cellular energetics**: Cancer cells often undergo metabolic changes that allow them to generate energy in ways that support rapid cell growth and survival.
- **Avoiding immune destruction**: Cancer cells can evade detection and destruction by the immune system, allowing them to grow and spread unchecked.

Causes and Risk Factors

The development of cancer is influenced by a combination of genetic, environmental, and lifestyle factors. Some of the key risk factors for cancer include:

- **Genetics**: Inherited mutations in certain genes can increase a person's risk of developing cancer. For example, mutations in the BRCA1 and BRCA2 genes are associated with a higher risk of breast and ovarian cancers.
- **Environmental factors**: Exposure to certain chemicals, radiation, and pollutants can increase the risk of cancer. For example, smoking is a major risk factor for lung cancer, and exposure to ultraviolet (UV) radiation from the sun is a significant risk factor for skin cancer.
- **Lifestyle factors**: Diet, physical activity, and alcohol consumption can all influence cancer risk. Diets high in red and processed meats, for example, are linked to colorectal cancer, while a diet rich in fruits and vegetables may reduce the risk of several types of cancer.
- **Hormones**: Hormonal factors, particularly those related to reproductive history, can influence cancer risk. For example, prolonged exposure to estrogen, such as in women who have had early menstruation or late menopause, is associated with an increased risk of breast cancer.

Diagnosis and Staging

Diagnosing cancer typically involves a combination of physical examinations, imaging studies, laboratory tests, and biopsies. A biopsy, in which a small sample of tissue is removed and examined under a microscope, is often the definitive test for diagnosing cancer.

Once cancer is diagnosed, it is important to determine the stage of the disease, which refers to the extent to which the cancer has spread in the body. Staging helps guide treatment decisions and provides an indication of prognosis. The most commonly used staging system is the TNM system, which assesses:

- **T (Tumor)**: The size and extent of the primary tumor.
- **N (Node)**: Whether the cancer has spread to nearby lymph nodes.
- **M (Metastasis)**: Whether the cancer has spread to distant parts of the body.

Based on these criteria, cancer is typically classified into stages I through IV, with stage I indicating localized disease and stage IV indicating advanced disease with distant metastasis.

Prevention and Early Detection

Preventing cancer involves reducing exposure to risk factors and adopting a healthy lifestyle. Some key strategies for cancer prevention include:

- **Avoiding tobacco**: Not smoking and avoiding exposure to secondhand smoke are the most important steps one can take to prevent cancer.
- **Maintaining a healthy diet**: A diet rich in fruits, vegetables, and whole grains with no consumption of animal products of any kind can help reduce the risk of cancer.

- **Exercising regularly**: Regular physical activity can help maintain a healthy weight and reduce the risk of several types of cancer.
- **Protecting against UV radiation**: Using sunscreen, wearing protective clothing, and avoiding tanning beds can help reduce the risk of skin cancer.
- **Regular screening**: Regular cancer screening tests, such as mammograms, Pap smears, and colonoscopies, can help detect cancer early when it is most treatable.

Genetic Mutations and Oncogenes

One of the primary drivers of cancer cell growth is the accumulation of genetic mutations. These mutations can activate oncogenes, which are genes that promote cell proliferation. In normal cells, these genes are tightly regulated to prevent uncontrolled growth. However, when mutations occur, they can lead to the constant activation of these genes, driving the unchecked proliferation of cancer cells.

Ras Pathway

The Ras family of proteins is one of the most well-known oncogene families involved in cancer. Ras proteins are small GTPases that play a crucial role in transmitting signals from cell surface receptors to the nucleus, promoting cell growth and survival. Mutations in Ras genes, particularly in KRAS, HRAS, and NRAS, are common in various cancers, including pancreatic, lung, and colorectal cancers.

When Ras proteins are mutated, they become constitutively active, meaning they are always "on," even in the absence of growth signals. This leads to continuous activation of downstream signaling pathways, such as the MAPK/ERK and PI3K/AKT pathways, which promote cell proliferation and survival.

PI3K/AKT/mTOR Pathway

The PI3K/AKT/mTOR pathway is another critical signaling cascade frequently altered in cancer. This pathway is involved in regulating cell growth, metabolism, and survival. PI3K (phosphoinositide 3-kinase) is activated by various growth factors and hormones, leading to the activation of AKT, a serine/threonine kinase.

Once activated, AKT can phosphorylate a range of downstream targets, including mTOR (mechanistic target of rapamycin), which is a central regulator of cell growth and metabolism. Mutations or amplifications in components of this pathway, such as PIK3CA (the gene encoding the p110α subunit of PI3K) or loss of the tumor suppressor PTEN, lead to hyperactivation of the pathway, promoting the growth and survival of cancer cells. This pathway is explained in more detail in the next section of this chapter.

Tumor Suppressor Genes

While oncogenes drive the proliferation of cancer cells, the inactivation of tumor suppressor genes removes critical barriers that normally prevent uncontrolled cell growth. Tumor suppressor genes, such as TP53, RB1, and BRCA1/2, play vital roles in regulating the cell cycle, repairing DNA damage, and inducing apoptosis. More on Tumor Suppressor Genes in Chapter 3.

p53 Pathway

The p53 protein, encoded by the TP53 gene, is often referred to as the "guardian of the genome" due to its role in maintaining genomic stability. In response to DNA damage or other cellular stress, p53 can induce cell cycle arrest, allowing time for DNA repair or triggering apoptosis if the damage is irreparable.

However, mutations in TP53 are common in many cancers, leading to the loss of its tumor-suppressive functions. Without functional p53, cells with DNA damage can continue to proliferate, accumulating further mutations that drive cancer progression. Additionally, mutant p53 can gain new functions that actively promote cancer growth, a phenomenon known as "gain-of-function" mutations.

RB1 Pathway

The RB1 gene encodes the retinoblastoma protein (pRB), a key regulator of the cell cycle. pRB controls the transition from the G1 to the S phase of the cell cycle by inhibiting the activity of E2F transcription factors, which are necessary for DNA replication.

When RB1 is mutated or inactivated, pRB can no longer suppress E2F activity, leading to uncontrolled cell cycle progression and proliferation. This loss of cell cycle control is a common feature in many cancers, including retinoblastoma, osteosarcoma, and breast cancer.

Epigenetic Alterations

In addition to genetic mutations, epigenetic changes also play a crucial role in the continuous growth of cancer cells. Epigenetic alterations refer to heritable changes in gene expression that do not involve changes to the underlying DNA sequence. These changes can include DNA methylation, histone modifications, and changes in non-coding RNA expression.

DNA Methylation

DNA methylation involves the addition of a methyl group to the cytosine residues of DNA, typically at CpG islands, which are regions of the genome rich in cytosine and guanine nucleotides. In normal cells, DNA methylation is a key mechanism for regulating gene expression, particularly in silencing genes that should not be expressed.

In cancer, aberrant DNA methylation patterns are common. Hypermethylation of tumor suppressor gene promoters can lead to their silencing, while hypomethylation of oncogenes can result in their overexpression. For example, hypermethylation of the CDKN2A promoter, which encodes the p16INK4a tumor suppressor protein, is frequently observed in various cancers, leading to the loss of cell cycle control.

Histone Modifications

Histone proteins help package DNA into a compact, organized structure called chromatin. The post-translational modification of histones, such as acetylation, methylation, and phosphorylation, plays a crucial role in regulating gene expression by altering chromatin structure.

Cancer cells often exhibit abnormal histone modification patterns that lead to the dysregulation of gene expression. For instance, the loss of histone acetylation can result in the silencing of tumor suppressor genes, while increased histone methylation at certain residues can promote oncogene expression. These epigenetic changes contribute to the continuous growth and survival of cancer cells by altering the expression of key genes involved in cell proliferation, apoptosis, and DNA repair.

The Role of the Tumor Microenvironment

The tumor microenvironment (TME) is the surrounding environment in which cancer cells exist, including stromal cells, immune cells, blood vessels, and extracellular matrix components. The TME plays a crucial role in cancer progression by providing signals that support the growth, survival, and metastasis of cancer cells.

Angiogenesis

Angiogenesis, the formation of new blood vessels, is a critical process that supplies nutrients and oxygen to the growing tumor. Cancer cells can secrete pro-angiogenic factors, such as vascular endothelial growth factor (VEGF), which stimulate the growth of new blood vessels from existing ones.

The PI3K/AKT/mTOR pathway, mentioned earlier, is one of the key regulators of VEGF expression. Hyperactivation of this pathway in cancer cells leads to increased VEGF production, promoting angiogenesis and supporting tumor growth. Additionally, hypoxia, or low oxygen levels within the tumor, can further drive VEGF expression through the stabilization of hypoxia-inducible factor 1-alpha (HIF-1α).

Immune Evasion

The immune system plays a vital role in identifying and eliminating cancer cells. However, cancer cells have evolved various mechanisms to evade immune detection and destruction. One such mechanism is the expression of immune checkpoint proteins, such as PD-L1, which bind to PD-1 receptors on T cells and inhibit their activity.

The interaction between PD-L1 and PD-1 suppresses the immune response against cancer cells, allowing them to survive and proliferate. Additionally, cancer cells can secrete immunosuppressive cytokines, such as transforming growth factor-beta (TGF-β) and interleukin-10 (IL-10), which further inhibit the activity of immune cells within the TME.

Inflammation

Chronic inflammation is a well-established risk factor for cancer development and progression. Inflammatory cells, such as macrophages and neutrophils, can produce reactive oxygen species (ROS) and pro-inflammatory cytokines that promote DNA damage, cell proliferation, and angiogenesis.

The nuclear factor-kappa B (NF-κB) pathway is a key regulator of inflammation and is often activated in cancer. NF-κB can induce the expression of pro-inflammatory cytokines, such as IL-6 and tumor necrosis factor-alpha (TNF-α), which promote tumor growth and survival. Additionally, NF-κB can inhibit apoptosis and enhance the expression of anti-apoptotic proteins, further contributing to the continuous growth of cancer cells.

Metabolic Reprogramming

Cancer cells undergo significant metabolic reprogramming to support their rapid growth and proliferation. This metabolic shift, often referred to as the "Warburg effect," involves a preference for glycolysis over oxidative phosphorylation, even in the presence of oxygen.

Aerobic Glycolysis

In normal cells, glucose is primarily metabolized through oxidative phosphorylation in the mitochondria to generate ATP. However, cancer cells preferentially utilize glycolysis, a less efficient process that produces lactate, to generate energy. This phenomenon, known as aerobic glycolysis, allows cancer cells to rapidly produce the building blocks needed for cell growth, such as nucleotides, amino acids, and lipids.

The PI3K/AKT/mTOR pathway and the MYC oncogene are key regulators of this metabolic shift. AKT promotes glucose uptake and glycolysis by increasing the expression of glucose transporters (GLUTs) and glycolytic enzymes. Meanwhile, MYC drives the expression of genes involved in glycolysis and glutamine metabolism, further supporting the biosynthetic needs of rapidly proliferating cancer cells.

Glutamine Metabolism

In addition to glucose, cancer cells rely heavily on glutamine, an amino acid that serves as a carbon and nitrogen source for various biosynthetic processes. Glutamine is converted into glutamate by the enzyme glutaminase, which can then enter the tricarboxylic acid (TCA) cycle to support energy production and biosynthesis.

The MYC oncogene plays a central role in regulating glutamine metabolism in cancer cells. MYC can increase the expression of glutaminase and other enzymes involved in glutamine metabolism, promoting the utilization of glutamine for anabolic processes. This dependence on glutamine, known as "glutamine addiction," is a hallmark of many cancers.

DNA Repair Defects

Cancer cells often exhibit defects in DNA repair mechanisms, leading to the accumulation of mutations that drive cancer progression. The inability to repair DNA damage effectively allows cancer cells to continue growing despite having a high mutational burden.

Homologous Recombination Deficiency (HRD)

Homologous recombination is a critical DNA repair pathway that fixes double-strand breaks (DSBs) in DNA. Mutations in genes involved in homologous recombination, such as BRCA1 and BRCA2, lead to homologous recombination deficiency (HRD), making cancer cells more susceptible to accumulating DNA damage.

While HRD can increase the mutation rate in cancer cells, it also creates a therapeutic vulnerability. PARP inhibitors, a class of drugs that target another DNA repair pathway called base excision repair (BER), are particularly effective in cancers with HRD, as they induce synthetic lethality by overwhelming the cancer cells' remaining DNA repair capacity.

Mismatch Repair Deficiency (MMR)

Mismatch repair (MMR) is another critical DNA repair pathway that corrects errors that occur during DNA replication. Defects in MMR, often due to mutations in MLH1, MSH2, MSH6, or PMS2, lead to microsatellite instability (MSI), a condition characterized by the accumulation of short, repetitive DNA sequences.

MSI-high cancers, such as colorectal and endometrial cancers, are prone to accumulating mutations in oncogenes and tumor suppressor genes, driving cancer progression. However, MMR deficiency also makes these cancers more immunogenic, as the high mutational burden can lead to the production of neoantigens that are recognized by the immune system. This has led to the success of immune checkpoint inhibitors in treating MSI-high cancers.

The Role of Stem Cells

Cancer stem cells (CSCs) are a subpopulation of cancer cells with the ability to self-renew and differentiate into various cell types within the tumor. CSCs are believed to be responsible for tumor initiation, progression, and resistance to therapy.

Wnt/β-Catenin Pathway

The Wnt/β-catenin signaling pathway plays a crucial role in maintaining the self-renewal and pluripotency of CSCs. In normal cells, Wnt signaling is tightly regulated to control cell fate decisions. However, in cancer, aberrant activation of the Wnt/β-catenin pathway leads to the expansion of CSCs and promotes tumor growth.

Mutations in components of the Wnt pathway, such as APC (adenomatous polyposis coli) or β-catenin, are common in colorectal cancer and other cancers with a high stem cell component. These mutations result in the accumulation of β-catenin in the nucleus, where it activates the transcription of genes that promote cell proliferation and survival.

Hedgehog Pathway

The Hedgehog signaling pathway is another critical regulator of CSCs. In normal development, Hedgehog signaling controls cell growth and differentiation. However, in cancer, aberrant activation of the Hedgehog pathway can lead to the expansion of CSCs and contribute to tumor progression.

Mutations in components of the Hedgehog pathway, such as PTCH1 (patched 1) or SMO (smoothened), can lead to constitutive activation of the pathway, promoting the growth of CSCs. This has been observed in basal cell carcinoma and medulloblastoma, among other cancers.

Resistance to Cell Death

One of the defining features of cancer cells is their ability to resist apoptosis, the programmed cell death that normally eliminates damaged or unneeded cells. This resistance to cell death allows cancer cells to survive despite the accumulation of mutations and other cellular stresses.

BCL-2 Family Proteins

The BCL-2 family of proteins plays a central role in regulating apoptosis by controlling the release of cytochrome c from the mitochondria, a key step in the activation of caspases, the enzymes that execute apoptosis.

In cancer, the balance between pro-apoptotic and anti-apoptotic BCL-2 family members is often disrupted. Overexpression of anti-apoptotic proteins, such as BCL-2, BCL-XL, and MCL-1, is a common feature in many cancers and contributes to resistance to apoptosis. This allows cancer cells to survive in the face of chemotherapy and other treatments that would normally induce cell death.

Autophagy

Autophagy is a cellular process that involves the degradation and recycling of damaged or unnecessary cellular components. While autophagy can act as a tumor suppressor by eliminating damaged organelles and proteins, it can also promote cancer cell survival under conditions of stress, such as nutrient deprivation or chemotherapy.

In cancer, the role of autophagy is complex and context-dependent. In some cases, increased autophagy supports cancer cell survival by providing energy and building blocks for growth. In other cases, inhibition of autophagy can sensitize cancer cells to treatment by preventing them from coping with stress.

Cancer is a complex and multifaceted disease that arises from the uncontrolled growth of abnormal cells in the body. It is influenced by a combination of genetic, environmental, and lifestyle factors, and its development involves a series of stages characterized by the accumulation of genetic mutations. While cancer remains one of the leading causes of death worldwide, advances in early detection, treatment, and prevention have significantly improved the outcomes for many patients.

Oxidative Stress

Oxidative stress is a physiological imbalance between the production of reactive oxygen species (ROS) and the body's ability to detoxify them, resulting in potential damage to biomolecules such as lipids, proteins, and nucleic acids. ROS, including free radicals and non-radical species, are natural byproducts of cellular metabolism and play crucial roles in various signaling pathways. However, when their production exceeds the cellular antioxidant capacity, oxidative stress occurs.

One major source of ROS production is the electron transport chain (ETC), a fundamental process in cellular respiration that takes place in the inner mitochondrial membrane. The ETC consists of a series of protein complexes, including NADH dehydrogenase (complex I), succinate dehydrogenase (complex II), cytochrome b-c1 complex (complex III), cytochrome c, and cytochrome c oxidase (complex IV). Electrons from donors, such as NADH and succinate, move through these complexes, ultimately reducing molecular oxygen to water.

During this electron transfer, some electrons leak prematurely, leading to the formation of superoxide radicals ($O_2^{\bullet-}$) primarily at complexes I and III. Superoxide radicals can further generate other ROS, creating a cascade of reactive species. The process is regulated by the redox potential of electron carriers within the complexes and the presence of specific antioxidant enzymes.

Mitochondrial antioxidants, like superoxide dismutase (SOD), catalase, and glutathione peroxidase, help neutralize superoxide radicals and other ROS. However, when ROS production overwhelms these defenses, oxidative stress ensues. This phenomenon has been implicated in numerous pathological conditions, including neurodegenerative diseases, cardiovascular disorders, and cancer.

Beyond the mitochondria, other cellular components, such as peroxisomes, endoplasmic reticulum, and plasma membrane, also contribute to ROS production. Enzymatic and non-enzymatic antioxidants in the cytoplasm and extracellular space further counterbalance this oxidative load.

Oxidative stress induces damage through several mechanisms. Lipid peroxidation, initiated by ROS attacking unsaturated fatty acids in cell membranes, results in the generation of lipid peroxides and other toxic byproducts. Protein oxidation, involving modifications to amino acid residues, can impair protein structure and function. DNA damage can occur through direct attack by ROS or indirectly through oxidative stress-induced inflammation.

The consequences of oxidative stress extend beyond cellular damage. Chronic oxidative stress is implicated in aging and age-related diseases. It can modulate signal transduction pathways, leading to altered gene expression and promoting inflammation. Additionally, ROS can activate stress-responsive kinases, such as mitogen-activated protein kinases (MAPKs) and nuclear factor-kappa B (NF-κB), amplifying the inflammatory response.

Oxidative stress can induce mutations in cells through various mechanisms. Reactive oxygen species (ROS), which are generated during oxidative stress, can directly damage DNA. Here's how it typically happens:

- DNA Base Modifications: ROS can interact with DNA and cause modifications to its bases. For example, guanine, one of the

DNA bases, is particularly susceptible to oxidative damage. This can result in the formation of modified bases like 8-oxoguanine.

- Single-Strand Breaks (SSBs): ROS can cause breaks in the sugar-phosphate backbone of DNA, resulting in single-strand breaks. Repair processes may introduce errors or mutations during the repair of these breaks.
- Double-Strand Breaks (DSBs): Prolonged or severe oxidative stress can lead to double-strand breaks in the DNA molecule. Incorrect repair of these breaks may introduce mutations.
- Indirect Effects: ROS can also indirectly contribute to mutagenesis by activating signaling pathways that influence cellular processes like proliferation and apoptosis. Dysregulation of these processes can favor the survival and proliferation of cells with genetic mutations.

Accumulation of mutations in critical genes can lead to uncontrolled cell growth, a hallmark of cancer. It's important to note that while oxidative stress is a natural part of cellular processes, excessive and prolonged oxidative stress, as seen in conditions like exposure to certain environmental toxins, can increase the risk of mutagenesis and contribute to various diseases, including cancer.

Oxidative stress is a complex physiological phenomenon arising from the imbalance between ROS production and antioxidant defenses. The electron transport chain, a vital component of cellular respiration, plays a central role in ROS generation. Mitochondrial and cellular antioxidant systems work together to mitigate the detrimental effects of oxidative stress, but when overwhelmed, it contributes to the pathogenesis of various diseases. Numerous studies have stated the importance of antioxidant-rich diets, including fruits and vegetables, in mitigating oxidative stress-related diseases.

Hydroxyl Radicals (•OH)

Hydroxyl radicals (•OH) are highly reactive molecules that play a critical role in biological processes, often acting as a double-edged sword. On the one hand, they are involved in normal physiological processes and defense mechanisms in cells. On the other hand, due to their potent oxidative capacity, they are implicated in various pathological conditions, particularly oxidative stress and cellular damage.

Introduction to Hydroxyl Radicals (•OH)

Hydroxyl radicals belong to the group of reactive oxygen species (ROS), a subset of free radicals generated naturally in the body. Unlike other ROS, such as superoxide ($O_2^{\bullet -}$) and hydrogen peroxide (H_2O_2), the hydroxyl radical is unique because of its extreme reactivity, making it a potent oxidizing agent. Its presence in cells is usually transient due to its high reactivity, meaning it can cause significant damage to biomolecules like DNA, proteins, and lipids.

The symbol •OH reflects the radical nature of the hydroxyl group, where the unpaired electron (•) in the molecule makes it highly unstable and reactive. Hydroxyl radicals are often produced during metabolic processes or as a by-product of external environmental stressors such as radiation, pollution, and toxins.

Function of Hydroxyl Radicals

Despite their notorious role in cellular damage, hydroxyl radicals have specific functional roles in biological systems, particularly related to cell signaling, immune responses, and pathogen defense.

Cell Signaling and Regulation

Although hydroxyl radicals are primarily associated with oxidative damage, they also participate in cell signaling pathways, particularly those involved in the regulation of apoptosis (programmed cell death) and cellular responses to stress. In small amounts, ROS, including •OH, act as signaling molecules that help maintain cellular homeostasis and respond to changes in the environment. Hydroxyl radicals can modify proteins, lipids, and DNA, thereby altering their structure and function in ways that influence cellular pathways.

In particular, hydroxyl radicals are involved in redox signaling, where the oxidation and reduction of molecules affect cellular function. Redox signaling is critical for the regulation of inflammatory responses, the defense against pathogens, and the activation of immune cells.

Role in Immune Responses

The immune system uses ROS, including hydroxyl radicals, as part of its defense mechanism against pathogens. During the respiratory burst in phagocytic cells such as neutrophils and macrophages, hydroxyl radicals are produced to help neutralize and destroy invading microorganisms. In this context, the hydroxyl radical acts as a crucial element in the body's innate immune response, breaking down cell walls of bacteria and other pathogens through oxidative damage.

Hydroxyl Radicals and Apoptosis

Apoptosis, or programmed cell death, is a highly regulated process necessary for maintaining cellular integrity and homeostasis. Hydroxyl radicals can contribute to the activation of apoptosis by causing oxidative damage to key cellular components such as DNA and mitochondria. If cellular repair mechanisms are overwhelmed by ROS damage, apoptosis may be initiated to prevent further harm. This process is critical in protecting against the development of cancer, where the failure of apoptosis can lead to uncontrolled cell growth.

However, while apoptosis is a normal physiological process, excessive production of hydroxyl radicals can lead to unwanted cell death, contributing to degenerative diseases like Alzheimer's, Parkinson's, and amyotrophic lateral sclerosis (ALS).

Production of Hydroxyl Radicals

Hydroxyl radicals are produced both endogenously and exogenously through several mechanisms. Their formation is mainly dependent on the availability of certain substrates, metal ions, and conditions that favor the Fenton and Haber-Weiss reactions.

The Fenton Reaction

The most well-known pathway for hydroxyl radical production is the Fenton reaction, named after Henry John Horstman Fenton. This reaction occurs when hydrogen peroxide (H_2O_2), a less reactive ROS, reacts with transition metals like ferrous iron (Fe_2^+) or copper (Cu+). The reaction produces the hydroxyl radical as follows:

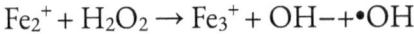

$Fe_2^+ + H_2O_2 \rightarrow Fe_3^+ + OH - + \bullet OH$

In this process, hydrogen peroxide is reduced by ferrous iron, generating hydroxyl radicals and ferric iron (Fe_3^+). Copper can also participate in similar reactions, contributing to •OH generation. The Fenton reaction is a critical contributor to oxidative stress because of the high reactivity of the resulting hydroxyl radical.

The Haber-Weiss Reaction

Another significant pathway for the production of hydroxyl radicals is the Haber-Weiss reaction, which involves the interaction of superoxide ($O_2^\bullet-$) and hydrogen peroxide (H_2O_2) to form hydroxyl radicals:

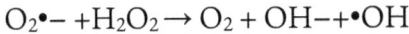

$O_2^\bullet- + H_2O_2 \rightarrow O_2 + OH - + \bullet OH$

This reaction proceeds in two steps. First, superoxide anion interacts with a transition metal ion (like Fe_3^+), producing O_2 and Fe_2^+. In the second step, Fe_2^+ reacts with H_2O_2 in the Fenton reaction, forming hydroxyl radicals. The Haber-Weiss reaction provides a pathway for hydroxyl radical production under conditions of elevated ROS.

Mitochondrial ROS Production

The mitochondria are the primary site of ROS generation in cells due to their role in oxidative phosphorylation. During electron transport, small amounts of oxygen are incompletely reduced, leading to the formation of superoxide anions ($O_2^\bullet-$). Through the mechanisms described above (Haber-Weiss and Fenton reactions), these anions can eventually lead to the production of hydroxyl radicals. Mitochondrial dysfunction or impairment can exacerbate this process, contributing to elevated levels of •OH, which can damage mitochondrial DNA (mtDNA), lipids, and proteins.

Exogenous Sources of Hydroxyl Radicals

While hydroxyl radicals are primarily produced endogenously, various environmental factors can also lead to their formation. Ultraviolet (UV) radiation, ionizing radiation, pollutants, and certain chemicals (e.g., tobacco smoke and pesticides) can generate ROS, including hydroxyl radicals. For example, ionizing radiation can cause water molecules in cells to split into hydroxyl radicals, contributing to oxidative damage that increases the risk of cancer.

Regulation of Hydroxyl Radicals

The high reactivity and potential for damage make the regulation of hydroxyl radicals critical to cellular health. Cells have evolved multiple antioxidant defense systems to neutralize ROS and prevent excessive hydroxyl radical formation. These regulatory mechanisms include both enzymatic and non-enzymatic components.

Antioxidant Enzymes

Several enzymes play crucial roles in the regulation and detoxification of ROS, helping to prevent the accumulation of hydroxyl radicals.

Superoxide Dismutase (SOD)

Superoxide dismutase is one of the first lines of defense against ROS, catalyzing the dismutation of superoxide anions ($O_2^{\bullet-}$) into hydrogen peroxide (H_2O_2) and oxygen (O_2). Although SOD does not directly neutralize hydroxyl radicals, it prevents their formation by removing the precursor superoxide anions that could otherwise participate in the Haber-Weiss reaction.

Catalase

Catalase is an enzyme that breaks down hydrogen peroxide into water and oxygen:

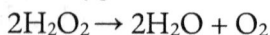

$$2H_2O_2 \rightarrow 2H_2O + O_2$$

By removing hydrogen peroxide, catalase limits the availability of this substrate for hydroxyl radical formation via the Fenton reaction. Catalase activity is found in peroxisomes, organelles specifically involved in detoxifying ROS.

Glutathione Peroxidase

Glutathione peroxidase is another key enzyme that protects cells from oxidative damage by reducing hydrogen peroxide and organic hydroperoxides using glutathione (GSH) as a cofactor:

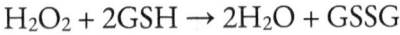

$$H_2O_2 + 2GSH \rightarrow 2H_2O + GSSG$$

This enzyme is particularly important in tissues with high oxidative stress, such as the liver, where detoxification of harmful substances is vital. By reducing hydrogen peroxide, glutathione peroxidase reduces the risk of hydroxyl radical formation.

Non-Enzymatic Antioxidants

In addition to enzymatic defense systems, the body employs several non-enzymatic antioxidants to neutralize ROS and reduce oxidative damage. These include vitamins, minerals, and other compounds that scavenge free radicals.

Vitamin C (Ascorbic Acid)

Vitamin C is a water-soluble antioxidant that directly scavenges ROS, including hydroxyl radicals. It donates electrons to neutralize free radicals, reducing oxidative damage. Vitamin C is particularly effective in extracellular fluids and can help regenerate other antioxidants, such as vitamin E.

Vitamin E (Tocopherol)

Vitamin E is a fat-soluble antioxidant that protects cell membranes from oxidative damage by scavenging lipid peroxyl radicals. While not directly involved in hydroxyl radical neutralization, it prevents the chain reaction of lipid peroxidation that hydroxyl radicals can initiate. By maintaining membrane integrity, vitamin E contributes to overall antioxidant defense.

Glutathione

Glutathione is a tripeptide composed of glutamine, cysteine, and glycine. It is one of the most important intracellular antioxidants, neutralizing ROS and maintaining cellular redox balance. In addition to its role as a cofactor for glutathione peroxidase, reduced glutathione (GSH) directly scavenges hydroxyl radicals, providing another layer of defense against oxidative damage.

Cellular Repair Mechanisms

In cases where hydroxyl radicals have already caused damage, cells employ repair mechanisms to fix damaged biomolecules. For example, DNA repair enzymes like base excision repair (BER) correct oxidative lesions in DNA caused by ROS. Similarly, damaged proteins are degraded by proteasomes, and lipid peroxidation products are removed or repaired by lipid-metabolizing enzymes.

Pathological Implications of Hydroxyl Radicals

When the balance between ROS production and antioxidant defenses is disrupted, oxidative stress occurs, leading to excessive hydroxyl radical production. This imbalance is implicated in several diseases.

Cancer

Hydroxyl radicals can cause mutations in DNA by inducing strand breaks and base modifications. If the damage is not repaired, these mutations can contribute to cancer initiation and progression. Oxidative stress is linked to various cancers, including lung, breast, and colon cancer.

Neurodegenerative Diseases

In diseases like Alzheimer's and Parkinson's, oxidative stress plays a key role in neuronal death. Hydroxyl radicals contribute to the accumulation of toxic protein aggregates and mitochondrial dysfunction, which further exacerbate oxidative damage.

Cardiovascular Disease

Oxidative stress is a major factor in the development of atherosclerosis, where hydroxyl radicals oxidize low-density lipoprotein (LDL), leading to plaque formation in blood vessels. This process increases the risk of heart attack and stroke.

Aging

The free radical theory of aging suggests that cumulative oxidative damage from ROS, including hydroxyl radicals, contributes to the aging process. Over time, the body's ability to repair oxidative damage declines, leading to the deterioration of cellular function and the onset of age-related diseases.

Hydroxyl radicals (•OH) are highly reactive molecules that play both beneficial and harmful roles in the body. While they are involved in immune responses, cell signaling, and apoptosis, their potential for causing oxidative damage makes their regulation critical for maintaining cellular health. Endogenously produced through reactions like the Fenton and Haber-Weiss processes and regulated by a network of antioxidant defenses, hydroxyl radicals must be tightly controlled to prevent disease. When regulation fails, excess hydroxyl radicals contribute to conditions such as cancer, neurodegenerative disorders, and cardiovascular disease. Understanding the intricate balance between ROS production and antioxidant defenses is key to mitigating the harmful effects of hydroxyl radicals while harnessing their beneficial roles.

PI3K/AKT/mTOR Pathway

The PI3K/AKT/mTOR pathway is a critical intracellular signaling pathway that plays a significant role in regulating various cellular processes, including growth, proliferation, survival, metabolism, and angiogenesis. This pathway is often dysregulated in many types of cancer and is a target for therapeutic interventions.

Overview of the PI3K/AKT/mTOR Pathway

The PI3K/AKT/mTOR pathway is a signal transduction pathway that begins with the activation of phosphoinositide 3-kinase (PI3K), which then leads to the activation of protein kinase B (AKT), and finally to the activation of the mammalian target of rapamycin (mTOR). The pathway is essential for the transmission of signals from extracellular growth factors to intracellular machinery that controls cell growth and survival.

Components of the Pathway

1. **PI3K (Phosphoinositide 3-Kinase):**
   - PI3K is a family of enzymes involved in cellular functions such as cell growth, proliferation, differentiation, motility, and survival.
   - PI3K is activated by various receptors, including receptor tyrosine kinases (RTKs), G-protein-coupled receptors (GPCRs), and integrins.
   - Upon activation, PI3K catalyzes the phosphorylation of phosphatidylinositol 4,5-bisphosphate (PIP2) to generate phosphatidylinositol 3,4,5-trisphosphate (PIP3), a key secondary messenger in the pathway.
2. **AKT (Protein Kinase B):**
   - AKT is a serine/threonine-specific protein kinase that plays a central role in the pathway.
   - It is recruited to the plasma membrane by binding to PIP3 and is subsequently activated by phosphorylation.
   - Activated AKT phosphorylates a wide range of downstream targets involved in cell survival, growth, and metabolism.

3. mTOR (Mammalian Target of Rapamycin):

- mTOR is a serine/threonine kinase that functions as a central regulator of cell growth, proliferation, and metabolism.
- mTOR exists in two distinct complexes: mTORC1 (mTOR Complex 1) and mTORC2 (mTOR Complex 2).
- mTORC1 is primarily involved in promoting protein synthesis and inhibiting autophagy, while mTORC2 is involved in regulating the cytoskeleton and activating AKT.

Activation and Regulation

The PI3K/AKT/mTOR pathway is activated by various extracellular signals, such as growth factors (e.g., insulin, IGF-1), cytokines, and hormones. These signals activate receptor tyrosine kinases (RTKs) or GPCRs, leading to the activation of PI3K. The pathway is tightly regulated by several mechanisms to ensure proper cellular function.

- **PTEN (Phosphatase and Tensin Homolog):** PTEN is a tumor suppressor that negatively regulates the pathway by dephosphorylating PIP3 back to PIP2, thus inhibiting AKT activation.
- **TSC1/TSC2 (Tuberous Sclerosis Complex):** TSC1/TSC2 complex acts as an upstream inhibitor of mTORC1 by inhibiting the GTPase Rheb, which is required for mTORC1 activation.
- **AMPK (AMP-activated Protein Kinase):** AMPK is an energy sensor that inhibits mTORC1 when cellular energy levels are low, thus preventing unnecessary cell growth under energy stress conditions.

Functions of the PI3K/AKT/mTOR Pathway

The PI3K/AKT/mTOR pathway is involved in regulating a multitude of cellular processes that are essential for normal cellular function and survival. The following sections detail the key functions of this pathway.

Cell Growth and Proliferation

One of the primary roles of the PI3K/AKT/mTOR pathway is to promote cell growth and proliferation. mTORC1, in particular, is a critical regulator of protein synthesis, which is necessary for cell growth.

- **mTORC1 and Protein Synthesis:** mTORC1 promotes protein synthesis by phosphorylating and activating S6K1 (ribosomal protein S6 kinase) and inhibiting 4E-BP1 (eukaryotic translation initiation factor 4E-binding protein 1). This leads to increased translation of mRNA into proteins, facilitating cell growth.
- **Regulation of Ribosome Biogenesis:** mTORC1 also regulates ribosome biogenesis, which is essential for protein synthesis. By controlling the production of ribosomal RNA (rRNA) and ribosomal proteins, mTORC1 ensures that cells have the capacity to produce the proteins required for growth and division.

Cell Survival and Apoptosis

The PI3K/AKT/mTOR pathway plays a crucial role in promoting cell survival and inhibiting apoptosis (programmed cell death).

- **AKT and Apoptosis Inhibition:** AKT promotes cell survival by phosphorylating and inactivating several pro-apoptotic factors, including BAD (Bcl-2-associated death promoter) and FOXO (Forkhead box O) transcription factors. By inactivating these factors, AKT prevents the initiation of apoptosis.
- **Regulation of Anti-apoptotic Proteins:** AKT also promotes the expression of anti-apoptotic proteins such as Bcl-2 and Mcl-1, further enhancing cell survival.

Metabolism

The pathway is intimately involved in regulating cellular metabolism to meet the energy and biosynthetic demands of cell growth and proliferation.

- **Glucose Metabolism:** AKT promotes glucose uptake by increasing the translocation of glucose transporter 4 (GLUT4) to the plasma membrane. It also enhances glycolysis by activating key glycolytic enzymes.
- **Lipid Metabolism:** AKT regulates lipid metabolism by promoting the synthesis of fatty acids and inhibiting fatty acid oxidation. This is achieved by phosphorylating and inhibiting acetyl-CoA carboxylase (ACC) and activating SREBP (sterol regulatory element-binding protein), which is involved in lipid biosynthesis.
- **Protein Metabolism:** mTORC1 regulates protein metabolism by promoting protein synthesis and inhibiting protein degradation through the autophagy pathway.

Angiogenesis

Angiogenesis, the formation of new blood vessels, is essential for supplying oxygen and nutrients to growing tissues and tumors. The PI3K/AKT/mTOR pathway is a key regulator of angiogenesis.

- **VEGF Production:** AKT promotes the production of vascular endothelial growth factor (VEGF), a potent angiogenic factor, by stabilizing hypoxia-inducible factor 1-alpha (HIF-1α). HIF-1α induces the expression of VEGF, leading to the formation of new blood vessels.
- **Endothelial Cell Function:** mTORC1 promotes the survival and proliferation of endothelial cells, which are essential for blood vessel formation. It also regulates the production of nitric oxide (NO), a molecule that promotes vasodilation and blood vessel permeability.

Dysregulation of the PI3K/AKT/mTOR Pathway in Disease

The PI3K/AKT/mTOR pathway is frequently dysregulated in various diseases, particularly cancer. Aberrations in this pathway can lead to uncontrolled cell growth, survival, and resistance to therapy, contributing to tumor development and progression.

Cancer

Dysregulation of the PI3K/AKT/mTOR pathway is one of the most common molecular alterations observed in cancer. Mutations, amplifications, and deletions in genes encoding components of the pathway can lead to its constitutive activation, promoting tumorigenesis.

- **PI3K Mutations:** Mutations in the PIK3CA gene, which encodes the p110α catalytic subunit of PI3K, are frequently observed in various cancers, including breast, colorectal, and endometrial cancers. These mutations result in the hyperactivation of PI3K, leading to increased PIP3 production and AKT activation.
- **PTEN Loss:** PTEN is one of the most commonly lost or mutated tumor suppressors in cancer. Loss of PTEN function leads to the accumulation of PIP3 and hyperactivation of AKT, promoting cell survival and growth.
- **AKT Amplification and Mutation:** Amplification or activating mutations in AKT can also lead to its constitutive activation, contributing to cancer progression.
- **mTOR Activation:** mTOR is often hyperactivated in cancer due to upstream mutations or alterations in its regulators, such as TSC1/TSC2. This leads to increased protein synthesis and cell growth, contributing to tumor development.

Other Roles of the PI3K/AKT/mTOR Pathway

Beyond its role in cancer, the PI3K/AKT/mTOR pathway is involved in various other physiological and pathological processes.

Metabolic Disorders

The PI3K/AKT/mTOR pathway is a key regulator of metabolic processes, and its dysregulation can contribute to metabolic disorders such as obesity and type 2 diabetes.

- **Insulin Signaling:** PI3K and AKT play critical roles in insulin signaling, promoting glucose uptake and metabolism in response to insulin. Dysregulation of this pathway can lead to insulin resistance, a hallmark of type 2 diabetes.
- **Obesity:** mTORC1 is involved in the regulation of adipogenesis (fat cell formation) and energy balance. Dysregulation of mTORC1 activity has been linked to obesity and related metabolic disorders.

Neurological Disorders

The PI3K/AKT/mTOR pathway is also implicated in the development and function of the nervous system, and its dysregulation is associated with various neurological disorders.

- **Neurodevelopment:** AKT signaling is important for neuronal survival, growth, and differentiation. Dysregulation of AKT signaling can lead to neurodevelopmental disorders such as autism and schizophrenia.
- **Neurodegeneration:** The pathway is involved in the regulation of autophagy, a process that clears damaged cellular components. Dysregulation of autophagy due to aberrant mTOR signaling is associated with neurodegenerative diseases such as Alzheimer's and Parkinson's disease.

The PI3K/AKT/mTOR pathway is a fundamental signaling pathway that regulates a wide range of cellular processes, including growth, proliferation, survival, metabolism, and angiogenesis. Its dysregulation is implicated in the development of various diseases, particularly cancer.

The RAS Pathway

The RAS pathway is one of the most well-studied signal transduction pathways in biology, with critical roles in regulating cell proliferation, differentiation, survival, and apoptosis. Mutations in the RAS pathway are implicated in various cancers and other diseases, making it a significant focus in both research and clinical settings.

Introduction to the RAS Pathway

The RAS pathway, often referred to as the RAS-MAPK (mitogen-activated protein kinase) pathway, is a critical signal transduction cascade that transmits signals from cell surface receptors to the nucleus. This pathway is involved in the regulation of a variety of cellular processes, including growth, survival, and differentiation. The name "RAS" is derived from the Rat Sarcoma virus, where the gene was first discovered. RAS proteins are small GTPases, enzymes that bind and hydrolyze GTP, acting as molecular switches to turn signaling pathways on and off.

Components of the RAS Pathway

The RAS pathway is composed of several key proteins and molecules that work together to transmit signals from the cell membrane to the nucleus. The main components include:

- **RAS Proteins**: These small GTPases (H-RAS, K-RAS, and N-RAS) are the central players in the pathway. They are activated by GTP binding and inactivated by GTP hydrolysis.
- **Growth Factor Receptors**: These are typically receptor tyrosine kinases (RTKs) located on the cell surface that initiate the signaling cascade when bound by growth factors.
- **Adaptor Proteins**: GRB2 (growth factor receptor-bound protein 2) is a key adaptor protein that links activated RTKs to the downstream signaling molecules.
- **SOS (Son of Sevenless)**: This is a guanine nucleotide exchange factor (GEF) that facilitates the exchange of GDP for GTP on RAS, thus activating it.
- **RAF Kinases**: RAF proteins (A-RAF, B-RAF, C-RAF) are serine/threonine kinases that are directly activated by RAS and, in turn, activate the downstream MAPK/ERK pathway.
- **MEK (MAPK/ERK Kinase)**: MEK1/2 are dual-specificity kinases that phosphorylate and activate ERK1/2.
- **ERK (Extracellular Signal-Regulated Kinase)**: ERK1/2 are critical kinases that enter the nucleus to regulate gene expression by phosphorylating various transcription factors.

Function of the RAS Pathway

The RAS pathway regulates multiple cellular processes, primarily through the activation of gene transcription that governs cell proliferation, differentiation, survival, and apoptosis. The key functions of the pathway include:

- **Cell Proliferation**: The pathway promotes the expression of genes that drive the cell cycle, leading to cell division. This function is critical during development and tissue regeneration but can lead to cancer if dysregulated.

- **Cell Differentiation**: By influencing the expression of specific sets of genes, the RAS pathway helps determine the fate of a cell, guiding it to differentiate into a particular cell type.
- **Cell Survival**: The pathway activates anti-apoptotic genes, helping cells resist programmed cell death under certain conditions, such as during growth or in response to survival signals.
- **Cell Migration**: The RAS pathway can influence the cytoskeleton and cell adhesion molecules, affecting how cells move and interact with their environment. This is particularly important during embryonic development and wound healing.

Production of RAS Proteins

RAS proteins are encoded by the RAS gene family, which includes HRAS, KRAS, and NRAS. These genes are expressed in various tissues and are responsible for producing the RAS proteins. The production of RAS proteins involves several steps:

- **Transcription**: The RAS genes are transcribed into mRNA in the nucleus. This process is regulated by transcription factors that respond to cellular signals.
- **Translation**: The mRNA is then translated into the RAS protein in the cytoplasm. Ribosomes facilitate this process by reading the mRNA and assembling the corresponding amino acid sequence.
- **Post-Translational Modifications**: Once synthesized, RAS proteins undergo several post-translational modifications that are critical for their function. These include:
  - **Prenylation**: The addition of a lipid group (farnesyl or geranylgeranyl) to the C-terminus of the RAS protein, which is essential for its attachment to the cell membrane.

- **Palmitoylation**: A reversible lipid modification that further anchors RAS to the membrane and regulates its localization.
- **Proteolysis**: The removal of a small C-terminal peptide to expose the prenylation site.
- **Methylation**: The addition of a methyl group to the prenylated cysteine, which is thought to play a role in membrane association.

These modifications ensure that RAS is properly localized to the plasma membrane, where it can interact with other components of the signaling pathway.

Activation and Deactivation of the RAS Pathway

The RAS pathway is tightly regulated by a cycle of activation and deactivation, ensuring that signals are transmitted only when appropriate.

- **Activation**: The pathway is activated when growth factors or other signaling molecules bind to receptor tyrosine kinases (RTKs) on the cell surface. This leads to the dimerization and autophosphorylation of the RTKs, creating docking sites for adaptor proteins like GRB2. GRB2 then recruits SOS, which acts as a guanine nucleotide exchange factor (GEF) to catalyze the exchange of GDP for GTP on RAS. GTP-bound RAS is the active form, which can then interact with and activate downstream effectors like RAF kinases.
- **Signal Propagation**: Once RAS is activated, it triggers a kinase cascade. RAS activates RAF, which then phosphorylates and activates MEK. MEK, in turn, phosphorylates ERK. Active ERK translocates to the nucleus, where it phosphorylates transcription factors, leading to changes in gene expression.
- **Deactivation**: RAS is inactivated by GTPase-activating proteins (GAPs), which accelerate the hydrolysis of GTP to GDP. The

GDP-bound form of RAS is inactive and unable to propagate the signal. This deactivation is crucial for preventing excessive or prolonged signaling that could lead to uncontrolled cell proliferation or other pathological conditions.

Regulation of the RAS Pathway

The RAS pathway is regulated at multiple levels to ensure that the appropriate cellular responses are elicited without leading to pathological conditions.

- **Regulation by Receptor Tyrosine Kinases (RTKs)**: The availability and activation state of RTKs directly influence the activation of the RAS pathway. RTKs are regulated by ligand availability, receptor dimerization, internalization, and degradation. Overexpression or mutations in RTKs can lead to aberrant activation of the RAS pathway.
- **GTPase-Activating Proteins (GAPs)**: GAPs play a critical role in turning off RAS signaling by enhancing its intrinsic GTPase activity. Mutations in GAPs, such as neurofibromin (NF1), a tumor suppressor, can lead to prolonged RAS activation and contribute to tumorigenesis.
- **Guanine Nucleotide Exchange Factors (GEFs)**: The activity of GEFs like SOS is also tightly regulated. SOS is recruited to the plasma membrane by interaction with GRB2 and phosphotyrosine residues on activated RTKs. Its activity is further modulated by phosphorylation and feedback mechanisms involving downstream signaling components.
- **Negative Feedback Loops**: The RAS pathway is subject to negative feedback regulation, where downstream components, such as ERK, can phosphorylate and inhibit upstream components, including RAF and SOS. This feedback ensures that the pathway is not overactivated.

- **Regulation by Phosphatases**: Phosphatases remove phosphate groups from proteins, counteracting the activity of kinases. For example, MAPK phosphatases (MKPs) dephosphorylate and inactivate ERK, providing another layer of regulation.
- **Subcellular Localization**: The localization of RAS and other pathway components is crucial for their function. RAS must be localized to the plasma membrane to interact with its effectors. Mislocalization of RAS, due to mutations in the prenylation or palmitoylation sites, can disrupt its signaling.
- **Oncogenic Mutations**: Mutations in RAS genes (particularly in KRAS) are among the most common oncogenic mutations in human cancers. These mutations often result in constitutive activation of RAS by impairing its GTPase activity, leading to continuous cell proliferation signals. Such mutations are challenging to target therapeutically, making them a major focus of cancer research.

Pathological Implications of Dysregulated RAS Signaling

Dysregulation of the RAS pathway is implicated in various diseases, particularly cancer. Oncogenic mutations in RAS genes (e.g., KRAS, NRAS, HRAS) are prevalent in many types of cancer, including pancreatic, colorectal, lung, and melanoma. These mutations typically result in constitutively active RAS that drives uncontrolled cell proliferation and survival.

- **Cancer**: Mutations in the RAS genes are found in approximately 30% of all human cancers. KRAS mutations are particularly common in pancreatic adenocarcinoma, colorectal cancer, and non-small cell lung cancer. These mutations often occur at codons 12, 13, or 61 and lead to the loss of GTPase activity, resulting in a RAS protein that is constantly active. The resulting hyperactivation of the downstream signaling pathways, particularly the

RAF-MEK-ERK and PI3K-AKT pathways, promotes oncogenesis by driving cell proliferation, survival, and metastasis.

- **Cardio-Facio-Cutaneous (CFC) Syndrome**: This is a rare genetic disorder caused by mutations in genes that encode components of the RAS-MAPK pathway, including KRAS, BRAF, and MEK1/2. CFC syndrome is characterized by cardiac defects, distinctive facial features, skin abnormalities, and developmental delays. The mutations lead to constitutive activation of the RAS-MAPK pathway, resulting in abnormal development.

- **Neurofibromatosis Type 1 (NF1)**: NF1 is an autosomal dominant genetic disorder caused by mutations in the NF1 gene, which encodes neurofibromin, a GAP that inactivates RAS. Loss of neurofibromin function leads to hyperactive RAS signaling, resulting in the development of benign and malignant tumors, particularly neurofibromas, and an increased risk of gliomas, pheochromocytomas, and other malignancies.

- **Noonan Syndrome**: Noonan syndrome is a developmental disorder caused by mutations in genes that encode components of the RAS-MAPK pathway, including PTPN11 (which encodes SHP2, a phosphatase that activates RAS signaling) and KRAS. It is characterized by distinctive facial features, short stature, heart defects, and an increased risk of leukemia. The mutations result in hyperactivation of the RAS-MAPK pathway, leading to abnormal growth and development.

- **Therapeutic Targeting of the RAS Pathway**: Given the central role of the RAS pathway in cancer, it has been a major target for drug development. However, targeting RAS directly has proven challenging due to its high affinity for GTP/GDP and the lack of suitable binding pockets for small molecules. Despite these challenges, recent advances have led to the development of inhibitors targeting specific mutations in KRAS (e.g., KRAS G12C inhibitors) and other components of the pathway (e.g., MEK and RAF inhibitors). Combination therapies targeting multiple points in the pathway, along with immunotherapy, are also being explored to overcome resistance mechanisms.

The RAS pathway is a crucial regulator of cellular processes, including proliferation, differentiation, survival, and apoptosis. Its proper function is essential for normal development and tissue homeostasis, while its dysregulation is a key driver of various diseases, particularly cancer. The pathway is tightly regulated at multiple levels, including through receptor tyrosine kinases, GTPase-activating proteins, and negative feedback mechanisms. Despite the challenges associated with targeting the RAS pathway therapeutically, ongoing research continues to provide new insights and potential strategies for treating RAS-driven diseases.

As our understanding of the RAS pathway deepens, it offers promising avenues for developing targeted therapies that can more effectively treat cancers and other disorders associated with dysregulated RAS signaling.

3

Tumor Suppressor Genes

Tumor suppressor genes play a critical role in maintaining cellular integrity by regulating cell division, repairing DNA errors, and ensuring that cells with damaged DNA do not proliferate uncontrollably. These genes are often referred to as the *"guardians of the genome"* because they protect cells from turning into cancerous cells. When tumor suppressor genes are mutated or inactivated, their protective functions are compromised, leading to increased risks of cancer development.

This chapter will provide a comprehensive overview of tumor suppressor genes, including their functions, mechanisms of action, the pathways they regulate, and their implications in cancer. Additionally, the chapter will explore the different types of tumor suppressor genes, and the processes through which they are inactivated.

The Role of Tumor Suppressor Genes in Cellular Function

Tumor suppressor genes are essential for regulating the cell cycle, ensuring that cells only divide when appropriate and that any genetic damage is repaired before cell division occurs. These genes can initiate apoptosis (programmed cell death) if the damage is irreparable, preventing the propagation of defective cells.

Key functions of tumor suppressor genes include:

1. **Cell Cycle Regulation**: Tumor suppressor genes like RB1 (Retinoblastoma 1) play a pivotal role in controlling the pro-

gression of the cell cycle, particularly the transition from the G1 phase to the S phase, where DNA replication occurs.

2. **DNA Repair**: Genes such as BRCA1 and BRCA2 are involved in the repair of DNA double-strand breaks, ensuring that genetic information is accurately passed on during cell division.

3. **Apoptosis Induction**: TP53, also known as the *"guardian of the genome,"* is crucial in triggering apoptosis in cells with significant DNA damage, preventing the survival and proliferation of potentially cancerous cells.

Mechanisms of Tumor Suppressor Gene Inactivation

Tumor suppressor genes can be inactivated through several mechanisms, which often lead to the onset of cancer. These mechanisms include:

1. **Mutations**: Point mutations, deletions, or insertions can result in a loss of function of tumor suppressor genes. For example, a mutation in the TP53 gene can lead to a defective p53 protein, which cannot effectively initiate apoptosis.

2. **Epigenetic Modifications**: DNA methylation and histone modification can silence tumor suppressor genes without altering the underlying DNA sequence. This epigenetic silencing is a common feature in many cancers.

3. **Loss of Heterozygosity (LOH)**: Tumor suppressor genes are often subject to LOH, where one allele of a gene is lost, leading to the complete inactivation of the gene if the remaining allele is already mutated or silenced.

4. **Chromosomal Deletions**: Large deletions in chromosomes can result in the loss of tumor suppressor genes. For example, deletions in chromosome 17p are often associated with the loss of TP53.

Major Tumor Suppressor Genes and Their Pathways

Several key tumor suppressor genes have been identified, each playing unique roles in cellular processes. This section will delve into the most well-studied tumor suppressor genes and their associated pathways:

1. **TP53 (p53 Pathway)**: TP53 is the most frequently mutated tumor suppressor gene in human cancers. The p53 protein it encodes is involved in DNA repair, apoptosis, and cell cycle arrest. The p53 pathway is activated in response to DNA damage, oncogene activation, or other cellular stressors, leading to the activation of target genes that mediate its effects.

2. **RB1 (Retinoblastoma Protein Pathway)**: The RB1 gene is crucial for controlling the cell cycle. The retinoblastoma protein (pRB) it encodes regulates the transition from the G1 to the S phase by inhibiting the activity of E2F transcription factors. Loss of RB1 function leads to unchecked cell proliferation.

3. **BRCA1 and BRCA2 (DNA Repair Pathway)**: BRCA1 and BRCA2 are involved in the homologous recombination repair of DNA double-strand breaks. Mutations in these genes are strongly associated with an increased risk of breast and ovarian cancers.

4. **APC (Wnt Signaling Pathway)**: The APC gene is a critical component of the Wnt signaling pathway, which regulates cell proliferation, differentiation, and apoptosis. Mutations in APC are commonly associated with colorectal cancer.

5. **PTEN (PI3K/AKT Pathway)**: PTEN is a phosphatase that negatively regulates the PI3K/AKT signaling pathway, which is involved in cell growth and survival. Loss of PTEN function leads to hyperactivation of this pathway, promoting cancer development.

Tumor Suppressor Gene Inactivation and Cancer

The inactivation of tumor suppressor genes is a hallmark of cancer. When these genes are no longer functional, cells lose critical regulatory controls, leading to unregulated cell growth, evasion of apoptosis, increased genomic instability, and other malignant behaviors.

This section will explore how the loss of function of specific tumor suppressor genes contributes to different types of cancer. For example:

- **Loss of TP53** is implicated in more than 50% of human cancers, including lung, colorectal, and breast cancers.
- **RB1 mutations** are associated with retinoblastoma, a rare childhood cancer, as well as other cancers such as osteosarcoma and small cell lung cancer.
- **BRCA1/2 mutations** significantly increase the risk of hereditary breast and ovarian cancers.

Tumor suppressor genes are fundamental to the prevention of cancer. Their inactivation represents a key step in tumorigenesis, and understanding the mechanisms by which these genes are silenced or mutated provides critical insights into cancer biology.

This chapter aims to equip readers with a thorough understanding of the complexity and significance of tumor suppressor genes, providing a foundation for further study and exploration in the field of cancer research.

TP53

The TP53 gene, also known as the guardian of the genome, plays a crucial role in regulating cell growth, maintaining genomic stability, and preventing tumorigenesis. As a central component of the cell's defense against cancer, TP53 is one of the most studied genes in molecular biology and oncology.

Function of TP53

TP53 encodes the p53 protein, a transcription factor that regulates the expression of various genes involved in cell cycle control, DNA repair, apoptosis (programmed cell death), and senescence (permanent cell cycle arrest). The primary function of p53 is to prevent the proliferation of cells with damaged DNA, thereby maintaining genomic integrity.

1. **Cell Cycle Arrest**: When DNA damage is detected, p53 can induce cell cycle arrest, primarily at the G1/S checkpoint, to allow time for DNA repair. This function is mediated by the transcriptional activation of the cyclin-dependent kinase inhibitor p21 (CDKN1A), which binds to and inhibits cyclin-CDK complexes, halting cell cycle progression.

2. **DNA Repair**: p53 also plays a role in DNA repair processes by upregulating genes involved in nucleotide excision repair, base excision repair, and homologous recombination. By facilitating these repair pathways, p53 ensures that cells can correct DNA damage before resuming proliferation.

3. **Apoptosis**: If the DNA damage is irreparable, p53 can initiate apoptosis to eliminate the damaged cell. This process involves the transcriptional activation of pro-apoptotic genes such as BAX, PUMA, and NOXA, which promote mitochondrial outer membrane permeabilization and the activation of caspases, leading to cell death.

4. **Senescence**: p53 can induce senescence, a state of permanent cell cycle arrest, in response to various stress signals, including oncogene activation and oxidative stress. Senescent cells no longer proliferate but remain metabolically active and secrete factors that can influence the tissue microenvironment.

5. **Angiogenesis Inhibition**: p53 also inhibits angiogenesis, the formation of new blood vessels, by downregulating pro-angiogenic factors such as vascular endothelial growth factor (VEGF) and upregulating anti-angiogenic factors like thrombospondin-1.

6. **Metabolic Regulation**: Recent research has uncovered a role for p53 in metabolic regulation, where it influences glycolysis, oxidative phosphorylation, and antioxidant defense, thus linking metabolic homeostasis with tumor suppression.

Production of TP53

The TP53 gene is located on chromosome 17p13.1 and spans approximately 20 kilobases of genomic DNA. It contains 11 exons and produces a 2.2-kilobase mRNA that is translated into the p53 protein. The p53 protein is composed of 393 amino acids and has a molecular weight of approximately 53 kDa.

The production of p53 is tightly regulated at multiple levels, including transcriptional, post-transcriptional, and post-translational mechanisms:

1. **Transcriptional Regulation**: The transcription of TP53 is controlled by various transcription factors, including Sp1 and E2F1, which bind to the TP53 promoter region to modulate its expression. Additionally, TP53 transcription can be influenced by cellular stress signals such as DNA damage, oxidative stress, and hypoxia.

2. **Post-Transcriptional Regulation**: TP53 mRNA stability and translation are regulated by RNA-binding proteins and microR-

NAs. For example, microRNA-504 has been shown to directly bind to TP53 mRNA, inhibiting its translation and reducing p53 protein levels.

3. **Post-Translational Modifications**: The activity of p53 is primarily regulated by post-translational modifications, including phosphorylation, acetylation, ubiquitination, sumoylation, and methylation. These modifications alter p53's stability, subcellular localization, DNA-binding affinity, and interaction with other proteins.

   • **Phosphorylation**: Phosphorylation of p53, particularly at serine and threonine residues, occurs in response to stress signals and enhances its stability by preventing interaction with its negative regulator, MDM2. Kinases such as ATM, ATR, Chk1, and Chk2 are responsible for p53 phosphorylation.

   • **Acetylation**: Acetylation of p53 by acetyltransferases such as p300/CBP and PCAF enhances its transcriptional activity by promoting the recruitment of coactivators and inhibiting its interaction with repressors.

   • **Ubiquitination**: Ubiquitination of p53, mediated primarily by MDM2, targets it for proteasomal degradation. MDM2 binds to the N-terminal domain of p53, facilitating its ubiquitination and subsequent degradation, thereby maintaining low basal levels of p53 in unstressed cells.

   • **Sumoylation and Methylation**: Sumoylation and methylation of p53 can modulate its activity by affecting its interaction with other proteins and its ability to bind DNA.

Regulation of TP53

The regulation of TP53 is complex and involves multiple feedback loops and regulatory proteins that ensure the appropriate cellular response to various stress signals. Key regulators of TP53 include MDM2, MDM4, ARF, and various post-translational modifications.

1. **MDM2 and MDM4**: The most well-characterized regulators of p53 are MDM2 and MDM4 (also known as MDMX). MDM2 is an E3 ubiquitin ligase that ubiquitinates p53, leading to its proteasomal degradation. MDM4, although structurally similar to MDM2, lacks ubiquitin ligase activity and primarily inhibits p53's transcriptional activity by binding to its transactivation domain.

   • **Negative Feedback Loop**: A critical regulatory mechanism involves a negative feedback loop between p53 and MDM2. p53 transcriptionally activates MDM2 expression, which in turn ubiquitinates p53, leading to its degradation. This feedback loop maintains low levels of p53 in unstressed cells and allows for rapid p53 accumulation in response to stress.

   • **Inhibition of MDM2/MDM4**: In response to stress signals such as DNA damage, the activity of MDM2 and MDM4 is inhibited, leading to the stabilization and activation of p53. This inhibition can occur through various mechanisms, including phosphorylation of p53 and MDM2, binding of ARF to MDM2, and disruption of the p53-MDM2/MDM4 interaction by small molecules or peptides.

2. **ARF (Alternative Reading Frame Protein)**: ARF is a tumor suppressor that antagonizes MDM2, thereby stabilizing p53. ARF binds to MDM2 and sequesters it in the nucleolus, preventing it from ubiquitinating p53. The ARF-MDM2-p53 pathway is a critical component of the cellular response to oncogene activation, as ARF is induced by hyperproliferative signals, leading to p53 activation and cell cycle arrest or apoptosis.

3. **Post-Translational Modifications**: As mentioned earlier, post-translational modifications such as phosphorylation, acetylation, and ubiquitination play a central role in regulating p53's stability, activity, and interactions. These modifications are often mediated by stress-activated kinases and other enzymes in response to DNA damage, oxidative stress, hypoxia, and other cellular stressors.

- **ATM/ATR and Chk1/Chk2 Kinases**: DNA damage activates the ATM and ATR kinases, which in turn phosphorylate and activate the Chk1 and Chk2 kinases. These kinases phosphorylate p53 at specific serine residues (e.g., Ser15 and Ser20), leading to its stabilization and activation.
- **p300/CBP and PCAF**: The acetyltransferases p300/CBP and PCAF acetylate p53 at lysine residues, enhancing its transcriptional activity. Acetylation promotes the recruitment of transcriptional coactivators and inhibits the binding of repressors such as MDM2.

4. **p53 Isoforms and Mutants**: TP53 can produce multiple isoforms through alternative splicing, alternative promoter usage, and alternative initiation of translation. These isoforms can have distinct or even opposing functions, adding another layer of complexity to p53 regulation. Moreover, mutations in TP53, particularly missense mutations in the DNA-binding domain, are common in various cancers and can lead to loss of p53 function or gain of oncogenic functions (e.g., promoting cell proliferation and survival).

TP53 Pathways and Their Role in Cancer Suppression

The TP53 gene is at the heart of several cellular pathways that collectively prevent the development of cancer. These pathways involve a network of genes and proteins that work together to maintain genomic stability, regulate cell growth, and eliminate damaged or potentially cancerous cells.

1. **DNA Damage Response Pathway**: One of the primary pathways involving p53 is the DNA damage response (DDR) pathway. When DNA damage is detected, sensors such as ATM and ATR are activated, leading to the phosphorylation and stabilization of p53. Activated p53 then induces the expression of genes involved in DNA repair, cell cycle arrest, and apoptosis.
   - **G1/S and G2/M Checkpoints**: p53-mediated cell cycle arrest occurs primarily at the G1/S checkpoint, allowing for DNA repair before the cell enters S phase (DNA synthesis). p53 can also induce cell cycle arrest at the G2/M checkpoint, preventing cells with damaged DNA from entering mitosis.
   - **p21 and Cyclin-CDK Inhibition**: The p21 protein, a downstream target of p53, inhibits cyclin-CDK complexes, thereby halting cell cycle progression. This allows the cell to repair its DNA or, if the damage is too severe, to undergo apoptosis or senescence.

2. **Apoptosis Pathway**: p53-induced apoptosis is a critical mechanism for eliminating damaged cells that could potentially become cancerous. p53 activates the transcription of pro-apoptotic genes such as BAX, PUMA, and NOXA, which promote the release of cytochrome c from mitochondria and the activation of caspases, leading to cell death.
   - **Intrinsic and Extrinsic Apoptosis Pathways**: p53 can initiate apoptosis through both the intrinsic (mitochondrial) and extrinsic (death receptor) pathways. In the intrinsic pathway, p53-induced BAX and PUMA promote mitochondrial outer membrane permeabilization, leading to cytochrome c release and caspase activation. In the extrinsic pathway, p53 can enhance the expression of death

receptors such as Fas, leading to caspase activation through death receptor signaling.

3. **Senescence Pathway**: p53-induced senescence is a tumor-suppressive mechanism that permanently arrests the cell cycle, preventing the proliferation of damaged or stressed cells. Senescence is characterized by the upregulation of cell cycle inhibitors such as p21 and p16, as well as changes in chromatin structure and gene expression.

   • **Senescence-Associated Secretory Phenotype (SASP)**: Senescent cells secrete various cytokines, growth factors, and proteases that can influence the surrounding tissue microenvironment. While SASP can have both pro-tumorigenic and anti-tumorigenic effects, p53-induced senescence generally serves as a barrier to cancer development.

4. **Metabolic Pathways**: p53 also regulates cellular metabolism by modulating the expression of genes involved in glycolysis, oxidative phosphorylation, and antioxidant defense. p53 can inhibit the Warburg effect, a metabolic shift commonly observed in cancer cells, by repressing glycolytic enzymes and promoting mitochondrial respiration.

   • **Antioxidant Defense**: p53 promotes the expression of antioxidant genes such as Sestrin1, Sestrin2, and TIGAR, which help to reduce reactive oxygen species (ROS) levels and prevent oxidative stress-induced DNA damage. By maintaining redox balance, p53 contributes to the prevention of oxidative stress-related tumorigenesis.

5. **Angiogenesis Inhibition Pathway**: p53 suppresses angiogenesis, the formation of new blood vessels, by downregulating pro-angiogenic factors like VEGF and upregulating anti-angiogenic factors such as thrombospondin-1. By inhibiting angiogenesis, p53 prevents the formation of new blood vessels that could supply nutrients and oxygen to growing tumors.

6. **Stem Cell Regulation Pathway**: Emerging evidence suggests that p53 plays a role in regulating stem cell function and preventing the expansion of cancer stem cells. p53 can influence the self-renewal and differentiation of stem cells, thereby limiting the pool of cells that can give rise to tumors.

   • **p53 and Cancer Stem Cells**: Cancer stem cells are a subpopulation of tumor cells with the ability to self-renew and differentiate into various cell types within a tumor. p53's role in suppressing cancer stem cells is an area of active research, with implications for cancer prevention.

TP53 Mutations and Cancer

Mutations in the TP53 gene are among the most common genetic alterations in human cancers, occurring in approximately 50% of all tumors. These mutations often result in the loss of normal p53 function, leading to uncontrolled cell proliferation, resistance to apoptosis, and increased genomic instability.

1. **Types of TP53 Mutations**: TP53 mutations can be classified into several categories, including missense mutations, nonsense mutations, frameshift mutations, and deletions. The most common type of TP53 mutation is a missense mutation in the DNA-binding domain, which impairs p53's ability to bind to its target genes and regulate their expression.

2. **Loss of Function**: Many TP53 mutations result in the loss of p53's tumor-suppressive functions, including cell cycle arrest, apoptosis, and DNA repair. Cells with mutated p53 are more likely to accumulate additional genetic alterations, leading to the development and progression of cancer.

3. **Gain of Function**: In some cases, TP53 mutations can confer gain-of-function (GOF) properties, where the mutant p53 protein acquires new oncogenic activities that promote tumorigen-

esis. GOF mutant p53 can enhance cell proliferation, invasion, metastasis, and resistance to chemotherapy.

4. **Dominant-Negative Effect**: Certain TP53 mutations exhibit a dominant-negative effect, where the mutant p53 protein interferes with the function of wild-type p53. This effect can occur when the mutant p53 forms complexes with wild-type p53, preventing it from binding to DNA and activating target genes.

The TP53 tumor suppressor gene is a critical regulator of cellular processes that maintain genomic integrity and prevent tumorigenesis. Through its roles in cell cycle control, DNA repair, apoptosis, senescence, and metabolic regulation, p53 acts as a central guardian against cancer development. However, mutations in TP53 are among the most common genetic alterations in human cancers, leading to the loss of p53's tumor-suppressive functions and the acquisition of oncogenic properties.

RB1

The RB1 tumor suppressor gene is one of the most studied and significant genes in the context of cancer biology. The RB1 gene encodes the retinoblastoma protein (pRB), which plays a crucial role in cell cycle regulation, differentiation, apoptosis, and genomic stability. Disruptions in the RB1 gene are closely linked to the development of various cancers, most notably retinoblastoma, but also many others, including breast cancer, lung cancer, and osteosarcoma.

Function of the RB1 Gene

The RB1 gene functions as a tumor suppressor by regulating the cell cycle, particularly the transition from the G1 phase to the S phase. The gene product, pRB, is a key player in this regulation. The protein operates by controlling the activity of E2F transcription factors, which are essential for the progression of the cell cycle. In its active, hypophosphorylated state, pRB binds to E2F transcription factors, preventing them from initiating the transcription of genes required for DNA synthesis and S phase entry.

When the cell is ready to progress to the S phase, pRB becomes phosphorylated by cyclin-dependent kinases (CDKs), leading to its inactivation. This phosphorylation causes pRB to release E2F transcription factors, thereby allowing the transcription of genes necessary for DNA replication and cell cycle progression. This regulatory mechanism ensures that cells only enter the S phase when appropriate signals are present, thereby preventing uncontrolled cell division.

Production of the RB1 Gene Product

The RB1 gene is located on chromosome 13q14.2 and consists of 27 exons. The gene spans approximately 200 kilobases and produces a 4.7 kb mRNA transcript that is translated into the pRB protein. The production of pRB is tightly regulated at the transcriptional, post-transcriptional, and post-translational levels to ensure proper cell cycle control.

Transcriptional Regulation

The transcription of the RB1 gene is controlled by various transcription factors, including E2F, Sp1, and AP-1, among others. E2F, despite being regulated by pRB, can also influence the transcription of the RB1 gene itself, creating a feedback loop. In the G0 and early G1 phases, pRB is hypophosphorylated and binds to E2F, inhibiting its activity. As cells progress through the cell cycle, pRB is phosphorylated, leading to the release of E2F, which can then promote the transcription of genes, including RB1, necessary for S phase entry and progression.

Post-Transcriptional Regulation

Post-transcriptional regulation of RB1 involves alternative splicing, mRNA stability, and microRNA (miRNA) interactions. Alternative splicing of RB1 mRNA can generate different isoforms of pRB with varying functions. The stability of RB1 mRNA is also subject to regulation by RNA-binding proteins and miRNAs. For example, miR-17-92 cluster miRNAs have been shown to target RB1 mRNA, leading to its degradation and reduced pRB levels, which can contribute to oncogenesis.

Post-Translational Regulation

The activity of pRB is primarily regulated by phosphorylation, as mentioned earlier. Cyclin D-CDK4/6 and cyclin E-CDK2 complexes phosphorylate pRB at multiple serine and threonine residues, leading to its inactivation and the subsequent release of E2F transcription factors. Dephosphorylation of pRB, mediated by protein phosphatases such as PP1, reactivates its tumor-suppressive functions. Additionally, pRB can be regulated by acetylation, ubiquitination, and other post-translational modifications that influence its stability and interaction with other proteins.

Regulation of the RB1 Pathway

The RB1 pathway is a critical component of cell cycle control and is regulated by a complex network of proteins that ensure proper cell proliferation and differentiation. Disruption of this pathway can lead to unchecked cell division and tumorigenesis. The key regulators of the RB1 pathway include CDKs, cyclins, CDK inhibitors, and various transcription factors.

Cyclins and CDKs

Cyclins are proteins that bind to CDKs, activating their kinase activity. Different cyclins are expressed at different stages of the cell cycle, ensuring that CDKs are active only at specific times. For example, cyclin D binds to CDK4/6 in the early G1 phase, leading to the initial phosphorylation of pRB. As the cell progresses through the G1 phase, cyclin E binds to CDK2, further phosphorylating pRB and driving the cell into the S phase. This stepwise phosphorylation of pRB is crucial for the precise control of the cell cycle.

CDK Inhibitors

CDK inhibitors (CKIs) are proteins that bind to and inhibit the activity of cyclin-CDK complexes, thereby preventing the phosphorylation of pRB. There are two main families of CKIs: the INK4 family (which includes p16INK4a, p15INK4b, p18INK4c, and p19INK4d) and the CIP/KIP family (which includes p21CIP1, p27KIP1, and p57KIP2). These inhibitors play a crucial role in preventing uncontrolled cell proliferation by maintaining pRB in its active, hypophosphorylated state.

E2F Transcription Factors

E2F transcription factors are the primary targets of pRB and are essential for the transcription of genes required for DNA replication and S phase entry. The E2F family consists of several members, some of which act as transcriptional activators (e.g., E2F1, E2F2, E2F3a) and others as repressors (e.g., E2F3b, E2F4, E2F5). The activity of E2F factors is tightly regulated by their interaction with pRB. When bound to pRB, E2F transcription factors are unable to promote gene expression, thereby inhibiting cell cycle progression.

pRB Interacting Proteins

In addition to E2F transcription factors, pRB interacts with a wide range of proteins that influence its function and stability. These include histone deacetylases (HDACs), chromatin remodeling factors, and other transcriptional regulators. Through these interactions, pRB can modulate chromatin structure and gene expression, contributing to its role in cell cycle control and differentiation.

Pathways Involving the RB1 Gene

The RB1 gene is involved in several key cellular pathways that regulate cell proliferation, apoptosis, and differentiation. These pathways include the p16INK4a-CDK4/6-pRB-E2F pathway, the p53-p21 pathway, and the TGF-β pathway, among others.

p16INK4a-CDK4/6-pRB-E2F Pathway

This pathway is central to the regulation of the cell cycle and is often referred to as the "RB pathway." The pathway is activated in response to various mitogenic signals that promote cell proliferation. Upon activation, cyclin D binds to CDK4/6, forming an active complex that phosphorylates pRB. Phosphorylated pRB releases E2F transcription factors, allowing the transcription of genes required for S phase entry.

The p16INK4a protein, a member of the INK4 family of CDK inhibitors, binds to CDK4/6 and prevents their association with cyclin D, thereby inhibiting pRB phosphorylation. This inhibition maintains pRB in its active, growth-suppressive state, preventing uncontrolled cell proliferation.

Mutations or deletions in the RB1 gene, as well as alterations in other components of this pathway (e.g., CDK4, p16INK4a), can disrupt the regulation of the cell cycle and contribute to tumorigenesis. For example, loss of p16INK4a function is commonly observed in cancers, leading to unchecked CDK4/6 activity and pRB inactivation.

p53-p21 Pathway

The p53 tumor suppressor protein is another key regulator of the cell cycle and apoptosis. In response to DNA damage or other cellular stresses, p53 is stabilized and activates the transcription of target genes, including p21CIP1. The p21CIP1 protein is a member of the CIP/KIP family of CDK inhibitors and functions to inhibit the activity of cyclin-CDK complexes, thereby preventing pRB phosphorylation and cell cycle progression.

The p53-p21 pathway acts as a safeguard against uncontrolled cell proliferation by ensuring that cells with damaged DNA do not proceed through the cell cycle. In cells with functional pRB, the p53-p21 pathway works in concert with the RB pathway to maintain cell cycle arrest in response to stress signals. Loss of p53 function, as observed in many cancers, can lead to a failure in this checkpoint, allowing cells with damaged DNA to proliferate and accumulate mutations.

TGF-β Pathway

The TGF-β (transforming growth factor-beta) pathway is involved in the regulation of cell proliferation, differentiation, and apoptosis. TGF-β signaling induces the expression of p15INK4b, another member of the INK4 family of CDK inhibitors, which inhibits CDK4/6 activity and prevents pRB phosphorylation. This pathway is particularly important in controlling cell growth and maintaining tissue homeostasis.

In addition to its role in cell cycle regulation, TGF-β signaling can also induce cell differentiation and apoptosis, processes in which pRB plays a crucial role. For example, during differentiation, pRB can promote the expression of genes involved in cell cycle exit and terminal differentiation. Disruption of the TGF-β pathway, as seen in some cancers, can lead to the loss of growth inhibition and contribute to tumorigenesis.

Implications of RB1 Dysfunction in Cancer

The RB1 gene is frequently altered in a wide range of cancers. These alterations can include point mutations, deletions, and promoter hypermethylation, leading to the loss of pRB function. The consequences of RB1 dysfunction are profound, as the loss of pRB leads to uncontrolled cell cycle progression, genomic instability, and an increased propensity for tumor development.

Retinoblastoma

Retinoblastoma is the most well-known cancer associated with RB1 mutations. This rare pediatric cancer arises from the retina and is typically diagnosed in children under the age of five. Retinoblastoma can occur in two forms: hereditary (bilateral) and sporadic (unilateral). In hereditary retinoblastoma, individuals inherit a germline mutation in one copy of the RB1 gene and acquire a second somatic mutation in the other copy, leading to the loss of pRB function and tumor development.

The study of retinoblastoma has provided crucial insights into the two-hit hypothesis of cancer development, proposed by Alfred Knudson. According to this hypothesis, both alleles of a tumor suppressor gene must be inactivated for cancer to develop. In the case of RB1, the first hit is often a germline mutation, while the second hit is a somatic mutation that occurs during retinal development.

Other Cancers

In addition to retinoblastoma, RB1 mutations and alterations are implicated in a variety of other cancers. For example, in breast cancer, RB1 inactivation is associated with resistance to certain therapies, such as CDK4/6 inhibitors. In lung cancer, RB1 mutations are often found in small cell lung carcinoma (SCLC), contributing to the aggressive nature of this cancer. Osteosarcoma, a bone cancer, also frequently harbors RB1 mutations, further highlighting the gene's role in tumor suppression.

The RB1 tumor suppressor gene plays a critical role in regulating the cell cycle, preventing uncontrolled cell proliferation, and maintaining genomic stability. The loss of RB1 function is a key event in the development of various cancers, most notably retinoblastoma. The regulation of the RB1 pathway is complex, involving multiple layers of control at the transcriptional, post-transcriptional, and post-translational levels.

BRCA1 and BRCA2

The BRCA1 and BRCA2 genes are crucial components of the human genome, playing significant roles in the maintenance of genetic stability. These genes are best known for their association with hereditary breast and ovarian cancers, but they also contribute to the suppression of other cancer types. Understanding the function, production, and regulation of BRCA1 and BRCA2 is essential for comprehending their roles in cancer prevention and the pathways involved in tumorigenesis when these genes are mutated.

Function of BRCA1 and BRCA2

BRCA1 (Breast Cancer gene 1) and BRCA2 (Breast Cancer gene 2) are tumor suppressor genes, which means they help prevent cells from growing and dividing too rapidly or in an uncontrolled way. Both genes produce proteins that are essential for repairing damaged DNA, thereby maintaining the integrity of the cell's genetic information. The primary function of BRCA1 and BRCA2 proteins is to repair double-strand breaks (DSBs) in DNA through a process known as homologous recombination (HR).

BRCA1 Function

BRCA1 is involved in several cellular processes, including DNA damage repair, transcriptional regulation, cell cycle checkpoint control, and maintaining genomic stability. BRCA1 is part of a large complex known as the BRCA1-associated genome surveillance complex (BASC), which is responsible for recognizing DNA damage and initiating the repair process.

1. **DNA Damage Repair**: BRCA1 plays a pivotal role in homologous recombination, a precise DNA repair mechanism. When double-strand breaks occur, BRCA1 is recruited to the site of damage, where it interacts with other proteins, such as RAD51, to facilitate the repair. This process is crucial for maintaining genomic integrity and preventing mutations that could lead to cancer.

2. **Transcriptional Regulation**: BRCA1 also regulates the transcription of various genes involved in cell cycle control and DNA

repair. It interacts with RNA polymerase II and other transcription factors to modulate the expression of genes that are critical for responding to DNA damage.

3. **Cell Cycle Control**: BRCA1 is involved in the regulation of the cell cycle, particularly at the G1/S and G2/M checkpoints. By controlling the progression of the cell cycle, BRCA1 ensures that cells do not replicate damaged DNA, which could lead to cancer.

4. **Genomic Stability**: By participating in DNA repair and transcriptional regulation, BRCA1 helps maintain genomic stability. Loss of BRCA1 function leads to chromosomal abnormalities and increased susceptibility to cancer.

BRCA2 Function

BRCA2, like BRCA1, is essential for the repair of DNA double-strand breaks through homologous recombination. However, BRCA2's role is more directly involved in the process of HR, particularly in mediating the function of RAD51, a protein that plays a critical role in the repair process.

1. **DNA Damage Repair**: BRCA2 directly interacts with RAD51 and helps load RAD51 onto the single-stranded DNA at the site of a double-strand break. This process is crucial for the accurate repair of DNA damage and the maintenance of genomic stability.

2. **Chromosomal Stability**: BRCA2 is vital for preserving chromosomal stability. It helps prevent chromosomal rearrangements and mutations that could lead to tumorigenesis. Cells deficient in BRCA2 are prone to chromosomal abnormalities, which increase the risk of cancer development.

3. **Cell Cycle Regulation**: BRCA2 also plays a role in cell cycle regulation, although its function in this area is less well-characterized compared to BRCA1. It is believed that BRCA2 may help regu-

late the G2/M checkpoint, ensuring that cells do not enter mitosis with damaged DNA.

Production of BRCA1 and BRCA2

The production of BRCA1 and BRCA2 proteins is a tightly regulated process, controlled at both the transcriptional and post-transcriptional levels. Mutations in these genes can lead to the production of truncated or non-functional proteins, which significantly increases the risk of cancer.

BRCA1 Production

1. **Gene Structure and Transcription**: The BRCA1 gene is located on chromosome 17q21 and spans approximately 81 kilobases of genomic DNA. It consists of 24 exons and produces a large mRNA transcript. The transcription of BRCA1 is regulated by various transcription factors, including estrogen receptor (ER), p53, and others involved in DNA damage response.

2. **Post-Transcriptional Regulation**: After transcription, BRCA1 mRNA undergoes splicing to produce different isoforms of the BRCA1 protein. The full-length BRCA1 protein consists of 1,863 amino acids. Post-translational modifications, such as phosphorylation, ubiquitination, and acetylation, regulate the stability, localization, and function of BRCA1. For example, phosphorylation of BRCA1 by ATM/ATR kinases in response to DNA damage is crucial for its role in DNA repair.

3. **Protein Complexes**: BRCA1 functions as part of multiple protein complexes. One of the key complexes is the BRCA1-associated RING domain (BARD1) complex, which is involved in ubiquitin ligase activity and DNA repair. The formation of these complexes is essential for BRCA1's tumor suppressor functions.

BRCA2 Production

1. **Gene Structure and Transcription**: The BRCA2 gene is located on chromosome 13q12.3 and spans approximately 84 kilobases of genomic DNA. It consists of 27 exons and produces a large mRNA transcript. The transcription of BRCA2 is also regulated by various transcription factors, including those involved in the DNA damage response.

2. **Post-Transcriptional Regulation**: BRCA2 mRNA is spliced to produce different isoforms of the BRCA2 protein. The full-length BRCA2 protein consists of 3,418 amino acids. Post-translational modifications, such as phosphorylation, also play a role in regulating the stability and function of BRCA2. BRCA2's interaction with other proteins, particularly RAD51, is crucial for its role in homologous recombination.

3. **Protein Complexes**: BRCA2 primarily functions through its interaction with RAD51. It also interacts with other proteins involved in DNA repair, such as PALB2, which acts as a bridge between BRCA1 and BRCA2, facilitating the formation of the DNA repair complex.

Regulation of BRCA1 and BRCA2

The regulation of BRCA1 and BRCA2 is complex and involves multiple layers of control, including transcriptional regulation, post-transcriptional modifications, and interactions with other proteins. Dysregulation of these genes can lead to genomic instability and an increased risk of cancer.

Transcriptional Regulation

1. **BRCA1 Transcriptional Regulation**: The expression of BRCA1 is tightly regulated by various factors, including hor-

mones, DNA damage signals, and transcription factors. For example, estrogen and progesterone can modulate BRCA1 expression through hormone receptor-mediated pathways. Additionally, transcription factors such as p53 and NF-κB play roles in the DNA damage-induced expression of BRCA1. Epigenetic modifications, such as DNA methylation and histone acetylation, also contribute to the regulation of BRCA1 expression.

2. **BRCA2 Transcriptional Regulation**: Like BRCA1, BRCA2 expression is regulated by DNA damage signals and transcription factors. The BRCA2 promoter is responsive to DNA damage, leading to increased expression of BRCA2 in response to genotoxic stress. Transcription factors such as p53 also play a role in regulating BRCA2 expression. Additionally, BRCA2 expression can be influenced by hormonal signals and epigenetic modifications.

Post-Transcriptional Regulation

1. **Alternative Splicing**: Both BRCA1 and BRCA2 undergo alternative splicing, which results in the production of different protein isoforms with distinct functions. This splicing is regulated by various splicing factors and is influenced by cellular stress, DNA damage, and other factors.

2. **Protein Stability and Degradation**: The stability of BRCA1 and BRCA2 proteins is regulated by post-translational modifications. For example, ubiquitination of BRCA1 can target it for degradation by the proteasome, thereby modulating its levels in the cell. Similarly, phosphorylation of BRCA1 and BRCA2 in response to DNA damage can affect their stability and activity.

3. **Protein-Protein Interactions**: The function and regulation of BRCA1 and BRCA2 are heavily dependent on their interactions with other proteins. For instance, BRCA1 interacts with BARD1, which stabilizes BRCA1 and enhances its ubiquitin lig-

ase activity. BRCA2's interaction with RAD51 is essential for its role in DNA repair.

Pathways Involving BRCA1 and BRCA2

BRCA1 and BRCA2 are involved in several key cellular pathways, most notably those related to DNA repair, cell cycle regulation, and apoptosis. Dysregulation of these pathways due to mutations in BRCA1 or BRCA2 can lead to tumorigenesis.

DNA Damage Response and Repair Pathways

1. **Homologous Recombination (HR) Pathway**: The HR pathway is the primary mechanism through which BRCA1 and BRCA2 maintain genomic stability. When a double-strand break occurs, BRCA1 is recruited to the site of damage, where it helps initiate the repair process. BRCA2 then facilitates the loading of RAD51 onto the single-stranded DNA, promoting strand invasion and homologous recombination. This pathway is crucial for the accurate repair of double-strand breaks, preventing chromosomal abnormalities and mutations.

2. **Non-Homologous End Joining (NHEJ) Pathway**: Although BRCA1 and BRCA2 primarily function in homologous recombination, they can also influence the non-homologous end joining (NHEJ) pathway, which is another mechanism for repairing double-strand breaks. NHEJ is a more error-prone repair mechanism, and the involvement of BRCA1 in this pathway helps ensure that DNA ends are processed correctly before ligation.

3. **Fanconi Anemia Pathway**: BRCA2 is involved in the Fanconi anemia (FA) pathway, a DNA repair pathway that repairs interstrand crosslinks. BRCA2 interacts with FANCD2, a key protein in this pathway, to promote the repair of crosslinks and maintain genomic stability.

Cell Cycle Regulation Pathways

1. **G1/S and G2/M Checkpoints**: BRCA1 plays a crucial role in regulating the G1/S and G2/M checkpoints of the cell cycle. In response to DNA damage, BRCA1 helps activate these checkpoints, preventing cells from progressing through the cell cycle with damaged DNA. This regulation is essential for preventing the accumulation of mutations and maintaining genomic stability.

2. **S Phase Progression**: BRCA2 is involved in the regulation of DNA replication during the S phase of the cell cycle. It helps ensure that replication forks are stabilized and that any DNA damage encountered during replication is repaired efficiently. This function is critical for preventing genomic instability during cell division.

Apoptosis Pathways

1. **p53-Mediated Apoptosis**: BRCA1 can influence the p53-mediated apoptosis pathway. In response to severe DNA damage, BRCA1 can help activate p53, leading to the induction of apoptosis. This function is important for eliminating cells with irreparable DNA damage, thereby preventing the development of cancer.

2. **Caspase Activation**: BRCA1 can also modulate apoptosis by influencing the activation of caspases, the enzymes responsible for executing apoptosis. Through its interactions with other proteins involved in the apoptotic pathway, BRCA1 can help determine whether a cell undergoes apoptosis in response to DNA damage.

Mutations in BRCA1 and BRCA2 and Cancer Risk

Mutations in BRCA1 and BRCA2 significantly increase the risk of developing several types of cancer, most notably breast and ovarian cancer. These mutations can be inherited in an autosomal dominant manner, meaning that a single copy of the mutated gene can increase cancer risk.

Types of Mutations

1. **Truncating Mutations**: Truncating mutations, which lead to the production of shortened, non-functional proteins, are among the most common types of mutations in BRCA1 and BRCA2. These mutations often result in a complete loss of function of the protein, leading to an inability to repair DNA damage effectively.
2. **Missense Mutations**: Missense mutations result in a single amino acid change in the protein, which can affect its function. Depending on the location of the mutation, it can either partially or completely disrupt the protein's ability to perform its role in DNA repair.
3. **Large Genomic Rearrangements**: In addition to point mutations, large genomic rearrangements, such as deletions or duplications of large sections of the gene, can also lead to a loss of function of BRCA1 or BRCA2.

Cancer Types Associated with BRCA1 and BRCA2 Mutations

1. **Breast Cancer**: Women with BRCA1 or BRCA2 mutations have a significantly increased risk of developing breast cancer. BRCA1 mutations are more commonly associated with triple-negative breast cancer, a particularly aggressive form of the disease. BRCA2 mutations are associated with an increased risk of both estrogen receptor-positive and triple-negative breast cancer.
2. **Ovarian Cancer**: Mutations in BRCA1 and BRCA2 also increase the risk of ovarian cancer. BRCA1 mutations are associ-

ated with a higher risk than BRCA2 mutations. These mutations lead to a loss of function in DNA repair pathways, resulting in the accumulation of mutations that can drive cancer development.

3. **Prostate Cancer**: Men with BRCA1 or BRCA2 mutations have an increased risk of developing prostate cancer. BRCA2 mutations, in particular, are associated with a higher risk of aggressive prostate cancer.

4. **Pancreatic Cancer**: Both BRCA1 and BRCA2 mutations are associated with an increased risk of pancreatic cancer. The loss of BRCA1/2 function in pancreatic cells can lead to genomic instability and the accumulation of mutations that drive cancer progression.

5. **Other Cancers**: Mutations in BRCA1 and BRCA2 have also been linked to an increased risk of other cancers, including melanoma and stomach cancer.

BRCA1 and BRCA2 are critical tumor suppressor genes that play essential roles in maintaining genomic stability through DNA repair, cell cycle regulation, and apoptosis. Mutations in these genes significantly increase the risk of several cancers, particularly breast and ovarian cancer.

APC

The Adenomatous Polyposis Coli (APC) gene is a critical tumor suppressor gene with essential roles in various cellular processes, most notably in the regulation of the Wnt signaling pathway, which is crucial for cell proliferation, differentiation, and apoptosis. Mutations in the APC gene are strongly associated with the development of colorectal cancer, particularly in the context of familial adenomatous polyposis (FAP), an inherited condition that significantly increases the risk of colon cancer.

Function of the APC Gene

The APC gene encodes a large multi-domain protein that plays a pivotal role in regulating several cellular processes, including cell cycle progression, apoptosis, and chromosomal stability. One of the primary functions of the APC protein is to regulate the Wnt signaling pathway, which is vital for maintaining the balance between cell proliferation and differentiation in various tissues.

1. Regulation of Wnt Signaling Pathway

The Wnt signaling pathway is a complex network of proteins that play a crucial role in embryonic development, cell proliferation, and differentiation. The APC protein is a key negative regulator of this pathway. In the absence of Wnt signaling, the APC protein forms a destruction complex with other proteins, including glycogen synthase kinase 3β (GSK-3β), Axin, and casein kinase 1α (CK1α). This complex targets β-catenin, a central effector of the Wnt pathway, for ubiquitination and subsequent degradation by the proteasome.

When the Wnt pathway is activated, Wnt ligands bind to Frizzled receptors on the cell surface, leading to the inhibition of the destruction complex. As a result, β-catenin accumulates in the cytoplasm and translocates to the nucleus, where it interacts with T-cell factor/lymphoid enhancer factor (TCF/LEF) transcription factors to promote the expression of Wnt target genes involved in cell proliferation and survival.

Mutations in the APC gene, particularly those leading to the truncation of the APC protein, result in the inability of the destruction complex to efficiently degrade β-catenin. Consequently, β-catenin accumulates in the nucleus, leading to the constitutive activation of Wnt target genes and uncontrolled cell proliferation, a hallmark of cancer development.

2. Role in Cell Migration and Adhesion

The APC protein is also involved in cell migration and adhesion, processes that are critical for maintaining tissue architecture and integrity. APC interacts with microtubules and actin filaments, contributing to cytoskeletal dynamics and cell polarity. Through its interaction with microtubules, APC plays a role in stabilizing the mitotic spindle during cell division, ensuring accurate chromosome segregation. This function is essential for maintaining genomic stability and preventing aneuploidy, a condition characterized by an abnormal number of chromosomes that is commonly observed in cancer cells.

In addition, APC regulates cell adhesion by interacting with β-catenin at the plasma membrane. APC promotes the formation of adherens junctions, which are essential for maintaining cell-cell adhesion and epithelial tissue integrity. Loss of APC function can disrupt cell adhesion, leading to increased cell motility and invasiveness, which are key features of cancer metastasis.

3. Role in Apoptosis

The APC protein is also involved in the regulation of apoptosis, a process of programmed cell death that is essential for maintaining tissue homeostasis and preventing the accumulation of damaged or abnormal cells. APC promotes apoptosis by interacting with proteins involved in the apoptotic pathway, including caspases and the Bcl-2 family of proteins. The loss of APC function can impair apoptosis, allowing cells with DNA damage or other abnormalities to survive and proliferate, contributing to tumor development.

Production of the APC Protein

The production of the APC protein is a tightly regulated process that involves the transcription of the APC gene, post-transcriptional modifications, and protein processing. The APC gene is located on chromosome 5q22.2 and consists of 15 exons that encode a protein of approximately 2,843 amino acids.

1. Transcriptional Regulation

The transcription of the APC gene is regulated by various transcription factors and epigenetic modifications. Several promoter regions have been identified in the APC gene, which are responsive to different transcription factors. For example, the transcription factor Sp1 has been shown to bind to the APC promoter and regulate its expression in a cell-type-specific manner.

Epigenetic modifications, such as DNA methylation and histone acetylation, also play a role in the regulation of APC gene expression. Hypermethylation of the APC promoter region has been observed in several types of cancer, including colorectal cancer, leading to the silencing of the APC gene and loss of APC protein expression.

2. Post-Transcriptional Regulation

After transcription, the APC mRNA undergoes several post-transcriptional modifications, including splicing, polyadenylation, and transport to the cytoplasm for translation. Alternative splicing of the APC mRNA can result in different isoforms of the APC protein, which may have distinct functions or subcellular localizations.

The stability of APC mRNA is also regulated by RNA-binding proteins and microRNAs (miRNAs). For example, miR-135a and miR-135b have been shown to target the 3' untranslated region (UTR) of APC mRNA, leading to its degradation and decreased APC protein levels in colorectal cancer cells.

3. Protein Processing and Post-Translational Modifications

The APC protein undergoes several post-translational modifications that are essential for its function and stability. These modifications include phosphorylation, ubiquitination, and acetylation. Phosphorylation of APC by GSK-3β and CK1α is critical for its interaction with β-catenin and the formation of the destruction complex.

Ubiquitination of APC can target the protein for degradation by the proteasome, thereby regulating its levels in the cell. The E3 ubiquitin ligase complex, including the APC/C complex (anaphase-promoting complex/cyclosome), plays a role in the ubiquitination and degradation of APC during the cell cycle.

Regulation of the APC Gene

The regulation of the APC gene and its protein product is a complex process involving multiple layers of control, including transcriptional, post-transcriptional, and post-translational mechanisms. Disruption of these regulatory processes can lead to the loss of APC function and contribute to tumorigenesis.

1. Regulation by the Wnt Signaling Pathway

The Wnt signaling pathway not only involves the APC protein in its regulation but also exerts feedback control on APC gene expression. The activation of Wnt signaling has been shown to downregulate APC expression, creating a feedback loop that modulates the intensity and duration of Wnt signaling.

2. Epigenetic Regulation

As mentioned earlier, epigenetic modifications such as DNA methylation and histone acetylation play a significant role in regulating APC gene expression. Hypermethylation of the APC promoter region is a common epigenetic alteration in cancer that leads to the silencing of the APC gene and loss of tumor suppressor function. Conversely, histone acetylation can enhance APC gene expression by promoting a more open chromatin structure that is accessible to transcription factors.

3. Regulation by Non-Coding RNAs

Non-coding RNAs, including miRNAs and long non-coding RNAs (lncRNAs), are important regulators of APC gene expression. As previously mentioned, miR-135a and miR-135b target the 3' UTR of APC mRNA, leading to its degradation and decreased APC protein levels. Other miRNAs, such as miR-27a and miR-494, have also been implicated in the regulation of APC expression in cancer.

LncRNAs can regulate APC gene expression through various mechanisms, including chromatin remodeling, transcriptional interference, and miRNA sponging. For example, the lncRNA HOTAIR has been shown to promote the silencing of the APC gene in colorectal cancer by recruiting the polycomb repressive complex 2 (PRC2) to the APC promoter region, leading to histone H3 lysine 27 trimethylation (H3K27me3) and transcriptional repression.

Pathways Involving the APC Gene

The APC gene is involved in several key signaling pathways that regulate cellular processes such as proliferation, differentiation, apoptosis, and migration. The dysregulation of these pathways due to mutations or loss of APC function is a critical event in the development of cancer, particularly colorectal cancer.

1. Wnt/β-Catenin Signaling Pathway

The Wnt/β-catenin signaling pathway is the most well-known pathway regulated by the APC protein. As previously discussed, APC is a central component of the destruction complex that targets β-catenin for degradation. In the absence of functional APC, β-catenin accumulates in the nucleus and activates the transcription of Wnt target genes that promote cell proliferation and survival.

Mutations in the APC gene, particularly those leading to the truncation of the APC protein, disrupt the destruction complex and result in the constitutive activation of the Wnt/β-catenin pathway. This leads to uncontrolled cell proliferation and the development of adenomas, which can progress to colorectal cancer.

2. APC and the Cell Cycle

The APC protein is involved in the regulation of the cell cycle, particularly during the transition from the G1 to the S phase. APC interacts with the anaphase-promoting complex/cyclosome (APC/C), a multi-subunit E3 ubiquitin ligase that targets cell cycle regulators for degradation. By promoting the degradation of cyclin B and securin, the APC/C complex ensures the proper progression of the cell cycle and prevents genomic instability.

In addition to its role in the APC/C complex, the APC protein is also involved in the regulation of the mitotic spindle and chromosome segregation. APC interacts with microtubules and is required for the proper attachment of spindle microtubules to kinetochores, ensuring accurate chromosome segregation during mitosis. Loss of APC function can lead to chromosomal instability and aneuploidy, both of which are common features of cancer cells.

3. APC and Cell Adhesion

The APC protein plays a role in regulating cell adhesion and maintaining the integrity of epithelial tissues. APC interacts with β-catenin at the plasma membrane and promotes the formation of adherens junctions, which are essential for maintaining cell-cell adhesion and tissue architecture.

In cancer, the loss of APC function can disrupt cell adhesion, leading to increased cell motility and invasiveness. This contributes to the epithelial-mesenchymal transition (EMT), a process in which epithelial cells lose their cell-cell adhesion properties and acquire a more migratory and invasive phenotype. EMT is a key step in cancer metastasis, allowing tumor cells to invade surrounding tissues and spread to distant organs.

4. APC and Apoptosis

The APC protein is involved in the regulation of apoptosis through its interaction with various components of the apoptotic machinery. APC has been shown to interact with caspases, a family of proteases that play a central role in the execution of apoptosis. By promoting the activation of caspases, APC contributes to the elimination of damaged or abnormal cells, preventing the accumulation of potentially cancerous cells.

In addition, APC interacts with members of the Bcl-2 family of proteins, which regulate the intrinsic pathway of apoptosis. APC has been shown to promote the pro-apoptotic activity of Bax and Bak, leading to the release of cytochrome c from mitochondria and the activation of caspase-9. The loss of APC function can impair apoptosis, allowing cells with DNA damage or other abnormalities to survive and proliferate, contributing to tumorigenesis.

Mutations in the APC Gene and Cancer

Mutations in the APC gene are one of the most common genetic alterations in colorectal cancer, particularly in the context of familial adenomatous polyposis (FAP), an inherited condition characterized by the development of hundreds to thousands of adenomatous polyps in the colon and rectum. FAP is caused by germline mutations in the APC gene, which are typically inherited in an autosomal dominant manner. Individuals with FAP have a nearly 100% lifetime risk of developing colorectal cancer if the polyps are not removed.

Most APC mutations in colorectal cancer are truncating mutations that result in the production of a truncated, non-functional APC protein. These mutations often occur in the mutation cluster region (MCR) of the APC gene, which is located between codons 1,280 and 1,510. Truncating mutations in this region lead to the loss of the β-catenin binding sites, preventing the formation of the destruction complex and resulting in the accumulation of β-catenin in the nucleus. This leads to the constitutive activation of the Wnt/β-catenin signaling pathway and uncontrolled cell proliferation.

In addition to truncating mutations, other types of APC mutations, such as missense mutations, small deletions, and insertions, have been identified in colorectal cancer. These mutations can also disrupt the function of the APC protein and contribute to tumorigenesis.

The APC gene is a critical tumor suppressor gene with essential roles in regulating the Wnt/β-catenin signaling pathway, cell cycle progression, apoptosis, and cell adhesion. Mutations in the APC gene are strongly associated with the development of colorectal cancer, particularly in the context of familial adenomatous polyposis (FAP). The loss of APC function leads to the constitutive activation of the Wnt/β-catenin pathway, resulting in uncontrolled cell proliferation and tumorigenesis.

WT1

The Wilms' Tumor 1 (WT1) gene plays a crucial role in development, cellular differentiation, and cancer suppression. Originally identified as a tumor suppressor gene associated with Wilms' tumor, a pediatric kidney cancer, WT1 has since been implicated in various biological processes and cancers.

Function of the WT1 Gene

1. Role in Development

The WT1 gene encodes a protein that is a critical regulator of development, particularly in the urogenital system. WT1 is expressed in several tissues, including the kidneys, gonads, and heart, and it plays a pivotal role in the formation of these organs. During kidney development, WT1 is essential for the induction and maintenance of the metanephric mesenchyme, which gives rise to the nephrons, the functional units of the kidney. The gene also influences the development of the gonads, where it is involved in sex determination and differentiation.

The WT1 protein functions as a transcription factor, binding to DNA and regulating the expression of target genes involved in cell proliferation, apoptosis, and differentiation. For example, WT1 regulates the expression of genes such as Pax2, Bcl2, and Pod1, which are crucial for kidney and gonadal development.

2. Tumor Suppression

As a tumor suppressor gene, WT1 helps prevent the formation of tumors by regulating cell growth and apoptosis. In its normal function, WT1 ensures that cells proliferate and differentiate in a controlled manner. Loss of WT1 function, due to mutations or deletions, can lead to uncontrolled cell growth, resulting in tumor formation. This is particularly evident in Wilms' tumor, where inactivating mutations in WT1 are frequently observed.

In addition to its role in Wilms' tumor, WT1 mutations have been implicated in other cancers, including leukemias, breast cancer, and mesothelioma. The WT1 protein's ability to regulate genes involved in apoptosis (e.g., Bcl2) and cell cycle control (e.g., p21) underscores its importance as a tumor suppressor.

3. Regulation of Gene Expression

WT1's role as a transcription factor involves the regulation of several target genes, both by activating and repressing their expression. This dual function is mediated by the different isoforms of the WT1 protein, which arise due to alternative splicing. Some isoforms contain a three-amino-acid insertion (KTS) between the third and fourth zinc fingers of the DNA-binding domain, which affects the protein's DNA-binding properties and its ability to regulate gene expression.

WT1's transcriptional activity is modulated by its interaction with other proteins, such as p53, a well-known tumor suppressor, and BASP1, a protein that enhances WT1's repressive functions. Through these interactions, WT1 can influence various cellular processes, including apoptosis, proliferation, and differentiation.

Production of WT1
1. Gene Structure and Isoforms

The WT1 gene is located on chromosome 11p13 and spans approximately 50 kilobases. It comprises 10 exons that encode the WT1 protein, which contains four zinc finger motifs at the C-terminus, characteristic of transcription factors. Alternative splicing of the WT1 pre-mRNA generates multiple isoforms of the WT1 protein, which differ in their functional properties.

There are four major isoforms of WT1, resulting from two alternative splicing events: the inclusion or exclusion of exon 5 (17 amino acids) and the inclusion or exclusion of three amino acids (KTS) between exons 9 and 10. These isoforms have distinct DNA-binding properties and transcriptional activities, allowing WT1 to regulate a wide array of target genes.

The WT1 protein is produced in various tissues during development, with particularly high expression in the kidneys, gonads, and heart. In the adult, WT1 expression is maintained in the kidney's podocytes, the testis's Sertoli cells, and certain other cell types, reflecting its continued role in tissue homeostasis.

2. Transcriptional Regulation of WT1

The expression of the WT1 gene is tightly regulated at the transcriptional level. Several transcription factors, including SP1, EGR1, and WT1 itself, have been shown to bind to the WT1 promoter and modulate its expression. WT1 is also subject to regulation by epigenetic mechanisms, such as DNA methylation and histone modification, which influence the accessibility of the WT1 promoter to the transcriptional machinery.

During development, WT1 expression is activated in response to signaling pathways, such as the Wnt/β-catenin pathway, which is essential for kidney development. The precise timing and location of WT1 expression are critical for its function, as aberrant expression can lead to developmental defects and tumorigenesis.

3. Post-Transcriptional Regulation

WT1 expression is also regulated at the post-transcriptional level through mechanisms such as alternative splicing, mRNA stability, and translation. The alternative splicing of WT1 pre-mRNA generates different isoforms, each with distinct functions. This splicing is tightly controlled by splicing factors, which ensure the production of the appropriate WT1 isoforms in different tissues and developmental stages.

MicroRNAs (miRNAs) also play a role in the post-transcriptional regulation of WT1 by targeting its mRNA for degradation or translational repression. For example, miR-125b has been shown to directly target WT1 mRNA, reducing WT1 protein levels and influencing cell differentiation and proliferation.

Regulation of WT1
1. Upstream Signaling Pathways

WT1 is regulated by various upstream signaling pathways that control its expression and activity. These pathways include the Wnt/β-catenin pathway, the Notch signaling pathway, and the Sonic Hedgehog (Shh) pathway.

- **Wnt/β-Catenin Pathway**: The Wnt/β-catenin pathway is a key regulator of WT1 expression during kidney development. Activation of this pathway leads to the stabilization of β-catenin, which translocates to the nucleus and activates the transcription of target genes, including WT1. This pathway is essential for the induction of the metanephric mesenchyme, where WT1 is highly expressed.
- **Notch Signaling Pathway**: The Notch signaling pathway also regulates WT1 expression, particularly in the context of kidney and heart development. Notch signaling influences the differentiation of progenitor cells and the maintenance of tissue-specific stem cells, processes in which WT1 plays a critical role.
- **Sonic Hedgehog (Shh) Pathway**: The Shh pathway is involved in the regulation of WT1 expression in the gonads and the central nervous system. Shh signaling controls the proliferation and differentiation of progenitor cells, with WT1 acting as a downstream effector of this pathway.

2. Interaction with Other Proteins

The WT1 protein interacts with several other proteins that modulate its function and stability. These interactions are crucial for WT1's role as a transcription factor and tumor suppressor.

- **p53**: WT1 interacts with p53, another tumor suppressor protein, to regulate the expression of genes involved in apoptosis and cell cycle control. The interaction between WT1 and p53 enhances the transcriptional activity of both proteins, promoting cell cycle arrest and apoptosis in response to DNA damage.
- **BASP1**: BASP1 is a co-repressor that interacts with WT1 and enhances its repressive function on target genes. BASP1 modulates

WT1's ability to repress genes involved in cell proliferation, such as cyclin D1, thereby contributing to its tumor suppressor function.

- **TLE1**: TLE1 is a transcriptional co-repressor that interacts with WT1 to regulate gene expression during development. The WT1-TLE1 complex represses genes involved in cell differentiation, maintaining progenitor cell populations in a proliferative state.

3. Epigenetic Regulation

Epigenetic mechanisms, such as DNA methylation and histone modification, play a significant role in the regulation of WT1 expression. In cancer, aberrant epigenetic modifications of the WT1 gene promoter can lead to its silencing, contributing to tumorigenesis.

- **DNA Methylation**: Hypermethylation of the WT1 promoter has been observed in various cancers, including leukemia and breast cancer. This epigenetic modification reduces WT1 expression, impairing its tumor suppressor function and allowing uncontrolled cell proliferation.
- **Histone Modification**: Histone modifications, such as acetylation and methylation, also influence WT1 expression by altering the chromatin structure and accessibility of the WT1 promoter. For example, histone acetylation is associated with active transcription, while histone methylation can either activate or repress gene expression depending on the specific modification.

Pathways Involving WT1
1. WT1 in the Wnt/β-Catenin Pathway

The Wnt/β-catenin pathway is a key regulator of WT1 expression, particularly during kidney development. Activation of this pathway leads to the stabilization and nuclear translocation of β-catenin, which interacts with transcription factors to activate target genes, including WT1. In the developing kidney, WT1 is required for the formation of the metanephric mesenchyme, a precursor to the nephrons.

Mutations in components of the Wnt/β-catenin pathway can disrupt WT1 expression and lead to developmental abnormalities and tumor formation. For example, mutations in β-catenin have been implicated in Wilms' tumor, highlighting the importance of this pathway in regulating WT1 expression.

2. WT1 in the Notch Signaling Pathway

The Notch signaling pathway plays a crucial role in cell fate determination and differentiation, processes in which WT1 is also involved. In the kidney and heart, Notch signaling regulates the expression of WT1, influencing the differentiation of progenitor cells into specific cell types.

WT1 acts as both a target and a regulator of Notch signaling. For example, in the developing heart, WT1 regulates the expression of genes involved in cardiac progenitor cell differentiation, a process modulated by Notch signaling. Disruption of this pathway can lead to congenital heart defects and contribute to the development of cancer.

3. WT1 in the Sonic Hedgehog Pathway

The Sonic Hedgehog (Shh) pathway is involved in the regulation of WT1 expression in the gonads and central nervous system. Shh signaling controls the proliferation and differentiation of progenitor cells, with WT1 acting as a downstream effector of this pathway.

In the gonads, WT1 regulates the expression of genes involved in sex determination and differentiation, processes that are influenced by Shh signaling. Mutations in the components of the Shh pathway can lead to abnormal WT1 expression and contribute to the development of disorders such as gonadal dysgenesis and cancer.

4. WT1 in Apoptosis and Cell Cycle Regulation

WT1 plays a critical role in regulating apoptosis and the cell cycle, processes that are essential for tumor suppression. As a transcription factor, WT1 regulates the expression of genes involved in these processes, including Bcl2, p21, and p53.

- **Bcl2**: WT1 regulates the expression of Bcl2, an anti-apoptotic protein that prevents cell death. In its tumor suppressor role, WT1 represses Bcl2 expression, promoting apoptosis in response to cellular stress or DNA damage. Loss of WT1 function can lead to increased Bcl2 expression and resistance to apoptosis, contributing to tumor formation.
- **p21**: WT1 also regulates the expression of p21, a cyclin-dependent kinase inhibitor that controls cell cycle progression. By inducing p21 expression, WT1 promotes cell cycle arrest, preventing uncontrolled cell proliferation. Mutations in WT1 that impair its ability to regulate p21 can lead to unchecked cell division and tumor growth.
- **p53**: The interaction between WT1 and p53 is critical for the regulation of apoptosis and the cell cycle. WT1 enhances p53's transcriptional activity, promoting the expression of pro-apoptotic genes and cell cycle inhibitors. This interaction is essential for the tumor suppressor functions of both WT1 and p53.

5. WT1 in Angiogenesis

WT1 is also involved in the regulation of angiogenesis, the process by which new blood vessels are formed. Angiogenesis is essential for tumor growth, as it provides the necessary oxygen and nutrients to the proliferating tumor cells.

WT1 regulates the expression of several angiogenic factors, including VEGF (vascular endothelial growth factor) and angiopoietin-1. By controlling the expression of these factors, WT1 can influence the formation of blood vessels in both normal and tumor tissues. In its tumor suppressor role, WT1 represses the expression of angiogenic factors, inhibiting the formation of blood vessels that would otherwise support tumor growth.

Pathological Implications of WT1
WT1 Mutations in Cancer

Mutations in the WT1 gene are frequently observed in various cancers, including Wilms' tumor, leukemia, breast cancer, and mesothelioma. These mutations can lead to the loss of WT1 function, contributing to uncontrolled cell proliferation, resistance to apoptosis, and tumor formation.

- **Wilms' Tumor**: Inactivating mutations in WT1 are a hallmark of Wilms' tumor, a pediatric kidney cancer. These mutations disrupt the normal function of WT1 in kidney development, leading to the formation of tumors. WT1 mutations in Wilms' tumor often involve point mutations, deletions, or insertions that affect the zinc finger domain, impairing WT1's ability to bind DNA and regulate target genes.
- **Leukemia**: WT1 mutations are also observed in acute myeloid leukemia (AML) and acute lymphoblastic leukemia (ALL). These mutations often result in the overexpression of WT1, which acts as an oncogene in this context, promoting the proliferation of leukemic cells.
- **Breast Cancer and Mesothelioma**: WT1 is overexpressed in certain breast cancers and mesothelioma, where it contributes to tumor progression by promoting cell proliferation and inhibiting apoptosis. In these cancers, WT1 acts as an oncogene, in contrast to its tumor suppressor role in other contexts.

The WT1 tumor suppressor gene is a critical regulator of development, cellular differentiation, and tumor suppression. Its functions are mediated through its role as a transcription factor, regulating the expression of genes involved in apoptosis, cell cycle control, and angiogenesis. The regulation of WT1 expression and activity involves complex interactions between signaling pathways, epigenetic modifications, and protein-protein interactions.

Mutations in WT1 are implicated in various cancers, including Wilms' tumor, leukemia, and breast cancer, highlighting its importance in maintaining cellular homeostasis.

VHL

The von Hippel-Lindau (VHL) tumor suppressor gene plays a crucial role in regulating cell growth, differentiation, and apoptosis. It is best known for its involvement in the VHL disease, a hereditary cancer syndrome that predisposes individuals to various types of tumors, particularly in the kidneys, adrenal glands, pancreas, and the central nervous system. The VHL gene encodes the VHL protein (pVHL), which is pivotal in cellular oxygen sensing and proteasomal degradation of hypoxia-inducible factors (HIFs).

Function of the VHL Tumor Suppressor Gene
Cellular Oxygen Sensing and HIF Regulation

One of the primary functions of the VHL gene is to regulate the cellular response to hypoxia (low oxygen levels). The VHL protein is a key component of the E3 ubiquitin ligase complex, which targets hypoxia-inducible factors (HIFs) for degradation under normoxic conditions (normal oxygen levels). HIFs are transcription factors that activate the expression of various genes involved in angiogenesis, erythropoiesis, and glycolysis, which are essential for cellular adaptation to hypoxia.

Under normoxia, pVHL recognizes and binds to hydroxylated proline residues on HIF-α subunits (HIF-1α, HIF-2α, and HIF-3α), which are hydroxylated by prolyl hydroxylase domain (PHD) enzymes. This binding leads to the ubiquitination of HIF-α by the E3 ubiquitin ligase complex, marking it for proteasomal degradation. Thus, under normal oxygen conditions, HIF-α levels remain low, preventing the expression of hypoxia-responsive genes.

In contrast, under hypoxic conditions, PHD enzymes are inactive, resulting in the stabilization of HIF-α subunits. These stabilized HIF-α subunits translocate to the nucleus, dimerize with HIF-β, and initiate the transcription of genes that promote angiogenesis (e.g., VEGF), erythropoiesis (e.g., EPO), and anaerobic metabolism (e.g., GLUT1).

Tumor Suppression

The VHL gene's role in tumor suppression is largely attributed to its ability to regulate HIF-α levels. Loss or inactivation of VHL leads to the accumulation of HIF-α even under normoxic conditions, driving the overexpression of hypoxia-inducible genes. This inappropriate activation of hypoxia-responsive pathways can lead to increased angiogenesis, cell proliferation, and survival, contributing to tumorigenesis.

VHL also interacts with various other proteins and signaling pathways that contribute to its tumor suppressor functions. For instance, pVHL has been shown to stabilize microtubules, regulate extracellular matrix (ECM) formation, and inhibit the nuclear factor-kappa B (NF-κB) signaling pathway, all of which play roles in maintaining normal cellular homeostasis and preventing uncontrolled cell growth.

Production of the VHL Tumor Suppressor Gene
Gene Structure and Expression

The VHL gene is located on the short arm of chromosome 3 (3p25-26) and spans approximately 10 kilobases. It consists of three exons and two introns, with exon 1 containing the translation start site. The gene is transcribed into a 4.5-kilobase mRNA, which is subsequently translated into the pVHL protein. There are two major isoforms of pVHL, arising from alternative splicing: pVHL30 and pVHL19, named based on their molecular weights of 30 kDa and 19 kDa, respectively. Both isoforms share a common domain structure, including the α-domain (responsible for binding HIF-α) and the β-domain (involved in interactions with elongin C and other components of the E3 ubiquitin ligase complex).

Protein Structure

The VHL protein has a highly conserved structure that is critical for its function. The α-domain contains two key motifs: the β-sheet domain, which interacts with elongin C, and the α-helical domain, which binds to HIF-α. The β-domain, on the other hand, is involved in the recognition of hydroxylated proline residues on HIF-α, facilitating its ubiquitination.

Regulation of the VHL Tumor Suppressor Gene
Transcriptional Regulation

The expression of the VHL gene is tightly regulated at the transcriptional level. Various transcription factors, including specificity protein 1 (Sp1) and nuclear factor Y (NF-Y), have been identified as regulators of VHL gene expression. Additionally, epigenetic modifications, such as DNA methylation and histone acetylation, play a role in controlling VHL transcription.

Hypoxia has been shown to downregulate VHL expression through the hypoxia-responsive element (HRE) in its promoter region. This feedback mechanism ensures that under hypoxic conditions, when HIF-α stabilization is necessary, VHL expression is reduced to allow for the appropriate cellular response.

Post-Translational Modifications

The activity of the VHL protein is modulated by several post-translational modifications. Phosphorylation, acetylation, and ubiquitination of pVHL can influence its stability, localization, and interactions with other proteins.

Phosphorylation of pVHL at serine and threonine residues has been reported to affect its ability to bind to HIF-α and other components of the E3 ubiquitin ligase complex. Acetylation of pVHL, particularly at lysine residues, can also modulate its interactions with other proteins and its subcellular localization.

Proteasomal Degradation

Like many other proteins, pVHL is subject to proteasomal degradation. The stability of pVHL is regulated by its own ubiquitination and subsequent degradation by the proteasome. This autoregulatory mechanism ensures that pVHL levels are tightly controlled, preventing excessive degradation of HIF-α under normoxic conditions.

Pathways Involving the VHL Tumor Suppressor Gene
The VHL-HIF Pathway

The VHL-HIF pathway is central to the gene's tumor suppressor function. As previously mentioned, under normoxic conditions, pVHL targets HIF-α subunits for degradation, thereby preventing the activation of hypoxia-responsive genes. Loss of VHL function disrupts this pathway, leading to the constitutive activation of HIFs, even in the presence of normal oxygen levels.

This aberrant activation of HIFs drives the expression of genes involved in angiogenesis, cell proliferation, and survival, contributing to tumorigenesis. For example, overexpression of VEGF (vascular endothelial growth factor) promotes the formation of new blood vessels, providing a blood supply to growing tumors. Similarly, increased expression of EPO (erythropoietin) can lead to polycythemia, a condition characterized by an increased number of red blood cells, which is often associated with VHL disease.

VHL and the mTOR Pathway

The mammalian target of rapamycin (mTOR) pathway is another key regulator of cell growth and metabolism that is influenced by VHL. Studies have shown that loss of VHL function can lead to the activation of the mTOR pathway, promoting cell growth and proliferation. This activation is mediated, in part, by the stabilization of HIF-α, which can upregulate the expression of genes involved in glucose metabolism and protein synthesis, both of which are critical for tumor growth.

Additionally, pVHL has been shown to interact with TSC2 (tuberous sclerosis complex 2), a key negative regulator of the mTOR pathway. Through this interaction, pVHL can inhibit mTOR signaling, thereby suppressing cell growth and proliferation. Loss of VHL function disrupts this inhibitory interaction, leading to unchecked mTOR activity and tumorigenesis.

VHL and ECM Regulation

The extracellular matrix (ECM) plays a crucial role in maintaining tissue architecture and regulating cell behavior. VHL has been implicated in the regulation of ECM components, particularly fibronectin, a glycoprotein involved in cell adhesion, migration, and differentiation.

pVHL interacts with fibronectin and promotes its assembly into the ECM. Loss of VHL function disrupts fibronectin assembly, leading to alterations in the ECM that can contribute to tumor progression. For example, disrupted fibronectin assembly can enhance cell migration and invasion, promoting metastasis.

VHL and Microtubule Stability

Microtubules are key components of the cytoskeleton that are involved in various cellular processes, including cell division, intracellular transport, and signal transduction. pVHL has been shown to stabilize microtubules by interacting with α-tubulin, a major component of microtubules.

This interaction promotes the polymerization of microtubules and helps maintain cellular architecture. Loss of VHL function can lead to microtubule destabilization, resulting in defects in cell division and increased genomic instability, both of which contribute to tumorigenesis.

VHL and NF-κB Signaling

The nuclear factor-kappa B (NF-κB) signaling pathway is a key regulator of inflammation, immune response, and cell survival. Aberrant activation of NF-κB has been implicated in various cancers, as it can promote cell proliferation, inhibit apoptosis, and enhance angiogenesis.

pVHL has been shown to inhibit NF-κB signaling by promoting the degradation of key components of the NF-κB pathway, such as IκBα. Loss of VHL function leads to increased NF-κB activity, which can contribute to tumorigenesis by promoting inflammation and cell survival.

Implications of VHL Dysfunction in Cancer
VHL Disease

VHL disease is a hereditary cancer syndrome caused by germline mutations in the VHL gene. Individuals with VHL disease are at increased risk of developing various tumors, particularly in the kidneys, adrenal glands, pancreas, and central nervous system. The most common tumors associated with VHL disease include renal cell carcinoma (RCC), pheochromocytoma, and hemangioblastomas of the brain, spinal cord, and retina.

The loss of VHL function in these tumors leads to the constitutive activation of HIFs, driving the expression of genes involved in angiogenesis, cell proliferation, and survival. As a result, VHL-associated tumors are highly vascularized and exhibit rapid growth.

Renal Cell Carcinoma

Renal cell carcinoma (RCC) is the most common type of kidney cancer, and VHL mutations are found in approximately 90% of sporadic clear cell RCC cases. Loss of VHL function leads to the stabilization of HIF-α and the overexpression of hypoxia-responsive genes, including VEGF, which promotes angiogenesis and tumor growth.

Pheochromocytoma and Paraganglioma

Pheochromocytomas are tumors of the adrenal gland, while paragangliomas are similar tumors that arise in the sympathetic and parasympathetic ganglia. Both types of tumors are associated with VHL mutations. The loss of VHL function in these tumors leads to the activation of HIF-α and the overexpression of catecholamine biosynthesis genes, resulting in excessive production of adrenaline and noradrenaline.

The excessive catecholamine production in pheochromocytoma and paraganglioma can lead to symptoms such as hypertension, palpitations, and headaches. Surgical removal of the tumor is the primary treatment, but targeted therapies that inhibit HIF-α or its downstream effectors are being investigated as potential treatments for unresectable or metastatic tumors.

Hemangioblastoma

Hemangioblastomas are benign tumors of the central nervous system, most commonly found in the cerebellum, spinal cord, and retina. These tumors are highly vascularized and are associated with VHL mutations. The loss of VHL function in hemangioblastomas leads to the overexpression of angiogenic factors, such as VEGF, which promotes the formation of new blood vessels and tumor growth.

Surgical resection is the primary treatment for hemangioblastomas.

The VHL tumor suppressor gene plays a critical role in regulating cellular oxygen sensing, maintaining cellular homeostasis, and preventing tumorigenesis. Through its regulation of the HIF pathway, mTOR signaling, ECM composition, microtubule stability, and NF-κB signaling, VHL exerts its tumor suppressor functions in various tissues. Dysfunction of the VHL gene, whether through inherited mutations or somatic alterations, leads to the development of various cancers, particularly those associated with VHL disease.

NF1

The NF1 gene, also known as neurofibromin 1, plays a crucial role as a tumor suppressor in the human body. It is responsible for producing a protein called neurofibromin, which is involved in the regulation of cell growth and division. Neurofibromin functions by inhibiting the activity of a protein called Ras, a critical regulator of cell proliferation and survival. Ras proteins belong to the family of small GTPases, which act as molecular switches within cells, toggling between an active (GTP-bound) and inactive (GDP-bound) state.

The primary function of the NF1 gene is to suppress the uncontrolled proliferation of cells by inactivating the Ras signaling pathway. Neurofibromin exerts its effects by acting as a GTPase-activating protein (GAP) for Ras. In this capacity, neurofibromin accelerates the conversion of Ras from its active GTP-bound form to its inactive GDP-bound form, thus downregulating the Ras-MAPK (mitogen-activated protein kinase) signaling pathway. By doing so, neurofibromin prevents excessive cell division and reduces the likelihood of tumor formation.

Mutations or deletions in the NF1 gene lead to a reduction or loss of neurofibromin activity, resulting in the uncontrolled activation of Ras signaling. This unchecked activation contributes to the development of various tumors, particularly those associated with neurofibromatosis type 1 (NF1), a genetic disorder characterized by the growth of benign and malignant tumors along nerves in the skin, brain, and other parts of the body.

Production of Neurofibromin

The NF1 gene is located on chromosome 17q11.2 and spans approximately 350 kilobases of DNA. It consists of 60 exons and encodes a large protein with a molecular weight of around 320 kDa. The production of neurofibromin begins with the transcription of the NF1 gene into messenger RNA (mRNA) within the cell nucleus. The mRNA is then transported to the cytoplasm, where it is translated into the neurofibromin protein by ribosomes.

Neurofibromin is composed of several functional domains, each contributing to its tumor suppressor activity. The central domain of neurofibromin contains a region known as the GAP-related domain (GRD), which is responsible for its GTPase-activating function. This domain interacts directly with Ras proteins, promoting the hydrolysis of GTP to GDP, thereby inactivating Ras and preventing the transmission of pro-growth signals within the cell.

The expression of the NF1 gene is regulated at multiple levels, including transcriptional, post-transcriptional, and post-translational modifications. The transcriptional regulation of NF1 involves a variety of transcription factors and regulatory elements within the promoter region of the gene. Additionally, alternative splicing of NF1 mRNA can produce different isoforms of neurofibromin, which may have distinct functions in different tissues.

Regulation of the NF1 Gene

The regulation of the NF1 gene is complex and involves multiple signaling pathways and regulatory mechanisms. One of the key regulatory mechanisms is the control of NF1 gene expression by various transcription factors. For example, the transcription factor p53, a well-known tumor suppressor, has been shown to directly bind to the NF1 promoter and activate its transcription in response to cellular stress and DNA damage. This regulation ensures that neurofibromin levels are increased when the cell needs to suppress excessive growth signals.

Another layer of regulation occurs at the post-transcriptional level, where microRNAs (miRNAs) can influence NF1 mRNA stability and translation. miRNAs are small non-coding RNAs that can bind to complementary sequences in the 3' untranslated region (UTR) of target mRNAs, leading to their degradation or inhibition of translation. Specific miRNAs have been identified that target NF1 mRNA, modulating neurofibromin levels in response to various cellular signals.

Additionally, neurofibromin activity is regulated by post-translational modifications, such as phosphorylation. Phosphorylation of neurofibromin by kinases, such as protein kinase A (PKA) or protein kinase C (PKC), can alter its activity, localization, and interactions with other proteins. These modifications allow for fine-tuning of neurofibromin's function in response to changes in the cellular environment.

Pathways Involving NF1
Ras-MAPK Pathway

The primary pathway regulated by the NF1 gene is the Ras-MAPK signaling pathway. This pathway is critical for controlling cell proliferation, differentiation, and survival. In normal cells, the binding of growth factors to receptor tyrosine kinases (RTKs) on the cell surface triggers the activation of Ras. Ras, in its active GTP-bound form, initiates a cascade of phosphorylation events involving the MAPK kinase (MEK) and extracellular signal-regulated kinase (ERK). The final step in this cascade is the phosphorylation and activation of transcription factors that promote the expression of genes involved in cell cycle progression and proliferation.

Neurofibromin, through its GAP activity, inactivates Ras by converting it to its GDP-bound form, thus terminating the Ras-MAPK signaling. In the absence of functional neurofibromin, Ras remains constitutively active, leading to continuous signaling through the MAPK pathway. This persistent activation can drive uncontrolled cell division and contribute to tumorigenesis, particularly in cells that are prone to other genetic alterations.

mTOR Pathway

In addition to the Ras-MAPK pathway, neurofibromin also influences the mammalian target of rapamycin (mTOR) signaling pathway. The mTOR pathway is a key regulator of cell growth, metabolism, and protein synthesis. It integrates signals from nutrients, growth factors, and energy status to control anabolic and catabolic processes within the cell.

Neurofibromin negatively regulates mTOR signaling by inhibiting the activity of Ras and its downstream effector, PI3K (phosphoinositide 3-kinase). PI3K activation leads to the production of phosphatidylinositol-3,4,5-trisphosphate (PIP3), which in turn activates AKT, a key kinase that promotes mTOR activation. By suppressing Ras and PI3K activity, neurofibromin reduces mTOR signaling, thereby preventing excessive cell growth and proliferation.

Loss of neurofibromin function, as seen in NF1-associated tumors, results in hyperactivation of the mTOR pathway. This contributes to the growth and survival of tumor cells by enhancing protein synthesis, nutrient uptake, and resistance to apoptosis.

cAMP Pathway

Neurofibromin also plays a role in the cyclic adenosine monophosphate (cAMP) signaling pathway. cAMP is a second messenger involved in the regulation of various cellular processes, including metabolism, gene expression, and cell proliferation. The cAMP pathway is activated by the binding of hormones or neurotransmitters to G protein-coupled receptors (GPCRs) on the cell surface, leading to the activation of adenylyl cyclase and the production of cAMP.

Neurofibromin has been shown to interact with components of the cAMP pathway, influencing the levels of cAMP within the cell. Specifically, neurofibromin can inhibit the activity of adenylyl cyclase, thereby reducing cAMP production. This regulation is important for maintaining the balance between cell proliferation and differentiation, particularly in neural cells.

In the context of NF1, loss of neurofibromin can lead to dysregulation of cAMP signaling, contributing to the development of tumors in the nervous system. Elevated cAMP levels can promote the growth of Schwann cells, which are the primary cell type affected in neurofibromatosis type 1.

NF1 and Neurofibromatosis Type 1

Neurofibromatosis type 1 (NF1) is a genetic disorder caused by mutations in the NF1 gene. It is one of the most common inherited neurological disorders, affecting approximately 1 in 3,000 individuals worldwide. NF1 is characterized by the development of multiple neurofibromas, which are benign tumors that arise from Schwann cells in the peripheral nervous system. In addition to neurofibromas, individuals with NF1 are at an increased risk of developing malignant tumors, such as malignant peripheral nerve sheath tumors (MPNSTs), gliomas, and pheochromocytomas.

The clinical manifestations of NF1 are highly variable, even among individuals with the same NF1 mutation. Common features of the disorder include café-au-lait spots (pigmented skin lesions), Lisch nodules (benign iris hamartomas), skeletal abnormalities, learning disabilities, and an increased risk of cardiovascular disease. The development of these symptoms is thought to result from the loss of neurofibromin function and the subsequent dysregulation of Ras signaling in various tissues.

Mutations in the NF1 gene can occur in any of the 60 exons, leading to a wide range of effects on neurofibromin function. These mutations can be inherited from an affected parent or arise de novo in the germline. The type and location of the mutation, as well as the presence of other genetic and environmental factors, contribute to the variability in disease severity and presentation.

The NF1 gene is a critical tumor suppressor that plays a vital role in regulating cell growth, proliferation, and differentiation through its effects on the Ras-MAPK, mTOR, and cAMP signaling pathways. Neurofibromin, the protein product of the NF1 gene, acts as a GTPase-activating protein that inactivates Ras, thereby preventing uncontrolled cell proliferation. Loss of neurofibromin function due to mutations in the NF1 gene leads to the development of neurofibromatosis type 1, a genetic disorder characterized by the formation of benign and malignant tumors in the nervous system.

NF2

The NF2 gene (Neurofibromatosis type 2) is a critical tumor suppressor gene that plays a vital role in cellular processes, particularly in the suppression of tumor formation. Mutations in this gene can lead to the development of a variety of tumors, most notably schwannomas, meningiomas, and ependymomas.

Function of the NF2 Gene

The NF2 gene encodes a protein known as merlin (or schwannomin), which is a member of the ERM (ezrin, radixin, moesin) family of proteins. Merlin is predominantly involved in the regulation of cell growth, proliferation, adhesion, and motility. It achieves this by interacting with various cellular structures and signaling pathways.

1. Cell Growth and Proliferation

Merlin is a crucial regulator of cell proliferation. It functions by inhibiting the activity of certain growth factor receptors, such as the epidermal growth factor receptor (EGFR), thereby preventing uncontrolled cell division. Merlin also interacts with the Hippo signaling pathway, which is a well-known regulator of organ size and tissue homeostasis. Through this pathway, merlin helps maintain appropriate cell numbers within tissues by promoting cell cycle exit and apoptosis in response to cellular crowding.

2. Cell Adhesion and Motility

Another vital function of merlin is in the regulation of cell adhesion and motility. Merlin stabilizes cell-cell junctions by interacting with the cytoskeleton and the cell membrane. This stabilization is crucial for maintaining tissue integrity and preventing cells from becoming invasive. By controlling cell motility, merlin reduces the likelihood of metastasis, where cancer cells spread to other parts of the body.

3. Interaction with Other Proteins

Merlin interacts with various proteins that are involved in signaling pathways related to tumorigenesis. For example, merlin binds to the cytoplasmic domain of certain transmembrane proteins, such as CD44, to regulate their activity. This interaction influences processes like cell growth, apoptosis, and cytoskeletal organization.

Production of the NF2 Gene

The production of the NF2 gene involves the transcription of DNA into mRNA, which is then translated into the merlin protein. This process is tightly regulated at multiple levels, including transcriptional, post-transcriptional, and post-translational modifications.

1. Transcriptional Regulation

The transcription of the NF2 gene is controlled by various transcription factors that bind to its promoter region. These transcription factors include members of the ETS family, which are known to regulate genes involved in cell growth and differentiation. Additionally, the NF2 gene promoter contains several CpG islands, which are regions of DNA where cytosine nucleotides are followed by guanine nucleotides. Methylation of these CpG islands can repress NF2 transcription, leading to reduced merlin levels and potential tumorigenesis.

2. Post-Transcriptional Regulation

After transcription, the NF2 mRNA undergoes several modifications before it is translated into protein. These include the addition of a 5′ cap and a poly-A tail, as well as splicing to remove introns. Alternative splicing of NF2 mRNA can produce different isoforms of merlin, which may have distinct functions in cells. The stability and translation efficiency of NF2 mRNA are also regulated by microRNAs (miRNAs), which can bind to the 3′ untranslated region (UTR) of the mRNA and inhibit its translation or promote its degradation.

3. Post-Translational Regulation

Once translated, merlin undergoes several post-translational modifications that are crucial for its function. Phosphorylation is one of the most significant modifications, as it regulates merlin's ability to bind to other proteins and its localization within the cell. Phosphorylated merlin is generally inactive and is found in the cytoplasm, while dephosphorylated merlin is active and associates with the cell membrane, where it can exert its tumor-suppressive effects. Ubiquitination, another post-translational modification, can target merlin for degradation by the proteasome, thereby regulating its levels in the cell.

Regulation of the NF2 Gene

The regulation of the NF2 gene and its protein product, merlin, is complex and involves multiple signaling pathways. Proper regulation is essential for maintaining cellular homeostasis and preventing tumor formation. Disruption of NF2 regulation can lead to unchecked cell growth and the development of tumors.

1. Hippo Signaling Pathway

One of the primary pathways through which NF2 exerts its tumor suppressive function is the Hippo signaling pathway. The Hippo pathway regulates cell proliferation, apoptosis, and stem cell renewal, and its dysregulation is implicated in various cancers.

Merlin acts as an upstream regulator of the Hippo pathway. It activates the core components of the Hippo pathway, such as the kinases MST1/2 (mammalian sterile 20-like kinases 1 and 2) and LATS1/2 (large tumor suppressor kinases 1 and 2). These kinases phosphorylate and inactivate the transcriptional co-activators YAP (Yes-associated protein) and TAZ (transcriptional coactivator with PDZ-binding motif), preventing them from entering the nucleus and promoting gene expression that leads to cell proliferation and survival. By maintaining the activity of the Hippo pathway, merlin helps to suppress inappropriate cell growth and tumor formation.

2. Rac1 Signaling Pathway

Merlin also interacts with the Rac1 signaling pathway, which is involved in regulating the cytoskeleton, cell shape, and cell migration. Rac1 is a small GTPase that promotes the formation of lamellipodia, cellular protrusions that drive cell movement. Merlin can inhibit Rac1 activity, thereby reducing cell motility and preventing the invasion of surrounding tissues by tumor cells.

3. mTOR Signaling Pathway

The mammalian target of rapamycin (mTOR) signaling pathway is another critical pathway regulated by NF2. The mTOR pathway controls cell growth, protein synthesis, and autophagy in response to nutrients, growth factors, and energy status. Merlin negatively regulates the mTOR pathway by interacting with components of the pathway, such as mTORC1 (mTOR complex 1), to inhibit its activity. This inhibition prevents excessive cell growth and proliferation, contributing to merlin's tumor suppressive function.

4. CD44-Merlin Interaction

Merlin's interaction with the transmembrane protein CD44 is another mechanism through which it regulates cell growth and adhesion. CD44 is a cell surface receptor involved in cell-cell and cell-matrix interactions. The CD44-merlin complex is important for organizing the cytoskeleton and maintaining contact inhibition, a process that stops cells from dividing when they come into contact with each other. Loss of merlin function disrupts this interaction, leading to uncontrolled cell proliferation and tumor development.

NF2-Related Pathways and Tumorigenesis

Mutations or loss of function of the NF2 gene can disrupt the pathways mentioned above, leading to tumorigenesis. The most common tumors associated with NF2 mutations are schwannomas, meningiomas, and ependymomas.

1. Schwannomas

Schwannomas are benign tumors that arise from Schwann cells, which form the myelin sheath around peripheral nerves. NF2-related schwannomas most commonly occur in the vestibular nerve, leading to hearing loss and balance problems. The loss of merlin function in Schwann cells leads to dysregulation of the Hippo pathway and other signaling pathways, resulting in uncontrolled cell proliferation and tumor formation.

2. Meningiomas

Meningiomas are tumors that develop from the meninges, the protective membranes that cover the brain and spinal cord. These tumors can be benign or malignant, and their development is also linked to NF2 mutations. Merlin's role in regulating cell proliferation and adhesion is crucial in preventing the formation of meningiomas. When NF2 is mutated, the resulting loss of merlin function leads to the disruption of cell-cell junctions and increased cell proliferation, contributing to tumor growth.

3. Ependymomas

Ependymomas are tumors that arise from ependymal cells, which line the ventricles of the brain and the central canal of the spinal cord. NF2 mutations are associated with a subset of ependymomas, particularly in the spinal cord. The exact mechanisms by which NF2 mutations contribute to ependymoma formation are not fully understood, but it is likely related to the disruption of merlin's regulatory functions in cell proliferation and adhesion.

The NF2 tumor suppressor gene plays a crucial role in regulating cell growth, proliferation, adhesion, and motility through its protein product, merlin. By interacting with various signaling pathways, such as the Hippo, Rac1, and mTOR pathways, merlin helps maintain cellular homeostasis and prevent tumor formation. Mutations or loss of function of the NF2 gene can lead to the development of tumors such as schwannomas, meningiomas, and ependymomas.

CDKN2A

The CDKN2A gene, located on chromosome 9p21, is one of the most important tumor suppressor genes in the human genome. It plays a critical role in regulating cell cycle progression and maintaining cellular homeostasis. The gene encodes two distinct proteins, p16INK4a and p14ARF, which are involved in different pathways leading to cell cycle arrest and apoptosis. Dysregulation or mutation of CDKN2A is commonly associated with various types of cancers, highlighting its importance in tumor suppression.

Function of CDKN2A

The CDKN2A gene is unique because it encodes two distinct tumor suppressor proteins through alternative reading frames: p16INK4a and p14ARF.

p16INK4a

p16INK4a is a cyclin-dependent kinase inhibitor that specifically inhibits CDK4 and CDK6. These kinases, when activated by cyclin D, phosphorylate the retinoblastoma protein (RB), leading to the release of E2F transcription factors, which then promote the transcription of genes necessary for the S phase of the cell cycle. By inhibiting CDK4/6, p16INK4a prevents RB phosphorylation, thereby maintaining RB in its active form, which sequesters E2F and halts the cell cycle in the G1 phase. This action effectively prevents uncontrolled cell proliferation, a hallmark of cancer development.

p14ARF

p14ARF functions in the p53 pathway, a major pathway involved in the response to cellular stress and DNA damage. p14ARF binds to and inhibits MDM2, an E3 ubiquitin-protein ligase that targets p53 for degradation. By inhibiting MDM2, p14ARF stabilizes p53, leading to the activation of p53 target genes involved in cell cycle arrest, DNA repair, and apoptosis. Thus, p14ARF serves as a critical regulator of the p53 tumor suppressor pathway, ensuring that cells with damaged DNA do not proceed to divide and potentially form tumors.

Production of CDKN2A

The production of p16INK4a and p14ARF from the CDKN2A gene is tightly regulated at both the transcriptional and post-transcriptional levels. The gene is transcribed into mRNA, which is then translated into the respective proteins. However, the mechanisms regulating the expression of these two proteins differ.

Transcriptional Regulation

The CDKN2A gene has two promoters: the P1 promoter drives the transcription of p16INK4a, while the P2 promoter initiates the transcription of p14ARF. The use of these promoters is regulated by various transcription factors that respond to different cellular signals.

For p16INK4a, transcription factors such as E2F1, ETS1, and SP1 have been shown to enhance its expression, particularly in response to oncogenic signals that drive cell cycle progression. Conversely, transcriptional repressors like BMI1 and EZH2, components of the Polycomb repressive complex 1 (PRC1) and 2 (PRC2) respectively, silence the p16INK4a promoter under normal conditions, thereby preventing premature cell cycle arrest.

For p14ARF, the transcription factors MYC and E2F1 are known to activate its transcription, especially in response to hyperproliferative signals. MYC, a potent oncogene, can upregulate p14ARF expression as a safeguard against unchecked proliferation, linking the regulation of p14ARF directly to oncogenic stress.

Post-Transcriptional Regulation

After transcription, the mRNA of CDKN2A can be further regulated by microRNAs (miRNAs) and RNA-binding proteins (RBPs). miRNAs such as miR-24 and miR-141 have been implicated in the post-transcriptional downregulation of p16INK4a mRNA, contributing to its degradation or preventing its translation. Similarly, p14ARF mRNA can be regulated by miRNAs like miR-221 and miR-222, which reduce its translation efficiency.

Regulation of CDKN2A Pathways

The regulation of CDKN2A involves complex interactions between various signaling pathways, epigenetic modifications, and feedback mechanisms. Key pathways that interact with CDKN2A include the RB pathway, the p53 pathway, and the PI3K/AKT pathway.

RB Pathway

The RB pathway is directly regulated by p16INK4a. In normal cells, p16INK4a inhibits CDK4/6, preventing RB phosphorylation and thus maintaining the cell cycle arrest at the G1 phase. However, in cancer cells with CDKN2A mutations or deletions, p16INK4a is lost, leading to uncontrolled CDK4/6 activity, RB inactivation, and unchecked cell cycle progression.

Mutations in the RB pathway components, including RB itself, can lead to resistance against p16INK4a-mediated cell cycle arrest, contributing to tumorigenesis. Additionally, overexpression of cyclin D1, a regulatory partner of CDK4/6, can overcome p16INK4a inhibition, further driving cell proliferation.

p53 Pathway

The p53 pathway is regulated by p14ARF, which stabilizes p53 by inhibiting MDM2. When the p53 pathway is activated, it can induce cell cycle arrest or apoptosis in response to DNA damage or oncogenic stress. In cells with CDKN2A deletions or mutations, p14ARF is lost, leading to MDM2-mediated degradation of p53 and impaired p53-dependent responses.

This loss of p53 function allows cells to evade apoptosis and continue dividing despite having DNA damage, contributing to tumorigenesis. Furthermore, p14ARF can also influence other p53 family members, such as p73, adding another layer of complexity to its role in tumor suppression.

PI3K/AKT Pathway

The PI3K/AKT pathway is a major pro-survival signaling pathway that is often upregulated in cancer. It negatively regulates p16^INK4a by promoting its degradation through the proteasome pathway. AKT phosphorylates MDM2, enhancing its ability to target p53 for degradation and thereby counteracting the effects of p14ARF.

In addition, the PI3K/AKT pathway can promote the expression of transcriptional repressors like EZH2, which silences the CDKN2A gene through histone methylation, further contributing to the downregulation of p16INK4a and p14ARF in cancer cells.

Epigenetic Regulation of CDKN2A

Epigenetic modifications play a crucial role in the regulation of CDKN2A expression. These modifications include DNA methylation, histone modifications, and chromatin remodeling, all of which can influence the accessibility of the CDKN2A locus to the transcriptional machinery.

DNA Methylation

Hypermethylation of the CDKN2A promoter region is a common mechanism by which the gene is silenced in cancer. This epigenetic alteration prevents the binding of transcription factors to the promoter, leading to reduced expression of both p16INK4a and p14ARF. Methylation of CDKN2A is frequently observed in various cancers, including melanoma, lung cancer, and pancreatic cancer, and is associated with poor prognosis.

Histone Modifications

Histone modifications, such as methylation and acetylation, also regulate CDKN2A expression. For example, the Polycomb repressive complex 2 (PRC2) catalyzes the trimethylation of histone H3 on lysine 27 (H3K27me3), a mark associated with gene repression. This modification is often found at the CDKN2A locus in cancer cells, leading to the silencing of the gene.

Conversely, histone acetylation, which is associated with active transcription, can promote the expression of CDKN2A. Histone deacetylase inhibitors (HDACi) have been shown to induce the expression of p16INK4a in cancer cells by preventing the removal of acetyl groups from histones, thereby increasing chromatin accessibility.

Mutations and Deletions in CDKN2A

Mutations and deletions in the CDKN2A gene are among the most common genetic alterations in cancer. These genetic changes often lead to the loss of function of p16INK4a and p14ARF, contributing to tumorigenesis.

Point Mutations

Point mutations in CDKN2A can lead to the production of nonfunctional or partially functional proteins. These mutations are commonly observed in familial melanoma and pancreatic cancer syndromes. For example, the p16INK4a R24P mutation, which disrupts its ability to bind and inhibit CDK4/6, has been identified in several melanoma-prone families.

Deletions

Homozygous deletions of CDKN2A are frequently observed in various cancers, including glioblastoma, bladder cancer, and non-small cell lung cancer. These deletions result in the complete loss of both p16INK4a and p14ARF, leading to the inactivation of the RB and p53 pathways, respectively.

CDKN2A Pathways: Detailed Analysis

The CDKN2A gene is involved in several critical pathways that regulate cell cycle progression, apoptosis, and cellular senescence. Here, we provide a detailed analysis of these pathways.

The RB-E2F Pathway

The RB-E2F pathway is one of the primary pathways regulated by p16INK4a. In its active state, RB binds to and sequesters E2F transcription factors, preventing them from promoting the transcription of genes required for the S phase of the cell cycle. The phosphorylation of

RB by CDK4/6 leads to the release of E2F, allowing the cell to progress from the G1 to the S phase.

p16INK4a inhibits CDK4/6, thereby preventing RB phosphorylation and maintaining cell cycle arrest. In cancer cells with CDKN2A mutations or deletions, p16INK4a is lost, leading to unchecked CDK4/6 activity, RB inactivation, and uncontrolled cell proliferation.

The p53-MDM2 Pathway

The p53-MDM2 pathway is regulated by p14ARF. Under normal conditions, MDM2 binds to p53 and targets it for ubiquitin-mediated degradation. p14ARF binds to MDM2, inhibiting its E3 ligase activity and stabilizing p53. Activated p53 can then induce the transcription of target genes involved in cell cycle arrest, DNA repair, and apoptosis.

In cells with CDKN2A deletions or mutations, p14ARF is lost, leading to MDM2-mediated degradation of p53 and impaired p53-dependent tumor suppressor functions. This allows cells with DNA damage or oncogenic stress to evade apoptosis and continue proliferating, contributing to tumorigenesis.

The PI3K/AKT Pathway

The PI3K/AKT pathway is a major pro-survival signaling pathway that is often upregulated in cancer. AKT phosphorylates and inactivates several targets, including p21 and p27, which are inhibitors of cyclin-CDK complexes. This promotes cell survival and proliferation.

AKT also phosphorylates MDM2, enhancing its nuclear localization and ability to degrade p53. This counteracts the effects of p14ARF and allows cancer cells to evade p53-mediated apoptosis. Additionally, the PI3K/AKT pathway can promote the expression of transcriptional repressors that silence CDKN2A, further downregulating p16INK4a and p14ARF in cancer cells.

The CDKN2A gene is a crucial tumor suppressor that regulates key pathways involved in cell cycle control, apoptosis, and senescence. Through its two distinct products, p16INK4a and p14ARF, CDKN2A plays a central role in maintaining cellular homeostasis and preventing tumorigenesis. The dysregulation of CDKN2A, whether through mutations, deletions, or epigenetic silencing, is a common event in cancer and has significant implications for cancer diagnosis, prognosis, and therapy.

The restoration of CDKN2A function in cancer cells, whether through the use of CDK4/6 inhibitors, epigenetic therapies, or other strategies, represents a promising avenue for cancer treatment.

PTEN

The PTEN (Phosphatase and Tensin Homolog) tumor suppressor gene is a crucial component in the regulation of cellular processes such as growth, proliferation, survival, and metabolism. It is one of the most frequently mutated genes in human cancers, underscoring its significance in maintaining cellular homeostasis. This article will explore the PTEN gene in detail, including its function, production, and regulation, as well as the pathways it influences.

Function of the PTEN Gene

The PTEN gene encodes a dual-specificity phosphatase that primarily acts as a lipid phosphatase, though it also has protein phosphatase activity. PTEN's primary role is to dephosphorylate the phosphatidylinositol-3,4,5-trisphosphate (PIP3) at the D3 position to generate phosphatidylinositol-4,5-bisphosphate (PIP2), thereby antagonizing the PI3K/AKT signaling pathway.

1. **Regulation of Cell Growth and Proliferation**: The PI3K/AKT pathway is a critical signaling pathway that promotes cell growth, proliferation, and survival. PTEN acts as a negative regulator of this pathway by converting PIP3 to PIP2, thus inhibit-

ing AKT activation. When PTEN function is lost, AKT remains constitutively active, leading to uncontrolled cell proliferation and survival, which are hallmarks of cancer.

2. **Cell Cycle Control**: PTEN also plays a role in regulating the cell cycle. By inhibiting the PI3K/AKT pathway, PTEN indirectly promotes the activity of cyclin-dependent kinase inhibitors such as p27Kip1 and p21Cip1, which are crucial for halting the cell cycle at various checkpoints. Loss of PTEN function can lead to unchecked progression through the cell cycle, contributing to tumorigenesis.

3. **Apoptosis**: PTEN promotes apoptosis, or programmed cell death, by antagonizing the survival signals mediated by the PI3K/AKT pathway. AKT activation inhibits apoptosis by phosphorylating and inactivating several pro-apoptotic factors, including Bad, a member of the Bcl-2 family, and the forkhead family transcription factors (FOXO), which are involved in the expression of pro-apoptotic genes. PTEN, by inhibiting AKT, facilitates the activation of these pro-apoptotic pathways.

4. **Cellular Metabolism**: PTEN is involved in the regulation of cellular metabolism by controlling the PI3K/AKT/mTOR pathway, which is central to cellular energy homeostasis. AKT activation promotes glucose uptake and glycolysis while inhibiting autophagy, a process where cells degrade and recycle components for energy. PTEN's inhibitory effect on AKT ensures that cells do not overconsume glucose and maintain a balance between energy production and consumption.

5. **Migration and Invasion**: PTEN also influences cell migration and invasion, processes critical in cancer metastasis. It negatively regulates focal adhesion kinase (FAK) and integrins, both of which are involved in cell movement. By inhibiting these molecules, PTEN reduces the ability of cancer cells to migrate and invade surrounding tissues.

Production of PTEN

The PTEN gene is located on chromosome 10q23.3 and consists of nine exons that encode a protein of 403 amino acids. The production of PTEN involves several key steps, including transcription, translation, and post-translational modifications.

1. **Transcription**: The transcription of PTEN is regulated by various transcription factors, including p53, EGR1 (early growth response 1), and PPARγ (peroxisome proliferator-activated receptor gamma). These transcription factors bind to specific sequences in the PTEN promoter region to initiate the transcription of PTEN mRNA.

2. **Translation**: After transcription, PTEN mRNA is translated into protein in the cytoplasm. The translation process is tightly regulated by various factors, including microRNAs (miRNAs), which can bind to the 3' untranslated region (UTR) of PTEN mRNA and inhibit its translation. Notable miRNAs that regulate PTEN expression include miR-21, miR-22, and miR-214.

3. **Post-Translational Modifications**: PTEN undergoes several post-translational modifications that influence its stability, localization, and activity. These modifications include phosphorylation, ubiquitination, acetylation, and oxidation.

   - **Phosphorylation**: PTEN is phosphorylated on its C-terminal tail, which helps stabilize the protein but also reduces its phosphatase activity. The phosphorylation state of PTEN is regulated by kinases such as CK2 and GSK3β.
   - **Ubiquitination**: PTEN can be ubiquitinated by E3 ubiquitin ligases like NEDD4-1, leading to its degradation by the proteasome. This process is crucial for maintaining the appropriate levels of PTEN in the cell.
   - **Acetylation**: PTEN acetylation can affect its phosphatase activity and stability. For instance, acetylation by p300/

CBP-associated factor (PCAF) increases PTEN stability but reduces its activity.

- **Oxidation**: PTEN contains a cysteine residue in its active site that is susceptible to oxidation. Oxidation of this residue can inactivate PTEN's phosphatase function, thereby promoting PI3K/AKT signaling.

Regulation of PTEN

The regulation of PTEN occurs at multiple levels, including transcriptional, post-transcriptional, and post-translational levels. Various factors and pathways are involved in this regulation.

1. **Transcriptional Regulation**: PTEN transcription is regulated by several transcription factors, as mentioned earlier. Additionally, epigenetic modifications, such as DNA methylation and histone modifications, play a significant role in regulating PTEN expression.
   - **DNA Methylation**: Hypermethylation of the PTEN promoter is a common mechanism of PTEN silencing in various cancers. DNA methyltransferases (DNMTs) add methyl groups to CpG islands in the PTEN promoter, preventing the binding of transcription factors and thereby reducing PTEN expression.
   - **Histone Modifications**: Histone modifications, such as acetylation and methylation, can either promote or repress PTEN transcription. For example, histone acetylation generally promotes gene expression by making the chromatin structure more accessible to transcription factors.

2. **Post-Transcriptional Regulation**: PTEN mRNA stability and translation are regulated by miRNAs, as previously discussed. Additionally, long non-coding RNAs (lncRNAs) and RNA-

binding proteins (RBPs) can influence PTEN mRNA stability and translation efficiency.

- **miRNAs**: miRNAs such as miR-21, miR-22, and miR-214 can bind to the 3' UTR of PTEN mRNA, leading to its degradation or translational repression. This post-transcriptional regulation is critical in various physiological and pathological processes, including cancer.
- **lncRNAs**: lncRNAs can act as molecular sponges for miRNAs, preventing them from binding to PTEN mRNA. For example, the lncRNA HOTAIR can sequester miR-21, thereby increasing PTEN expression.
- **RBPs**: RBPs such as HuR can bind to PTEN mRNA and protect it from degradation, thereby enhancing PTEN expression.

3. **Post-Translational Regulation**: PTEN activity and stability are regulated by various post-translational modifications, including phosphorylation, ubiquitination, and oxidation.

- **Phosphorylation**: PTEN phosphorylation by kinases such as CK2 and GSK3β stabilizes the protein but reduces its phosphatase activity. Dephosphorylation of PTEN, on the other hand, increases its activity but makes it more susceptible to degradation.
- **Ubiquitination**: PTEN ubiquitination by E3 ubiquitin ligases like NEDD4-1 targets the protein for proteasomal degradation. The balance between ubiquitination and deubiquitination is crucial for maintaining appropriate PTEN levels in the cell.
- **Oxidation**: PTEN oxidation at its active site cysteine residue inactivates its phosphatase function. Antioxidant systems, such as the glutathione system, can reverse this oxidation and restore PTEN activity.

PTEN-Related Pathways

PTEN is involved in several critical signaling pathways that regulate cellular processes such as growth, proliferation, survival, and metabolism. Below, we will explore the major pathways influenced by PTEN.

1. **PI3K/AKT/mTOR Pathway**: The PI3K/AKT/mTOR pathway is the most well-known pathway regulated by PTEN. As a lipid phosphatase, PTEN dephosphorylates PIP3 to PIP2, thereby inhibiting the activation of AKT. AKT is a serine/threonine kinase that promotes cell survival, growth, and proliferation by phosphorylating various downstream targets, including mTOR, GSK3β, and FOXO transcription factors. By inhibiting AKT activation, PTEN acts as a brake on the PI3K/AKT/mTOR pathway, thereby preventing uncontrolled cell growth and proliferation.

2. **Focal Adhesion Kinase (FAK) Pathway**: PTEN negatively regulates the FAK pathway, which is involved in cell adhesion, migration, and survival. FAK is a non-receptor tyrosine kinase that is activated by integrin signaling and is crucial for the formation of focal adhesions, which are contact points between cells and the extracellular matrix (ECM). PTEN dephosphorylates focal adhesion components, thereby inhibiting FAK activation and reducing cell migration and invasion. This function is particularly important in preventing cancer metastasis.

3. **MAPK/ERK Pathway**: PTEN indirectly influences the MAPK/ERK pathway, which is involved in regulating cell proliferation, differentiation, and survival. The MAPK/ERK pathway is activated by receptor tyrosine kinases (RTKs) and involves a cascade of phosphorylation events leading to the activation of ERK1/2. PTEN, by inhibiting PI3K/AKT signaling, can reduce the activation of RTKs and thereby modulate the MAPK/ERK pathway. Additionally, PTEN can interact with the scaffolding

protein β-arrestin, which is involved in MAPK/ERK signaling, further influencing this pathway.

4. **Wnt/β-catenin Pathway**: The Wnt/β-catenin pathway is involved in regulating cell proliferation, differentiation, and migration. PTEN negatively regulates this pathway by inhibiting AKT, which in turn prevents the stabilization and nuclear translocation of β-catenin. β-catenin is a transcription factor that promotes the expression of genes involved in cell proliferation and survival. By inhibiting β-catenin, PTEN acts as a tumor suppressor in tissues where the Wnt/β-catenin pathway is active.

5. **p53 Pathway**: PTEN can also interact with the p53 tumor suppressor pathway. p53 is a transcription factor that regulates the expression of genes involved in cell cycle arrest, apoptosis, and DNA repair. PTEN can stabilize p53 by inhibiting MDM2, a ubiquitin ligase that targets p53 for degradation. Additionally, PTEN can enhance p53 transcriptional activity by promoting the acetylation of p53. This interaction between PTEN and p53 is crucial for maintaining genomic stability and preventing tumorigenesis.

6. **TGF-β/Smad Pathway**: PTEN modulates the TGF-β/Smad pathway, which is involved in regulating cell growth, differentiation, and apoptosis. PTEN inhibits the PI3K/AKT pathway, which can enhance TGF-β signaling by promoting the nuclear translocation of Smad2/3. Smad2/3 are transcription factors that mediate the effects of TGF-β by regulating the expression of target genes involved in cell cycle arrest and apoptosis. This crosstalk between PTEN and the TGF-β/Smad pathway is important for maintaining tissue homeostasis and preventing cancer progression.

7. **NF-κB Pathway**: The NF-κB pathway is involved in regulating immune responses, inflammation, and cell survival. PTEN negatively regulates this pathway by inhibiting AKT, which in turn prevents the activation of IKK (IκB kinase). IKK phosphorylates

IκB, leading to its degradation and the release of NF-κB, which then translocates to the nucleus to promote the expression of pro-survival and inflammatory genes. By inhibiting NF-κB activation, PTEN plays a role in preventing chronic inflammation and cancer.

The PTEN tumor suppressor gene is a central regulator of numerous cellular processes, including growth, proliferation, survival, and metabolism. Through its lipid and protein phosphatase activities, PTEN acts as a brake on several key signaling pathways, including the PI3K/AKT/mTOR pathway, the FAK pathway, and the MAPK/ERK pathway. The regulation of PTEN occurs at multiple levels, including transcriptional, post-transcriptional, and post-translational levels, and involves various factors such as transcription factors, miRNAs, and post-translational modifications. Given its critical role in maintaining cellular homeostasis, it is not surprising that PTEN is one of the most frequently mutated genes in human cancers.

SMAD4

SMAD4, also known as DPC4 (Deleted in Pancreatic Carcinoma, locus 4), is a critical tumor suppressor gene involved in various cellular processes, including signal transduction, cell cycle regulation, apoptosis, and DNA repair. Mutations or deletions in SMAD4 are commonly associated with several forms of cancer, particularly pancreatic and colorectal cancers.

Function of SMAD4

SMAD4 is a central mediator in the transforming growth factor-beta (TGF-β) signaling pathway, which plays a pivotal role in regulating cell growth, differentiation, apoptosis, and extracellular matrix production. TGF-β signaling is crucial for maintaining tissue homeostasis and preventing uncontrolled cell proliferation. SMAD4 acts as a signal transducer that transmits signals from the cell membrane to the nucleus, where it influences the transcription of target genes involved in these processes.

TGF-β/SMAD Signaling Pathway

The TGF-β/SMAD signaling pathway is initiated when TGF-β ligands bind to their respective receptors on the cell surface. This binding activates the receptor, leading to the phosphorylation of receptor-regulated SMADs (R-SMADs), specifically SMAD2 and SMAD3. These phosphorylated R-SMADs then form a complex with SMAD4, which translocates to the nucleus. In the nucleus, the SMAD4 complex regulates the transcription of target genes by interacting with various transcription factors and co-factors.

SMAD4 functions as a co-mediator that is essential for the proper transcriptional regulation of TGF-β-responsive genes. The loss or mutation of SMAD4 disrupts this signaling pathway, leading to unregulated cell proliferation, resistance to apoptosis, and other hallmarks of cancer.

Production of SMAD4

SMAD4 is encoded by the SMAD4 gene located on chromosome 18q21.1. The gene consists of 11 exons that encode a protein of 552 amino acids. The SMAD4 protein contains two highly conserved domains: the MH1 (MAD homology 1) domain at the N-terminus and the MH2 (MAD homology 2) domain at the C-terminus. The MH1 domain is involved in DNA binding, while the MH2 domain is responsible for protein-protein interactions, including the formation of complexes with R-SMADs.

Transcriptional Regulation of SMAD4

The expression of SMAD4 is tightly regulated at the transcriptional level. Several transcription factors have been identified that bind to the promoter region of the SMAD4 gene and regulate its expression. These include SP1, AP-1, and p53, among others. The promoter region of SMAD4 also contains CpG islands, which are subject to methylation. Hypermethylation of these CpG islands can lead to the silencing of SMAD4 expression, contributing to the loss of its tumor suppressor function in cancer.

Regulation of SMAD4

SMAD4 activity is regulated at multiple levels, including post-translational modifications, protein-protein interactions, and subcellular localization. These regulatory mechanisms ensure that SMAD4 functions appropriately in response to cellular signals and that its activity is tightly controlled to prevent aberrant signaling.

Post-Translational Modifications

SMAD4 undergoes various post-translational modifications that regulate its stability, activity, and interactions with other proteins. These modifications include phosphorylation, ubiquitination, sumoylation, and acetylation.

- **Phosphorylation:** Phosphorylation of SMAD4 can either enhance or inhibit its activity depending on the specific residues that are modified. For example, phosphorylation of serine residues in the MH2 domain can promote the formation of SMAD complexes, while phosphorylation of the linker region between the MH1 and MH2 domains can inhibit nuclear translocation.
- **Ubiquitination:** SMAD4 is subject to ubiquitination by E3 ubiquitin ligases, which targets it for degradation by the protea-

some. The ubiquitination of SMAD4 is a key regulatory mechanism that controls its protein levels in the cell.

- **Sumoylation:** Sumoylation of SMAD4 has been shown to enhance its transcriptional activity by promoting its interaction with transcriptional co-activators. This modification occurs on lysine residues in the MH1 domain.
- **Acetylation:** Acetylation of SMAD4 by acetyltransferases can increase its DNA binding affinity and transcriptional activity. Deacetylation by histone deacetylases (HDACs) can reverse this effect, leading to a reduction in SMAD4 activity.

Protein-Protein Interactions

SMAD4 interacts with various proteins that modulate its function. These interactions can either enhance or inhibit SMAD4-mediated transcriptional regulation.

- **Co-activators and Co-repressors:** SMAD4 forms complexes with co-activators such as p300/CBP and co-repressors such as TGIF to regulate the transcription of target genes. The balance between these interactions determines the outcome of TGF-β signaling.
- **Inhibitory SMADs (I-SMADs):** SMAD4 is negatively regulated by inhibitory SMADs (I-SMADs), such as SMAD6 and SMAD7. These I-SMADs can prevent the formation of SMAD complexes by binding to R-SMADs or SMAD4, thereby blocking their nuclear translocation and transcriptional activity.

Subcellular Localization

The subcellular localization of SMAD4 is a critical aspect of its regulation. SMAD4 must translocate to the nucleus to exert its transcriptional effects. This translocation is tightly regulated by various signaling pathways and cellular conditions.

- **Nuclear Import:** SMAD4 is imported into the nucleus by binding to R-SMADs that have been phosphorylated by activated TGF-β receptors. The nuclear import of SMAD4 is facilitated by nuclear localization signals (NLS) present in the MH2 domain.
- **Nuclear Export:** The nuclear export of SMAD4 is mediated by exportins, which recognize nuclear export signals (NES) in the SMAD4 protein. The balance between nuclear import and export determines the steady-state localization of SMAD4 and, consequently, its activity.

Pathways Involving SMAD4

SMAD4 is involved in multiple signaling pathways, most notably the TGF-β/SMAD pathway. However, SMAD4 also participates in other pathways that contribute to its tumor suppressor function and influence cancer development.

TGF-β/SMAD Pathway

The TGF-β/SMAD pathway is the primary signaling cascade involving SMAD4. This pathway is critical for controlling cell growth, differentiation, and apoptosis. The disruption of SMAD4 in this pathway can lead to uncontrolled cell proliferation and tumorigenesis.

1. **TGF-β Ligand Binding:** The TGF-β pathway begins with the binding of TGF-β ligands (TGF-β1, TGF-β2, TGF-β3) to type II TGF-β receptors (TGFBR2) on the cell surface.
2. **Receptor Activation:** Upon ligand binding, TGFBR2 recruits and phosphorylates type I TGF-β receptors (TGFBR1). This activation leads to the phosphorylation of R-SMADs (SMAD2 and SMAD3).
3. **SMAD Complex Formation:** Phosphorylated SMAD2/3 forms a complex with SMAD4, which then translocates to the nucleus.

4. **Transcriptional Regulation:** The SMAD4 complex binds to specific DNA sequences in the promoter regions of target genes, recruiting co-activators or co-repressors to regulate gene transcription.
5. **Target Gene Expression:** The expression of TGF-β-responsive genes leads to various cellular outcomes, including growth inhibition, apoptosis, and extracellular matrix production.

Disruption of SMAD4 in this pathway can result in the loss of TGF-β-mediated growth inhibition, leading to increased cell proliferation and tumor development.

BMP/SMAD Pathway

Bone morphogenetic proteins (BMPs) are another group of TGF-β superfamily ligands that signal through the SMAD pathway. The BMP/SMAD pathway is essential for bone formation, embryonic development, and tissue homeostasis.

1. **BMP Ligand Binding:** BMP ligands bind to type II BMP receptors (BMPR2) on the cell surface.
2. **Receptor Activation:** BMPR2 phosphorylates type I BMP receptors (BMPR1), leading to the phosphorylation of SMAD1, SMAD5, and SMAD8 (R-SMADs specific to BMP signaling).
3. **SMAD Complex Formation:** Phosphorylated SMAD1/5/8 forms a complex with SMAD4, which translocates to the nucleus.
4. **Transcriptional Regulation:** The SMAD4 complex regulates the transcription of BMP-responsive genes, leading to cellular outcomes such as osteoblast differentiation and bone formation.

SMAD4 is essential for the proper transmission of BMP signals. Mutations in SMAD4 can impair BMP signaling, contributing to developmental abnormalities and cancer.

Wnt/SMAD Crosstalk

The Wnt signaling pathway is another crucial pathway that interacts with SMAD4. Wnt signaling plays a vital role in embryonic development, stem cell maintenance, and cancer. The crosstalk between Wnt and SMAD4 pathways can modulate cellular responses to TGF-β and BMP signaling.

- **Wnt Activation:** Wnt ligands bind to Frizzled receptors, leading to the stabilization of β-catenin, which translocates to the nucleus and regulates gene expression.
- **Crosstalk with SMAD4:** β-catenin can interact with SMAD4 in the nucleus, influencing the transcriptional outcomes of TGF-β and BMP signaling. This crosstalk is critical for balancing cell proliferation and differentiation.

Disruption of SMAD4 can alter Wnt signaling, contributing to the development of cancer by promoting uncontrolled cell proliferation and invasion.

p53/SMAD Interaction

The tumor suppressor protein p53 is another key player that interacts with SMAD4. p53 is involved in the regulation of cell cycle arrest, apoptosis, and DNA repair in response to cellular stress. The interaction between p53 and SMAD4 can enhance the tumor-suppressive effects of both proteins.

- **p53 Activation:** In response to DNA damage or oncogenic stress, p53 is activated and can bind to the SMAD4 complex in the nucleus.
- **Transcriptional Synergy:** The p53/SMAD4 complex can synergistically regulate the expression of genes involved in cell cycle arrest and apoptosis, enhancing the tumor suppressor function.

Loss of SMAD4 can impair p53-mediated tumor suppression, leading to the survival of cells with DNA damage and the progression of cancer.

SMAD4 and Cancer

The loss or mutation of SMAD4 is associated with the development of various cancers, particularly pancreatic, colorectal, and gastric cancers. SMAD4 mutations are also implicated in juvenile polyposis syndrome (JPS), a hereditary condition that predisposes individuals to gastrointestinal polyps and cancer.

Pancreatic Cancer

SMAD4 is frequently inactivated in pancreatic ductal adenocarcinoma (PDAC), one of the most aggressive forms of cancer. Approximately 50% of PDAC cases harbor SMAD4 mutations or deletions.

- **Role in Tumorigenesis:** The loss of SMAD4 in pancreatic cells disrupts TGF-β signaling, leading to uncontrolled cell proliferation, invasion, and metastasis. SMAD4 deficiency also contributes to the resistance of pancreatic cancer cells to apoptosis.
- **Clinical Implications:** SMAD4 status is used as a prognostic marker in pancreatic cancer. Patients with SMAD4-deficient tumors typically have a poorer prognosis and reduced overall survival.

Colorectal Cancer

SMAD4 mutations are also common in colorectal cancer, particularly in the late stages of tumor progression.

- **Tumor Suppression:** In colorectal cancer, the loss of SMAD4 leads to the disruption of TGF-β signaling, allowing for the unchecked growth of malignant cells. SMAD4 deficiency is associated with increased tumor invasiveness and metastasis.

- **Microsatellite Instability:** SMAD4 mutations are often found in colorectal cancers with microsatellite instability (MSI), a form of genetic hypermutability. MSI-high tumors are more likely to exhibit loss of SMAD4, contributing to their aggressive behavior.

Gastric Cancer

SMAD4 mutations have been identified in a subset of gastric cancers, particularly in diffuse-type gastric carcinoma.

- **Loss of Function:** The inactivation of SMAD4 in gastric cancer cells leads to the disruption of TGF-β signaling, promoting the survival and proliferation of cancer cells. SMAD4 loss is also associated with increased resistance to chemotherapy.
- **Prognostic Marker:** Similar to pancreatic and colorectal cancers, SMAD4 status is considered a prognostic marker in gastric cancer. Loss of SMAD4 expression is associated with poor prognosis and shorter survival.

Juvenile Polyposis Syndrome (JPS)

Juvenile polyposis syndrome (JPS) is a hereditary condition characterized by the development of multiple gastrointestinal polyps and an increased risk of colorectal cancer. SMAD4 mutations are responsible for approximately 20-30% of JPS cases.

- **Germline Mutations:** Individuals with JPS harbor germline mutations in the SMAD4 gene, leading to haploinsufficiency and the development of polyps. These polyps have a high risk of progressing to malignant tumors.
- **Genetic Testing:** Genetic testing for SMAD4 mutations is recommended for individuals with a family history of JPS or multiple juvenile polyps. Early detection and monitoring can help manage the risk of cancer in these patients.

The SMAD4 tumor suppressor gene plays a critical role in regulating cellular processes through its involvement in the TGF-β/SMAD signaling pathway. The loss or mutation of SMAD4 is a common event in several forms of cancer, including pancreatic, colorectal, and gastric cancers.

TP73

The TP73 gene, a member of the p53 family, plays a crucial role in cellular development, differentiation, and apoptosis. It encodes for the p73 protein, which, like its p53 counterpart, is involved in the regulation of cell cycle and apoptosis, acting as a tumor suppressor. However, TP73 also has distinct functions that are not entirely shared by p53, making it a unique player in the maintenance of cellular integrity and the prevention of tumorigenesis.

Function of TP73
Role in Tumor Suppression
TP73 primarily functions as a tumor suppressor, similar to p53, by regulating the cell cycle and promoting apoptosis in response to DNA damage. It activates transcription of genes involved in cell cycle arrest, such as p21, and pro-apoptotic genes like BAX, thereby preventing the propagation of damaged cells that might otherwise lead to tumor formation.

Distinction Between TAp73 and ΔNp73
TP73 generates multiple isoforms through alternative splicing, the most prominent being TAp73 and ΔNp73. TAp73 acts as a tumor suppressor by inducing apoptosis and cell cycle arrest, while ΔNp73 antag-

onizes the functions of both TAp73 and p53, promoting cell survival and proliferation. This dual functionality underlines the complexity of TP73's role in cellular homeostasis.

Involvement in Neural Development

In addition to its role in tumor suppression, TP73 is critical for normal neural development. Mice lacking p73 exhibit severe neurodevelopmental defects, including hippocampal dysgenesis, hydrocephalus, and cortical dysplasia. This indicates that TP73 is essential for the survival and maintenance of neural progenitor cells during brain development.

Production of TP73

Gene Structure and Expression

The TP73 gene is located on chromosome 1p36.3, a region frequently deleted in various cancers, suggesting its role as a tumor suppressor gene. The gene spans approximately 82 kilobases and consists of 14 exons, with multiple promoters leading to the production of different isoforms. TAp73 is transcribed from the P1 promoter, while ΔNp73 is transcribed from the P2 promoter.

Alternative Splicing and Isoform Diversity

TP73 undergoes extensive alternative splicing, resulting in multiple isoforms with distinct functions. The full-length TAp73 contains the transactivation domain necessary for its tumor suppressor activities, while ΔNp73 lacks this domain and acts as a dominant-negative inhibitor of both TAp73 and p53. The diversity of TP73 isoforms allows for a finely tuned regulation of its functions in different tissues and under various physiological conditions.

Regulation of TP73 Expression

The expression of TP73 is tightly regulated at multiple levels, including transcriptional, post-transcriptional, and post-translational mechanisms. Transcriptional regulation involves both positive and negative feedback loops, with factors like E2F1 promoting TP73 expression and ΔNp73 providing a negative feedback to inhibit its own expression and that of TAp73.

Regulation of TP73
Transcriptional Regulation

TP73 expression is controlled by several transcription factors, including E2F1, p53, and C-Myb. E2F1 is a key regulator of TP73, especially in response to DNA damage. It binds to the TP73 promoter and enhances its transcription, leading to the production of TAp73, which can induce apoptosis and cell cycle arrest. p53 also contributes to the regulation of TP73, although indirectly, by modulating the levels of E2F1 and other factors.

Post-transcriptional Regulation

MicroRNAs (miRNAs) play a significant role in the post-transcriptional regulation of TP73. For instance, miR-193a targets the 3' untranslated region (UTR) of TP73 mRNA, leading to its degradation and reduced protein expression. This regulation is particularly important in the context of cancer, where altered miRNA expression can lead to dysregulation of TP73 and contribute to tumorigenesis.

Post-translational Regulation

TP73 is also subject to various post-translational modifications that influence its stability and activity. These include phosphorylation, ubiquitination, and acetylation. Phosphorylation of TP73 by kinases such as c-Abl enhances its pro-apoptotic functions, while ubiquitination by MDM2 targets it for proteasomal degradation, thereby regulating its levels in the cell.

Pathways Involving TP73
TP73 and the p53 Pathway

TP73 is a member of the p53 family and shares significant homology with p53 in its DNA-binding domain. It can activate many of the same target genes as p53, including those involved in cell cycle arrest and apoptosis. However, TP73 also regulates unique sets of genes that are not influenced by p53, reflecting its distinct roles in cellular processes beyond tumor suppression.

TP73 in the DNA Damage Response

In response to DNA damage, TP73 is upregulated and contributes to the activation of the DNA damage response (DDR). It induces the expression of genes involved in DNA repair, such as GADD45 and RAD51, as well as pro-apoptotic genes like PUMA and NOXA. This ensures that cells with severe DNA damage are eliminated, preventing the accumulation of mutations that could lead to cancer.

TP73 in Apoptosis

TP73 plays a central role in the intrinsic pathway of apoptosis. It activates the transcription of pro-apoptotic BCL-2 family members, including BAX and BAK, which promote mitochondrial outer membrane permeabilization (MOMP) and the release of cytochrome c. This leads to the activation of caspases and the execution of apoptosis. The balance between TAp73 and ΔNp73 is crucial in determining whether a cell undergoes apoptosis or survives.

TP73 and Neural Development Pathways

Beyond its role in apoptosis, TP73 is essential for normal neural development. It regulates the expression of genes involved in neural progenitor cell maintenance and differentiation, including SOX2 and PAX6. TP73 also interacts with the Notch signaling pathway, which is critical for the regulation of neural stem cell fate decisions. The loss of TP73 disrupts these pathways, leading to neurodevelopmental defects.

TP73 and Cell Cycle Regulation

TP73 regulates the cell cycle by inducing the expression of p21, a cyclin-dependent kinase inhibitor that enforces G1 phase arrest. This prevents the progression of damaged cells through the cell cycle, allowing time for DNA repair. In the absence of TP73, cells may continue to proliferate despite the presence of DNA damage, increasing the risk of tumorigenesis.

TP73 in Immune Response

Recent studies have uncovered a role for TP73 in the regulation of immune responses. TP73 has been shown to influence the expression of cytokines and other immune-related genes, which can modulate the activity of immune cells in the tumor microenvironment. This suggests that TP73 may have a broader role in cancer biology, influencing not only the behavior of tumor cells but also their interaction with the immune system.

Pathological Implications of TP73 Dysregulation
TP73 in Cancer

The TP73 gene is frequently dysregulated in various cancers. This can occur through multiple mechanisms, including loss of heterozygosity (LOH) at the TP73 locus, hypermethylation of its promoter, and overexpression of the ΔNp73 isoform. These alterations can disrupt the balance between TAp73 and ΔNp73, leading to reduced tumor suppressor activity and increased cell survival and proliferation.

TP73 in Neurological Disorders

Given its role in neural development, TP73 dysregulation has been implicated in several neurological disorders. For example, mutations in TP73 have been associated with neurodegenerative diseases such as Alzheimer's disease, where the loss of TP73 function may contribute to the degeneration of neural cells. Additionally, TP73 has been linked to the development of certain neuroblastomas, further underscoring its importance in neural cell biology.

The TP73 gene is a multifaceted player in cellular homeostasis, with critical roles in tumor suppression, neural development, and cell cycle regulation. Its complex regulation through alternative splicing, post-transcriptional, and post-translational modifications allows for precise control of its functions in different cellular contexts. Dysregulation of TP73 is implicated in various cancers and neurological disorders, highlighting its importance in maintaining cellular integrity.

CDH1

The CDH1 gene, encoding the protein E-cadherin, is a critical player in maintaining cell adhesion and tissue architecture. Mutations or loss of function in CDH1 are associated with several types of cancer, particularly gastric and lobular breast cancers.

Function of CDH1

The primary function of the CDH1 gene is to encode E-cadherin, a calcium-dependent cell-cell adhesion glycoprotein. E-cadherin is essential in maintaining epithelial integrity and tissue architecture by mediating homophilic interactions between cells. It plays a crucial role in the formation of adherens junctions, which are necessary for maintaining epithelial layers and cellular polarity.

E-cadherin's role in cellular adhesion is vital for suppressing metastasis in epithelial cancers. By holding cells together within tissues, E-cadherin prevents cells from detaching and invading surrounding tissues, a key step in metastasis. E-cadherin also influences intracellular signaling pathways, such as the Wnt/β-catenin pathway, by sequestering β-catenin at the cell membrane. This action prevents β-catenin from translocating to the nucleus and activating transcription of oncogenic genes.

Additionally, E-cadherin is involved in maintaining epithelial-mesenchymal transition (EMT) status. EMT is a process by which epithelial cells lose their adhesion properties and gain migratory and invasive capabilities, transforming into mesenchymal cells. Downregulation or mutation of E-cadherin is often a trigger for EMT, contributing to cancer progression and metastasis.

Production of CDH1

The CDH1 gene is located on chromosome 16q22.1 and spans approximately 100 kilobases. It contains 16 exons, with exon 1 being noncoding and the remaining exons coding for the E-cadherin protein. The gene is transcribed into mRNA, which is then translated into a 120-kDa precursor protein. This precursor undergoes post-translational modifications, including glycosylation, before being processed into the mature 97-120 kDa E-cadherin protein.

The mature E-cadherin protein comprises several distinct domains:

1. **Extracellular Domain**: This domain contains five cadherin repeats (EC1-EC5) that mediate homophilic binding with E-cadherin molecules on adjacent cells.
2. **Transmembrane Domain**: This domain anchors E-cadherin in the cell membrane, facilitating its role in cell adhesion.
3. **Intracellular Domain**: This domain interacts with catenins (e.g., β-catenin, p120-catenin), linking E-cadherin to the actin cytoskeleton and mediating signal transduction.

The expression of CDH1 is tissue-specific, with high levels in epithelial tissues such as the skin, breast, gastrointestinal tract, and urogenital system. E-cadherin is crucial for the structural integrity and function of these tissues, and its loss or mutation is closely associated with tumorigenesis in these areas.

Regulation of CDH1

CDH1 expression and function are tightly regulated at multiple levels, including transcriptional, post-transcriptional, and post-translational mechanisms.

1. Transcriptional Regulation

CDH1 transcription is regulated by a combination of transcription factors, epigenetic modifications, and signaling pathways. Key factors include:

• **Transcription Factors**: Several transcription factors, such as SNAIL, SLUG, ZEB1, and ZEB2, repress CDH1 transcription by binding to its promoter region. These factors are often upregulated during EMT, leading to the downregulation of E-cadherin and promoting cancer metastasis. Conversely, transcription factors like KLF4 and FOXP3 can activate CDH1 expression, maintaining epithelial characteristics and inhibiting EMT.

- **Epigenetic Modifications**: The CDH1 promoter region is subject to epigenetic modifications, including DNA methylation and histone modifications, which can either silence or activate gene expression. Hypermethylation of the CDH1 promoter is a common mechanism of gene silencing in cancers, particularly in gastric cancer, where it contributes to the loss of E-cadherin expression and tumor progression.
- **Signaling Pathways**: Various signaling pathways, including the Wnt/β-catenin, TGF-β, and Notch pathways, influence CDH1 transcription. For example, activation of the Wnt/β-catenin pathway leads to the nuclear accumulation of β-catenin, which can interact with TCF/LEF transcription factors to repress CDH1 expression, promoting EMT and metastasis.

2. Post-Transcriptional Regulation

CDH1 mRNA is subject to post-transcriptional regulation by microRNAs (miRNAs) and RNA-binding proteins. Specific miRNAs, such as miR-9 and miR-200 family members, have been shown to target CDH1 mRNA, leading to its degradation or translational repression. These miRNAs are often upregulated in cancers, contributing to the downregulation of E-cadherin and promoting cancer progression.

3. Post-Translational Regulation

E-cadherin is regulated post-translationally through several mechanisms:

- **Phosphorylation**: Phosphorylation of E-cadherin and its associated catenins can modulate the stability and function of adherens junctions. For instance, phosphorylation of β-catenin can promote its dissociation from E-cadherin, leading to the disruption of cell adhesion and facilitating cancer cell invasion.

- **Proteolytic Cleavage**: E-cadherin is subject to proteolytic cleavage by several enzymes, including matrix metalloproteinases (MMPs), ADAM family proteases, and γ-secretase. Cleavage of E-cadherin generates soluble E-cadherin fragments, which can act as signaling molecules or decoys, further disrupting cell adhesion and promoting tumorigenesis.

- **Ubiquitination and Degradation**: E-cadherin can be ubiquitinated and targeted for degradation by the proteasome or lysosome. The E3 ubiquitin ligase Hakai, for example, ubiquitinates E-cadherin, leading to its internalization and degradation. This process is often upregulated in cancers, contributing to the loss of E-cadherin-mediated cell adhesion.

Pathways Involving CDH1

CDH1 is a central component of several cellular pathways that regulate cell adhesion, motility, and survival. Key pathways include:

1. Wnt/β-Catenin Pathway

The Wnt/β-catenin pathway plays a critical role in embryonic development, cell proliferation, and differentiation. E-cadherin regulates this pathway by sequestering β-catenin at the cell membrane, preventing its translocation to the nucleus. In the absence of Wnt signaling, β-catenin is degraded by the proteasome. However, when Wnt signaling is activated, β-catenin accumulates in the cytoplasm and translocates to the nucleus, where it interacts with TCF/LEF transcription factors to activate target genes.

Loss of E-cadherin disrupts this regulatory mechanism, leading to the accumulation of β-catenin in the nucleus and the activation of oncogenic transcription programs. This process is a key driver of EMT and cancer progression in epithelial tumors.

2. Hippo-YAP/TAZ Pathway

The Hippo pathway is a tumor suppressor pathway that regulates organ size, cell proliferation, and apoptosis. E-cadherin interacts with the

Hippo pathway by sequestering YAP/TAZ transcriptional co-activators at the cell membrane. When E-cadherin is lost or downregulated, YAP/TAZ translocate to the nucleus, where they interact with TEAD transcription factors to promote the expression of genes involved in cell proliferation and survival.

The loss of E-cadherin-mediated Hippo pathway regulation contributes to the unchecked growth and survival of cancer cells, promoting tumorigenesis and metastasis.

3. PI3K/AKT Pathway

The PI3K/AKT pathway is a key regulator of cell survival, growth, and metabolism. E-cadherin interacts with this pathway by modulating the localization and activity of PI3K. In normal cells, E-cadherin-mediated cell adhesion inhibits PI3K activation, leading to the suppression of the AKT signaling cascade. However, in cancer cells with reduced or lost E-cadherin expression, PI3K is aberrantly activated, leading to increased AKT signaling and enhanced cell survival and proliferation.

The activation of the PI3K/AKT pathway in the context of E-cadherin loss is a common feature of many epithelial cancers and contributes to the aggressive phenotype of these tumors.

4. TGF-β Signaling Pathway

The TGF-β signaling pathway plays a dual role in cancer, acting as a tumor suppressor in early stages and a tumor promoter in later stages. E-cadherin interacts with TGF-β signaling by modulating the activity of SMAD transcription factors. In normal epithelial cells, E-cadherin-mediated cell adhesion inhibits TGF-β-induced EMT by preventing the nuclear accumulation of SMADs.

However, in cancer cells, the loss of E-cadherin disrupts this regulation, leading to the activation of TGF-β signaling and the promotion of EMT, invasion, and metastasis.

CDH1 Mutations and Cancer

Mutations in the CDH1 gene are strongly associated with hereditary diffuse gastric cancer (HDGC) and lobular breast cancer. Germline mutations in CDH1 lead to the loss of E-cadherin function, resulting in increased susceptibility to these cancers. HDGC is an autosomal dominant syndrome characterized by an increased risk of diffuse gastric cancer, with a lifetime risk of approximately 70% for carriers of CDH1 mutations.

In addition to germline mutations, somatic mutations in CDH1 are frequently observed in sporadic cancers, particularly in lobular breast cancer and gastric cancer. These mutations result in the loss of E-cadherin expression, contributing to tumor progression, invasion, and metastasis.

The loss of E-cadherin function due to CDH1 mutations leads to the disruption of cell-cell adhesion, increased cellular motility, and enhanced invasive potential of cancer cells. This loss also triggers EMT, a process that is critical for cancer metastasis. As a result, CDH1 mutations are considered a key driver of tumorigenesis in epithelial cancers.

The CDH1 gene, through its product E-cadherin, plays a crucial role in maintaining epithelial integrity and preventing cancer metastasis. Its regulation involves a complex interplay of transcriptional, post-transcriptional, and post-translational mechanisms. Mutations or loss of function in CDH1 are associated with several types of cancer, particularly those of epithelial origin.

DCC

The Deleted in Colorectal Carcinoma (DCC) gene is a well-studied tumor suppressor gene initially identified in the context of colorectal cancer. It encodes a protein that plays a critical role in cellular processes such as apoptosis, cell adhesion, and axonal guidance. The DCC gene's function, production, regulation, and involvement in various biological pathways highlight its importance in maintaining cellular homeostasis and preventing tumorigenesis.

Function of the DCC Gene

The DCC gene encodes a netrin-1 receptor, a protein crucial for mediating various cellular processes. Netrin-1 is a secreted molecule that acts as a guidance cue for axonal migration during nervous system development. The DCC protein is a transmembrane receptor that belongs to the immunoglobulin superfamily, and it plays a pivotal role in cell signaling related to axon guidance, apoptosis, and cell adhesion.

1. **Axon Guidance**: The primary function of the DCC gene is related to axon guidance, where it interacts with netrin-1 to direct the growth of axons during neural development. Netrin-1 can attract or repel axons, depending on the receptor it interacts with, and DCC is one of the main receptors that mediate this guidance. The DCC protein is essential for proper neural circuit formation, contributing to the development of the central nervous system.

2. **Apoptosis**: The DCC protein also functions as a dependence receptor, which means it can induce apoptosis in the absence of its ligand, netrin-1. This feature is crucial for maintaining cellular homeostasis and preventing uncontrolled cell proliferation, which can lead to tumorigenesis. When netrin-1 binds to DCC, it inhibits apoptosis, allowing cells to survive and grow. However, in the absence of netrin-1, DCC promotes cell death, acting as a safeguard against potential malignancies.

3. **Cell Adhesion**: DCC plays a role in cell adhesion, which is essential for maintaining tissue architecture and cellular communication. The protein facilitates interactions between cells and the extracellular matrix, contributing to the structural integrity of tissues. This function is particularly important in the context of tumor suppression, as loss of cell adhesion can lead to metastasis, where cancer cells spread to other parts of the body.

Production of the DCC Protein

The production of the DCC protein begins with the transcription of the DCC gene, located on chromosome 18q21.3. The gene spans approximately 1.4 Mb and contains 29 exons, which are transcribed into a pre-mRNA molecule. This pre-mRNA undergoes splicing to remove introns, resulting in a mature mRNA that is translated into the DCC protein.

1. **Transcription**: The transcription of the DCC gene is tightly regulated by various transcription factors and epigenetic modifications. Promoter regions upstream of the gene contain binding sites for transcription factors that either enhance or suppress transcription. Epigenetic modifications, such as DNA methylation and histone acetylation, also play a role in regulating DCC gene expression. Hypermethylation of the DCC promoter region is often observed in colorectal cancer and other malignancies, leading to gene silencing and loss of protein expression.

2. **Translation**: After transcription, the mature mRNA is transported from the nucleus to the cytoplasm, where it is translated into the DCC protein by ribosomes. The DCC protein is synthesized as a precursor molecule that undergoes post-translational modifications, including glycosylation, which is essential for its proper folding and function. The mature DCC protein is then integrated into the cell membrane, where it can interact with its ligand, netrin-1, and other cellular components.

3. **Post-Translational Modifications**: The DCC protein undergoes various post-translational modifications that are critical for its function. Glycosylation, for instance, is necessary for proper folding and stability of the protein. Additionally, phosphorylation of the DCC protein can modulate its signaling capabilities, influencing its role in apoptosis and cell adhesion.

Regulation of the DCC Gene

The regulation of the DCC gene is complex and involves multiple layers of control, including transcriptional, post-transcriptional, and post-translational mechanisms. This regulation is crucial for ensuring that the DCC protein is produced in appropriate amounts and functions correctly in different cellular contexts.

1. **Transcriptional Regulation**: The transcription of the DCC gene is regulated by various transcription factors, including p53, a well-known tumor suppressor. p53 can bind to the promoter region of the DCC gene and enhance its transcription, particularly in response to DNA damage or cellular stress. This regulation links the function of DCC with the broader network of tumor suppressor pathways, contributing to its role in preventing cancer.

2. **Epigenetic Regulation**: Epigenetic modifications, such as DNA methylation and histone modifications, play a significant role in regulating DCC expression. In many cancers, the DCC gene is silenced through hypermethylation of its promoter region, leading to a loss of protein expression and contributing to tumorigenesis. This epigenetic silencing is reversible, and therapies targeting DNA methylation are being explored as potential treatments to restore DCC expression in cancer cells.

3. **Post-Transcriptional Regulation**: The stability and translation of DCC mRNA are also regulated by microRNAs (miRNAs). miRNAs are small non-coding RNAs that can bind to complementary sequences in the 3' untranslated region (UTR) of target mRNAs, leading to their degradation or inhibition of translation. Several miRNAs have been identified that target DCC mRNA, modulating its expression and influencing cellular processes such as apoptosis and cell adhesion.

4. **Post-Translational Regulation**: The activity of the DCC protein is further regulated by post-translational modifications, such as phosphorylation. These modifications can alter the protein's conformation, stability, and interaction with other cellular components. For example, phosphorylation of DCC by kinases such as Src can enhance its ability to mediate apoptosis, while dephosphorylation may reduce its tumor-suppressive functions.

Pathways Involving the DCC Gene

The DCC gene is involved in several signaling pathways that are crucial for cellular homeostasis, development, and tumor suppression. Understanding these pathways provides insight into how DCC functions in normal physiology and how its dysregulation can contribute to cancer.

1. **Netrin-1/DCC Signaling Pathway**: The primary pathway involving DCC is the netrin-1/DCC signaling pathway, which plays a critical role in axon guidance and apoptosis. In the presence of netrin-1, DCC activates signaling cascades that promote cell survival and axon extension. This process involves the activation of downstream effectors such as focal adhesion kinase (FAK) and extracellular signal-regulated kinase (ERK), which mediate cytoskeletal reorganization and cell migration. In the absence of netrin-1, DCC functions as a dependence receptor, triggering apoptosis through the activation of caspases, particularly caspase-9 and caspase-3. This dual role of DCC in promoting survival or apoptosis depending on ligand availability is crucial for maintaining cellular balance and preventing uncontrolled proliferation.

2. **p53/DCC Pathway**: The tumor suppressor p53 can regulate DCC expression, linking the DCC gene to broader tumor suppressive networks. In response to cellular stress or DNA damage,

p53 is activated and can enhance the transcription of DCC, lead-ing to increased apoptosis in cells that lack netrin-1. This pathway is particularly important in the context of cancer, as the loss of p53 function or DCC silencing can lead to reduced apoptosis and increased tumorigenesis.

3. **Src Kinase Pathway**: Src is a non-receptor tyrosine kinase that can phosphorylate DCC, modulating its signaling capabilities. Phosphorylation by Src enhances DCC's ability to mediate apop-tosis and suppress tumor growth. This interaction highlights the complex regulation of DCC by different kinases and its integra-tion into various signaling networks within the cell.

4. **Integrin Signaling Pathway**: DCC is also involved in cell ad-hesion through its interaction with integrins, which are trans-membrane receptors that mediate cell-extracellular matrix interactions. The DCC protein can influence integrin signaling, affecting cell migration, adhesion, and survival. This function is particularly relevant in the context of metastasis, where loss of cell adhesion contributes to the spread of cancer cells to distant or-gans.

5. **Wnt/β-catenin Pathway**: Although DCC is not a direct com-ponent of the Wnt/β-catenin pathway, its function is influenced by this signaling cascade. The Wnt/β-catenin pathway is involved in cell proliferation and differentiation, and its dysregulation is common in colorectal cancer. Loss of DCC expression can lead to increased Wnt/β-catenin signaling, promoting tumorigenesis. Conversely, restoring DCC function can inhibit this pathway, highlighting its potential role in regulating cell proliferation and differentiation.

6. **Caspase-Mediated Apoptosis Pathway**: In the absence of netrin-1, DCC induces apoptosis through the activation of cas-pases, a family of proteases that play a central role in the execution of programmed cell death. The DCC-induced apoptotic pathway primarily involves the activation of caspase-9, which in turn ac-

tivates caspase-3, leading to the cleavage of cellular components and cell death. This pathway is essential for eliminating damaged or abnormal cells, preventing the development of tumors.

DCC in Cancer

The loss of DCC expression is associated with the development and progression of various cancers, particularly colorectal cancer. The DCC gene was initially identified due to its frequent deletion in colorectal cancer, and subsequent studies have demonstrated its role as a tumor suppressor in other malignancies as well.

1. **Colorectal Cancer**: The DCC gene is often deleted or silenced in colorectal cancer, leading to reduced apoptosis and increased tumor growth. The loss of DCC expression is associated with poor prognosis and increased metastasis. Restoring DCC function in colorectal cancer cells has been shown to inhibit tumor growth and induce apoptosis, highlighting its potential as a therapeutic target.

2. **Gastric Cancer**: Similar to colorectal cancer, DCC expression is frequently lost in gastric cancer due to promoter hypermethylation or chromosomal deletions. The loss of DCC is associated with increased cell proliferation, invasion, and metastasis. Targeting the pathways regulated by DCC, such as the netrin-1/DCC signaling axis, is being explored as a potential therapeutic strategy in gastric cancer.

3. **Breast Cancer**: The role of DCC in breast cancer is less well-defined, but studies have shown that loss of DCC expression is associated with poor prognosis and increased metastasis. The interaction between DCC and integrins may play a role in regulating cell adhesion and migration in breast cancer, making it a potential target for therapeutic intervention.

4. **Lung Cancer**: In lung cancer, the loss of DCC expression is linked to increased tumor aggressiveness and reduced survival. The DCC gene may interact with other tumor suppressor pathways, such as p53, to regulate apoptosis and cell adhesion. Restoring DCC function in lung cancer cells has been shown to inhibit tumor growth and induce apoptosis.

5. **Other Cancers**: The loss of DCC expression has also been observed in other cancers, including pancreatic, esophageal, and prostate cancers. In each case, the loss of DCC contributes to reduced apoptosis, increased proliferation, and metastasis. The role of DCC as a tumor suppressor across multiple cancer types underscores its importance in maintaining cellular homeostasis and preventing tumorigenesis.

The DCC tumor suppressor gene plays a critical role in regulating apoptosis, cell adhesion, and axon guidance, making it a key player in maintaining cellular homeostasis and preventing tumorigenesis. The loss of DCC expression is associated with the development and progression of various cancers, highlighting its importance as a tumor suppressor.

MEN1

The MEN1 gene, which stands for Multiple Endocrine Neoplasia type 1, is a critical tumor suppressor gene located on chromosome 11q13. This gene encodes the protein menin, a nuclear protein that plays a pivotal role in regulating gene transcription, DNA repair, cell proliferation, and apoptosis. Mutations in the MEN1 gene are linked to a hereditary syndrome called Multiple Endocrine Neoplasia type 1 (MEN1), which predisposes individuals to develop tumors in multiple endocrine glands, including the parathyroid glands, pancreatic islet cells, and the anterior pituitary.

Function of the MEN1 Tumor Suppressor Gene

The primary function of the MEN1 gene is to encode the menin protein, which acts as a tumor suppressor by interacting with various transcription factors and chromatin remodeling proteins to regulate gene expression. Menin's involvement in multiple cellular pathways emphasizes its crucial role in maintaining cellular homeostasis and preventing uncontrolled cell growth.

1. **Regulation of Gene Transcription**: Menin is known to interact with transcription factors such as JunD, NF-kB, and Smad3. By binding to these factors, menin modulates their transcriptional activity, influencing the expression of target genes involved in cell proliferation and apoptosis. For example, menin represses JunD-mediated transcription, which in turn inhibits cell proliferation and promotes apoptosis.

2. **Chromatin Remodeling**: Menin also associates with chromatin remodeling complexes, such as the histone methyltransferase complexes, including MLL (mixed lineage leukemia) complexes. These complexes are involved in the methylation of histone H3 on lysine 4 (H3K4), a marker associated with active gene transcription. By interacting with these complexes, menin helps regulate the expression of genes involved in cell cycle control, differentiation, and proliferation.

3. **DNA Repair**: Another crucial function of menin is its role in DNA repair. Menin is involved in the homologous recombination repair (HRR) pathway, a critical mechanism for repairing double-strand breaks (DSBs) in DNA. This function is essential

for maintaining genomic stability and preventing mutations that could lead to cancer development.

4. **Cell Cycle Regulation**: Menin influences cell cycle regulation by modulating the activity of cyclin-dependent kinase inhibitors, such as p18INK4C and p27Kip1. These inhibitors play a role in controlling the progression of the cell cycle, particularly at the G1/S transition, thereby preventing uncontrolled cell proliferation.

Production of Menin Protein

The production of the menin protein is a tightly regulated process that begins with the transcription of the MEN1 gene. The MEN1 gene is composed of 10 exons that encode a protein of 610 amino acids. The production of menin involves several key steps:

1. **Transcription of MEN1 mRNA**: The MEN1 gene is transcribed into messenger RNA (mRNA) in the nucleus. The transcription of the MEN1 gene is regulated by various transcription factors, including Sp1 and NF-Y, which bind to specific promoter regions of the MEN1 gene.

2. **mRNA Processing**: The primary transcript of MEN1 mRNA undergoes processing, including the addition of a 5' cap, splicing of introns, and polyadenylation of the 3' end. This processed mRNA is then transported out of the nucleus into the cytoplasm for translation.

3. **Translation of Menin Protein**: In the cytoplasm, the MEN1 mRNA is translated into the menin protein by ribosomes. The resulting menin protein is then imported back into the nucleus, where it exerts its tumor suppressor functions.

Regulation of MEN1 Gene Expression

The expression of the MEN1 gene is tightly regulated at multiple levels, including transcriptional, post-transcriptional, and post-translational mechanisms. These regulatory mechanisms ensure that menin levels are appropriately maintained to prevent tumorigenesis.

1. **Transcriptional Regulation**: Transcriptional regulation of the MEN1 gene is primarily mediated by the binding of transcription factors to the MEN1 promoter region. Factors such as Sp1, NF-Y, and E2F1 have been shown to regulate MEN1 transcription. Additionally, epigenetic modifications, such as DNA methylation and histone acetylation, play a role in controlling MEN1 gene expression.

2. **Post-Transcriptional Regulation**: Post-transcriptional regulation of MEN1 involves mechanisms that influence the stability and translation of MEN1 mRNA. MicroRNAs (miRNAs) have been identified as regulators of MEN1 mRNA stability. For example, miR-24 has been shown to target MEN1 mRNA, leading to its degradation and reduced menin protein levels.

3. **Post-Translational Regulation**: Post-translational modifications (PTMs) of the menin protein, such as phosphorylation, acetylation, and ubiquitination, are critical for modulating its activity, stability, and subcellular localization. For instance, phosphorylation of menin by protein kinase C (PKC) has been shown to affect its nuclear localization and interaction with other proteins.

Pathways Involving MEN1 Gene

Menin, the protein encoded by the MEN1 gene, is involved in several key signaling pathways that regulate cell growth, proliferation, and apoptosis. Dysregulation of these pathways due to MEN1 mutations can lead to tumorigenesis. Below are the major pathways in which menin plays a critical role:

1. **TGF-β/Smad Pathway**: Menin is known to interact with Smad3, a critical mediator of the TGF-β (Transforming Growth Factor-beta) signaling pathway. The TGF-β pathway plays a dual role in cancer, acting as a tumor suppressor in the early stages and promoting tumor progression in the later stages. Menin enhances the transcriptional activity of Smad3, thereby promoting the expression of genes involved in growth inhibition and apoptosis. Loss of menin function can impair this pathway, leading to uncontrolled cell growth and tumor formation.

2. **Wnt/β-catenin Pathway**: The Wnt/β-catenin signaling pathway is crucial for cell proliferation, differentiation, and stem cell maintenance. Menin has been shown to interact with components of the Wnt/β-catenin pathway, influencing the transcription of Wnt target genes. Aberrant activation of the Wnt/β-catenin pathway due to MEN1 mutations can contribute to tumorigenesis by promoting cell proliferation and inhibiting apoptosis.

3. **Hedgehog Pathway**: Menin also plays a role in the Hedgehog signaling pathway, which is involved in embryonic development and the regulation of stem cell populations. Menin interacts with Gli1, a transcription factor activated by Hedgehog signaling, to modulate the expression of target genes. Dysregulation of this pathway due to MEN1 mutations can lead to the development of endocrine and non-endocrine tumors.

4. **mTOR Pathway**: The mTOR (mechanistic Target of Rapamycin) pathway is a central regulator of cell growth, metabolism, and survival. Menin has been implicated in the regulation of the mTOR pathway through its interaction with the TSC1/TSC2 complex, which negatively regulates mTOR activity. Loss

of menin function can lead to hyperactivation of the mTOR pathway, promoting cell growth and tumor development.

5. **p53 Pathway**: Menin is involved in the p53 signaling pathway, which plays a critical role in maintaining genomic stability and preventing tumorigenesis. Menin enhances the transcriptional activity of p53, promoting the expression of genes involved in cell cycle arrest and apoptosis. Mutations in the MEN1 gene can impair the function of p53, leading to the accumulation of genetic mutations and the development of cancer.

Clinical Implications of MEN1 Gene Mutations

Mutations in the MEN1 gene are associated with Multiple Endocrine Neoplasia type 1 (MEN1), a hereditary cancer syndrome characterized by the development of tumors in multiple endocrine glands. The most common tumors associated with MEN1 include:

1. **Parathyroid Tumors**: Hyperparathyroidism is the most common manifestation of MEN1, occurring in approximately 90% of affected individuals. Parathyroid tumors result in the overproduction of parathyroid hormone (PTH), leading to hypercalcemia. MEN1 mutations are often found in these tumors, and loss of menin function is thought to contribute to their development.

2. **Pancreatic Neuroendocrine Tumors (PanNETs)**: PanNETs are another common feature of MEN1, occurring in 30-80% of patients. These tumors arise from the pancreatic islet cells and can secrete hormones such as insulin, gastrin, and glucagon. The loss of menin function due to MEN1 mutations is believed to promote the development of PanNETs by disrupting normal cell cycle regulation and apoptosis.

3. **Pituitary Adenomas**: Pituitary adenomas occur in approximately 30-40% of individuals with MEN1. These tumors arise from the anterior pituitary gland and can secrete various hor-

mones, including prolactin, growth hormone, and ACTH. MEN1 mutations are commonly found in these tumors, and loss of menin function is thought to contribute to their pathogenesis by altering hormone regulation and cell proliferation.

4. **Thymic and Bronchial Carcinoids**: Thymic and bronchial carcinoids are less common but can occur in individuals with MEN1. These tumors are derived from neuroendocrine cells and can produce various hormones and neuropeptides. The role of MEN1 mutations in the development of these tumors is less well understood, but it is believed that the loss of menin function contributes to their growth.

5. **Adrenocortical Tumors**: Adrenocortical tumors can also occur in individuals with MEN1, although they are less common than other endocrine tumors. These tumors arise from the adrenal cortex and can produce excess cortisol, leading to Cushing's syndrome. The role of MEN1 mutations in the development of adrenocortical tumors is still being investigated, but it is believed that the loss of menin function plays a role.

The MEN1 tumor suppressor gene plays a critical role in regulating various cellular processes, including gene transcription, chromatin remodeling, DNA repair, and cell cycle regulation. Menin, the protein encoded by the MEN1 gene, interacts with numerous signaling pathways, such as the TGF-β/Smad, Wnt/β-catenin, Hedgehog, mTOR, and p53 pathways, to maintain cellular homeostasis and prevent tumorigenesis. Mutations in the MEN1 gene can lead to the development of Multiple Endocrine Neoplasia type 1 (MEN1), a hereditary cancer syndrome characterized by the development of tumors in multiple endocrine glands.

TSC1 and TSC2

Tuberous Sclerosis Complex (TSC) is a genetic disorder characterized by the growth of benign tumors in various organs, including the brain, kidneys, heart, eyes, lungs, and skin. The disorder is caused by mutations in two genes: TSC1 and TSC2. These genes encode for proteins that form a complex, acting as a tumor suppressor by inhibiting the mammalian target of rapamycin (mTOR) pathway, which is crucial for cell growth and proliferation.

Function of TSC1 and TSC2 Genes

The TSC1 gene is located on chromosome 9q34 and encodes a protein called hamartin. The TSC2 gene, located on chromosome 16p13.3, encodes tuberin. Hamartin and tuberin interact to form a functional complex known as the TSC1-TSC2 complex. This complex plays a critical role in the regulation of cell growth, proliferation, and survival by inhibiting the mTOR pathway.

TSC1 (Hamartin)

Hamartin, the protein encoded by the TSC1 gene, is a 130-kDa protein that functions as a stabilizer for tuberin. It ensures that tuberin maintains its conformation and is capable of inhibiting the mTOR pathway. Hamartin also has roles in cell adhesion and maintaining the integrity of the cytoskeleton, which is crucial for cellular stability and function.

TSC2 (Tuberin)

Tuberin, the protein encoded by the TSC2 gene, is a 200-kDa protein with GTPase-activating protein (GAP) activity. Tuberin acts on a small GTPase called Rheb (Ras homolog enriched in brain), converting it from its active GTP-bound state to its inactive GDP-bound state. This inactivation of Rheb is essential for the suppression of mTORC1 (mTOR complex 1) activity, thus preventing uncontrolled cell growth and proliferation.

Production of TSC1 and TSC2 Proteins

The production of TSC1 and TSC2 proteins is regulated at both the transcriptional and post-translational levels.

Transcriptional Regulation

The transcription of TSC1 and TSC2 genes is regulated by various transcription factors that respond to cellular signals. One of the key regulators is p53, a well-known tumor suppressor protein. In response to cellular stress or DNA damage, p53 can upregulate the transcription of TSC2, thereby enhancing its tumor-suppressive effects. Other factors, such as E2F1 and FOXO, also play roles in the transcriptional regulation of these genes.

Post-Translational Modifications

After translation, the TSC1 and TSC2 proteins undergo various post-translational modifications that affect their stability, localization, and activity. Phosphorylation is one of the most significant modifications, with multiple kinases involved in this process. For instance, the AMP-activated protein kinase (AMPK) phosphorylates TSC2, enhancing its activity and promoting the inhibition of mTORC1. On the other hand, AKT (also known as protein kinase B) phosphorylates TSC2 at different sites, leading to its inactivation and promoting mTORC1 activation.

Regulation of TSC1 and TSC2 Genes

The regulation of TSC1 and TSC2 genes is complex, involving multiple signaling pathways and feedback mechanisms. This regulation is crucial for maintaining cellular homeostasis and preventing tumorigenesis.

mTOR Pathway

The mTOR pathway is a central regulator of cell growth, metabolism, and survival. The TSC1-TSC2 complex inhibits the mTOR pathway by inactivating Rheb, a small GTPase that directly activates mTORC1. When the TSC1-TSC2 complex is functional, mTORC1 activity is suppressed, preventing excessive cell growth and proliferation.

However, when there are mutations in TSC1 or TSC2, this inhibition is lost, leading to hyperactivation of mTORC1 and uncontrolled cell growth, which can result in tumor formation.

AMPK Pathway

AMPK is an energy sensor that regulates cellular metabolism. Under conditions of low energy (high AMP/ATP ratio), AMPK is activated and phosphorylates TSC2, enhancing its ability to inhibit mTORC1. This pathway links cellular energy status to cell growth, ensuring that cells only grow when sufficient energy is available. Dysregulation of this pathway can contribute to tumorigenesis, particularly in the context of TSC1 or TSC2 mutations.

PI3K/AKT Pathway

The PI3K/AKT pathway is another key regulator of the TSC1-TSC2 complex. Growth factors, such as insulin, activate the PI3K/AKT pathway, leading to the phosphorylation and inactivation of TSC2. This inactivation allows for the activation of mTORC1, promoting cell growth and proliferation. In cases where the PI3K/AKT pathway is hyperactivated, such as in certain cancers, mTORC1 is persistently active, contributing to tumor growth. Mutations in TSC1 or TSC2 can exacerbate this effect by further reducing the inhibition of mTORC1.

Detailed Pathways Involving TSC1 and TSC2

The TSC1 and TSC2 genes are involved in several signaling pathways that regulate cell growth, metabolism, and survival. Understanding these pathways is crucial for elucidating the role of TSC1 and TSC2 in tumorigenesis and other diseases.

mTORC1 Signaling Pathway

The mTORC1 signaling pathway is the primary pathway regulated by the TSC1-TSC2 complex. mTORC1 is a key regulator of protein synthesis, lipid biosynthesis, and autophagy. The activation of mTORC1 promotes anabolic processes, leading to cell growth and proliferation.

1. **Activation of mTORC1**: mTORC1 is activated by the small GTPase Rheb, which is in turn regulated by the TSC1-TSC2 complex. When Rheb is in its active GTP-bound state, it directly interacts with mTORC1, leading to its activation. The TSC1-TSC2 complex inhibits Rheb by converting it to its inactive GDP-bound state, thus preventing mTORC1 activation.

2. **Role of Growth Factors**: Growth factors, such as insulin and IGF-1, activate the PI3K/AKT pathway, which leads to the phosphorylation and inactivation of TSC2. This inactivation allows Rheb to remain in its active state, thereby activating mTORC1 and promoting cell growth.

3. **Energy and Nutrient Sensing**: AMPK and the Rag GTPases are involved in the regulation of mTORC1 in response to cellular energy levels and nutrient availability. AMPK activates TSC2 in response to low energy levels, inhibiting mTORC1. Conversely, the Rag GTPases activate mTORC1 in response to amino acid availability, promoting anabolic processes.

4. **Autophagy Regulation**: mTORC1 also plays a crucial role in the regulation of autophagy, a process by which cells degrade and recycle damaged or unnecessary components. Under conditions of nutrient abundance, mTORC1 inhibits autophagy, promoting cell growth. However, when nutrients are scarce, mTORC1 is inhibited, allowing autophagy to proceed, which helps maintain cellular homeostasis.

Regulation by Hypoxia

Hypoxia, or low oxygen levels, is another condition that can regulate the activity of the TSC1-TSC2 complex. Under hypoxic conditions, the protein REDD1 (regulated in development and DNA damage responses 1) is upregulated. REDD1 inhibits the activity of mTORC1 by promoting the formation of the TSC1-TSC2 complex, thereby preventing cell growth in low-oxygen environments. This regulation is crucial for adapting to hypoxic conditions and preventing excessive cell proliferation under stress.

TGF-β Signaling Pathway

The TGF-β (transforming growth factor-beta) signaling pathway also interacts with the TSC1-TSC2 complex. TGF-β is a cytokine that regulates cell proliferation, differentiation, and apoptosis. In some contexts, TGF-β can activate the TSC1-TSC2 complex, leading to the inhibition of mTORC1 and promoting cell cycle arrest and apoptosis. This pathway highlights the role of TSC1 and TSC2 in responding to extracellular signals and maintaining tissue homeostasis.

Pathological Implications of TSC1 and TSC2 Mutations

Mutations in TSC1 and TSC2 are associated with several pathological conditions, most notably Tuberous Sclerosis Complex (TSC) and certain types of cancers. These mutations lead to the loss of function of the TSC1-TSC2 complex, resulting in the hyperactivation of mTORC1 and uncontrolled cell growth.

Tuberous Sclerosis Complex (TSC)

TSC is a genetic disorder characterized by the formation of benign tumors in multiple organs, including the brain, kidneys, heart, and skin. These tumors, known as hamartomas, are the result of excessive cell growth due to the loss of TSC1 or TSC2 function. The clinical manifestations of TSC are highly variable and can include seizures, intellectual disability, autism spectrum disorder, and skin abnormalities.

1. **Genetic Basis**: TSC is caused by mutations in either the TSC1 or TSC2 gene. These mutations are typically inherited in an autosomal dominant manner, meaning that a single copy of the mutated gene is sufficient to cause the disorder. However, in some cases, the mutations occur de novo, with no family history of the disease.

2. **Tumor Formation**: The loss of TSC1 or TSC2 function leads to the hyperactivation of mTORC1, resulting in increased cell

growth and proliferation. This unchecked cell growth leads to the formation of hamartomas, which can cause organ dysfunction depending on their size and location.

3. **Neurological Symptoms**: One of the most significant aspects of TSC is its impact on the brain. The formation of cortical tubers, subependymal nodules, and subependymal giant cell astrocytomas (SEGAs) can lead to seizures, developmental delays, and neuropsychiatric disorders. The exact mechanisms by which TSC1 and TSC2 mutations lead to these neurological symptoms are not fully understood, but they likely involve dysregulation of mTORC1 signaling in neurons and glial cells.

4. **Renal Manifestations**: Renal angiomyolipomas are another common feature of TSC. These benign tumors consist of blood vessels, smooth muscle cells, and fat cells. While usually asymptomatic, they can cause complications such as bleeding, hypertension, and renal failure if they grow large enough.

Cancer

While TSC is typically associated with benign tumors, there is also evidence that mutations in TSC1 and TSC2 can contribute to the development of malignant cancers. This is particularly true for certain types of brain, kidney, and lung cancers.

1. **Brain Cancer**: Mutations in TSC1 and TSC2 have been implicated in the development of certain brain cancers, such as glioblastoma. The loss of TSC1 or TSC2 function leads to the hyperactivation of mTORC1, promoting the growth and survival of cancerous cells.

2. **Renal Cell Carcinoma (RCC)**: TSC1 and TSC2 mutations are also associated with an increased risk of renal cell carcinoma, particularly the chromophobe subtype. In these cases, the loss of TSC1 or TSC2 function contributes to the hyperactivation of

mTORC1, driving the proliferation of cancerous cells in the kidney.

3. **Lymphangioleiomyomatosis (LAM)**: LAM is a rare lung disease that primarily affects women and is characterized by the proliferation of abnormal smooth muscle-like cells in the lungs. This proliferation is driven by mutations in TSC2, leading to the hyperactivation of mTORC1. LAM is considered a low-grade neoplasm and shares many similarities with TSC, including the presence of angiomyolipomas.

The TSC1 and TSC2 genes play a crucial role in regulating cell growth, proliferation, and survival through their inhibition of the mTOR pathway. Mutations in these genes lead to the development of Tuberous Sclerosis Complex and are associated with an increased risk of certain cancers.

STK11

The STK11 gene, also known as LKB1 (liver kinase B1), encodes a serine/threonine kinase that plays a critical role in cellular energy homeostasis, metabolism, and tumor suppression. Mutations in STK11 are implicated in several types of cancer, making it a crucial gene in the study of cancer biology.

Function of STK11 (LKB1)

STK11/LKB1 is a tumor suppressor gene that encodes a protein kinase involved in several key cellular processes. The STK11 protein plays a crucial role in regulating cell polarity, metabolism, and the response to cellular stress. It acts as a master kinase, activating a number of downstream kinases that are involved in various cellular functions.

1. **Cellular Metabolism and Energy Homeostasis**: The STK11 protein is essential in maintaining cellular energy balance. It activates AMP-activated protein kinase (AMPK), a critical energy sensor in cells. When cellular energy levels are low, AMPK is activated, leading to a series of metabolic changes that conserve energy and restore ATP levels. STK11 phosphorylates and activates AMPK, which in turn regulates pathways involved in glucose uptake, fatty acid oxidation, and mitochondrial biogenesis.

2. **Regulation of Cell Polarity**: STK11 plays a significant role in maintaining cell polarity, which is crucial for tissue organization and function. It does this by activating a group of kinases known as the Par-1/MARK family. These kinases are involved in establishing and maintaining the polarity of epithelial cells, neurons, and other cell types. Loss of STK11 function can lead to disruptions in cell polarity, contributing to tumorigenesis.

3. **Tumor Suppression**: As a tumor suppressor, STK11 is involved in preventing uncontrolled cell growth and proliferation. It exerts its tumor-suppressive effects by regulating processes such as apoptosis (programmed cell death), cell cycle arrest, and cellular senescence. Mutations in STK11 lead to the loss of these regulatory functions, which can contribute to the development and progression of cancer.

Production of STK11 (LKB1)

The STK11 gene is located on chromosome 19p13.3 and consists of nine exons. It is expressed in various tissues throughout the body, with particularly high expression levels in the liver, pancreas, testes, and brain. The STK11 protein is produced through the following process:

1. **Transcription**: The process begins with the transcription of the STK11 gene, where the DNA sequence is transcribed into messenger RNA (mRNA) in the cell nucleus. Transcription factors, such as SP1 and C/EBP, bind to the promoter region of the STK11 gene to initiate transcription.

2. **mRNA Processing**: The primary mRNA transcript undergoes processing, including the addition of a 5′ cap, splicing to remove introns, and the addition of a poly-A tail at the 3′ end. These modifications are necessary for the stability and translation of the mRNA.

3. **Translation**: The processed mRNA is then transported to the cytoplasm, where it is translated into the STK11 protein by ribosomes. The STK11 protein consists of 433 amino acids and has a molecular weight of approximately 48 kDa. The protein contains a kinase domain that is essential for its enzymatic activity.

4. **Post-translational Modifications**: After translation, the STK11 protein undergoes post-translational modifications, such as phosphorylation, which are crucial for its activation and function. These modifications allow STK11 to interact with other proteins and participate in various signaling pathways.

Regulation of STK11 (LKB1)

The activity of STK11 is tightly regulated at multiple levels, including transcriptional, post-transcriptional, and post-translational mechanisms. Proper regulation of STK11 is critical for maintaining normal cellular function and preventing tumorigenesis.

1. **Transcriptional Regulation**: The expression of STK11 is regulated by several transcription factors, including SP1, C/EBP, and NF-κB. These factors bind to the promoter region of the STK11 gene and either enhance or repress its transcription. For example, the transcription factor NF-κB has been shown to repress STK11

expression under certain conditions, which can contribute to the development of cancer.

2. **Post-transcriptional Regulation**: STK11 mRNA stability and translation can be influenced by various microRNAs (miRNAs) and RNA-binding proteins. For instance, miR-451 has been identified as a negative regulator of STK11, as it binds to the 3′ untranslated region (UTR) of STK11 mRNA, leading to its degradation. Dysregulation of these miRNAs can result in altered STK11 expression, contributing to tumorigenesis.

3. **Post-translational Regulation**: The activity of the STK11 protein is regulated by post-translational modifications such as phosphorylation, acetylation, and ubiquitination. For example, phosphorylation of STK11 by upstream kinases, such as PKA and PKC, enhances its kinase activity and promotes its tumor suppressor functions. Conversely, ubiquitination of STK11 by specific E3 ligases targets it for proteasomal degradation, leading to a decrease in its activity.

Pathways Involving STK11 (LKB1)

STK11/LKB1 is involved in several key signaling pathways that regulate cellular metabolism, growth, and survival. The loss of STK11 function disrupts these pathways, contributing to the development of cancer.

1. **AMPK Pathway**: One of the most well-characterized pathways regulated by STK11 is the AMPK pathway. Upon activation by STK11, AMPK phosphorylates and inhibits the activity of acetyl-CoA carboxylase (ACC), reducing fatty acid synthesis and promoting fatty acid oxidation. AMPK also inhibits mTOR (mechanistic target of rapamycin), a key regulator of cell growth and proliferation. By inhibiting mTOR, AMPK reduces protein

synthesis and cell growth, contributing to the tumor suppressor functions of STK11.

2. **mTOR Pathway**: The mTOR pathway is a central regulator of cell growth and metabolism. Under conditions of low energy, STK11 activates AMPK, which inhibits mTORC1 (mTOR complex 1) by phosphorylating TSC2 (tuberous sclerosis complex 2) and Raptor (regulatory-associated protein of mTOR). This inhibition of mTORC1 leads to a reduction in protein synthesis and cell growth, preventing uncontrolled proliferation and tumorigenesis.

3. **p53 Pathway**: STK11 also interacts with the p53 pathway, which is a critical regulator of the cellular response to stress and DNA damage. STK11 has been shown to stabilize p53 by promoting its phosphorylation and preventing its degradation. This interaction enhances p53-mediated cell cycle arrest and apoptosis, contributing to the tumor suppressor functions of STK11 .

4. **Wnt/β-catenin Pathway**: The Wnt/β-catenin signaling pathway is involved in the regulation of cell proliferation, differentiation, and migration. STK11 has been shown to inhibit the Wnt/β-catenin pathway by promoting the phosphorylation and degradation of β-catenin. This inhibition prevents the accumulation of β-catenin in the nucleus, where it would otherwise promote the expression of genes involved in cell proliferation and tumorigenesis.

5. **Autophagy Pathway**: STK11 plays a role in regulating autophagy, a process by which cells degrade and recycle damaged organelles and proteins. By activating AMPK, STK11 promotes the initiation of autophagy, which helps to maintain cellular homeostasis under conditions of stress. Autophagy can act as a tumor suppressive mechanism by preventing the accumulation of damaged cellular components that could otherwise contribute to cancer development.

STK11 (LKB1) in Cancer

Mutations or loss of function in the STK11 gene are associated with several types of cancer, including Peutz-Jeghers syndrome (PJS), lung cancer, and pancreatic cancer. The loss of STK11 function leads to the disruption of the pathways mentioned above, contributing to uncontrolled cell growth, proliferation, and tumorigenesis.

1. **Peutz-Jeghers Syndrome (PJS)**: PJS is a rare inherited disorder characterized by the development of benign polyps in the gastrointestinal tract and an increased risk of developing various cancers. PJS is caused by germline mutations in the STK11 gene, leading to the loss of its tumor suppressor functions. Individuals with PJS have a significantly increased risk of developing cancers of the gastrointestinal tract, pancreas, lung, breast, and reproductive organs.

2. **Lung Cancer**: STK11 mutations are frequently observed in non-small cell lung cancer (NSCLC), particularly in lung adenocarcinoma. The loss of STK11 function in lung cancer is associated with poor prognosis and resistance to certain therapies, such as immune checkpoint inhibitors. The loss of STK11 leads to the activation of mTOR and other pro-growth pathways, contributing to the aggressive behavior of lung tumors.

3. **Pancreatic Cancer**: Pancreatic ductal adenocarcinoma (PDAC) is another cancer type frequently associated with STK11 mutations. The loss of STK11 function in pancreatic cancer leads to dysregulation of the AMPK and mTOR pathways, promoting tumor growth and resistance to apoptosis. STK11 mutations in pancreatic cancer are associated with a poor prognosis and limited treatment options.

4. **Breast Cancer**: While less common, STK11 mutations have also been observed in breast cancer. The loss of STK11 function in breast cancer is associated with the disruption of cell polarity and

the activation of pro-survival pathways, contributing to tumor progression and metastasis.

The STK11 (LKB1) gene plays a vital role in maintaining cellular homeostasis, regulating energy metabolism, and suppressing tumorigenesis. Its functions are mediated through several key pathways, including the AMPK, mTOR, p53, Wnt/β-catenin, and autophagy pathways. Mutations or loss of function in STK11 are associated with several types of cancer, including Peutz-Jeghers syndrome, lung cancer, pancreatic cancer, and breast cancer.

Targeting the pathways regulated by STK11, such as AMPK and mTOR, represents a promising approach for the treatment of STK11-deficient cancers.

FHIT

The FHIT (Fragile Histidine Triad) gene is a critical tumor suppressor gene involved in maintaining cellular integrity and preventing malignant transformation. First identified in the mid-1990s, FHIT has since been recognized as a key player in various cancer types, including lung, breast, and gastrointestinal cancers. The gene is located on chromosome 3p14.2, a region frequently associated with chromosomal aberrations in cancer cells.

Function of the FHIT Gene
Tumor Suppressor Role

FHIT is primarily known for its role as a tumor suppressor gene. It functions by regulating cell cycle progression and apoptosis, two fundamental processes that, when dysregulated, contribute to the development of cancer. FHIT's tumor suppressor function is mediated through several mechanisms:

- **Apoptosis Induction**: FHIT promotes apoptosis by activating caspase-dependent pathways. It sensitizes cells to apoptotic signals, particularly in response to DNA damage. The loss or reduction of FHIT expression is associated with a decreased apoptotic response, allowing for the survival and proliferation of cells with genomic instability.
- **Inhibition of Cell Proliferation**: FHIT negatively regulates cell proliferation by modulating key signaling pathways, including the PI3K/AKT pathway. By inhibiting this pathway, FHIT reduces cell growth and proliferation, which is critical in preventing the unchecked cell division characteristic of cancer.
- **DNA Damage Response**: FHIT is involved in the cellular response to DNA damage. It helps maintain genomic integrity by participating in DNA repair processes. Cells deficient in FHIT show increased susceptibility to DNA damage and chromosomal instability, leading to tumorigenesis.

Interaction with Other Tumor Suppressor Genes

FHIT interacts with other tumor suppressor genes, including p53 and BRCA1, to coordinate the cellular response to stress and DNA damage. For instance, FHIT can enhance the pro-apoptotic function of p53, thereby amplifying the tumor suppressor effects of both proteins. Additionally, FHIT's interaction with BRCA1, a gene involved in DNA repair, suggests a synergistic role in maintaining genomic stability.

Role in Signal Transduction

FHIT is also involved in signal transduction pathways that regulate cellular stress responses. By modulating the activity of various signaling proteins, FHIT influences processes such as cell cycle arrest and apoptosis. The loss of FHIT expression disrupts these signaling pathways, leading to the promotion of tumorigenesis.

Production of the FHIT Protein
Gene Structure and Transcription

The FHIT gene spans approximately 1.1 megabases of DNA on chromosome 3p14.2. It consists of 10 exons, with the protein-coding sequence located in exons 5 through 9. The gene's large size and the presence of numerous fragile sites within its sequence make it particularly susceptible to deletions and rearrangements, which are common in cancer cells.

FHIT transcription is regulated by several promoter elements and transcription factors. The core promoter region contains binding sites for transcription factors such as Sp1, which is crucial for initiating transcription. Additionally, enhancers and silencers located upstream and downstream of the gene modulate its transcriptional activity.

mRNA Processing

The primary transcript of FHIT undergoes splicing to remove introns and produce a mature mRNA. This mRNA is then exported to the cytoplasm, where it is translated into the FHIT protein. The splicing process is tightly regulated, and alternative splicing events can lead to the production of different FHIT isoforms, which may have distinct functions.

Protein Translation and Post-Translational Modifications

The FHIT protein is synthesized on ribosomes in the cytoplasm. It is a 147 amino acid protein that contains a histidine triad motif, which is critical for its enzymatic activity. Post-translational modifications, such as phosphorylation, acetylation, and ubiquitination, play a significant role in regulating the stability, localization, and activity of the FHIT protein.

- **Phosphorylation**: Phosphorylation of FHIT by kinases such as ATM (ataxia-telangiectasia mutated) enhances its pro-apoptotic function. Phosphorylated FHIT is more effective in inducing apoptosis in response to DNA damage.

- **Ubiquitination**: Ubiquitination of FHIT targets it for degradation by the proteasome. This process is tightly controlled, and dysregulation of FHIT ubiquitination can lead to either its excessive degradation or accumulation, both of which are associated with cancer.

Regulation of FHIT Gene Expression
Transcriptional Regulation

FHIT gene expression is regulated at the transcriptional level by various transcription factors and epigenetic modifications. Several factors influence FHIT transcription, including:

- **Transcription Factors**: Factors such as Sp1, p53, and E2F1 directly bind to the FHIT promoter and regulate its transcription. Sp1 is particularly important for basal FHIT expression, while p53 enhances FHIT transcription in response to DNA damage.
- **Epigenetic Modifications**: DNA methylation and histone modifications also play a crucial role in regulating FHIT expression. Hypermethylation of the FHIT promoter is commonly observed in cancer cells and is associated with reduced FHIT expression. This epigenetic silencing of FHIT contributes to tumorigenesis by allowing cells to evade apoptosis and proliferate uncontrollably.

Post-Transcriptional Regulation

Post-transcriptional regulation of FHIT involves mechanisms that affect mRNA stability, localization, and translation. MicroRNAs (miRNAs) are key regulators of FHIT mRNA. For example, miR-92a has been shown to target FHIT mRNA for degradation, leading to reduced FHIT protein levels in certain cancers.

Additionally, RNA-binding proteins (RBPs) interact with FHIT mRNA to regulate its stability and translation efficiency. Dysregulation of these post-transcriptional mechanisms can lead to altered FHIT expression and contribute to tumorigenesis.

Pathways Involving FHIT
FHIT and the Apoptotic Pathway
The role of FHIT in apoptosis is well established. FHIT can activate both intrinsic and extrinsic apoptotic pathways, depending on the type of cellular stress. In the intrinsic pathway, FHIT interacts with components of the mitochondrial apoptosis pathway, such as Bax and Bak, promoting the release of cytochrome c and the activation of caspase-9. In the extrinsic pathway, FHIT enhances the activation of death receptors, such as Fas, leading to the activation of caspase-8 and subsequent apoptosis.

FHIT and the DNA Damage Response Pathway
FHIT plays a significant role in the DNA damage response (DDR) pathway. It is involved in the recognition and repair of DNA double-strand breaks (DSBs), a critical form of DNA damage. FHIT interacts with the MRN complex (MRE11-RAD50-NBS1), which is essential for the detection and repair of DSBs. By facilitating the recruitment of repair proteins to sites of damage, FHIT helps maintain genomic stability.

Furthermore, FHIT is phosphorylated by ATM in response to DNA damage, enhancing its pro-apoptotic function. This phosphorylation event is crucial for the activation of downstream DDR pathways, including the p53 pathway, which leads to cell cycle arrest and apoptosis.

FHIT and the PI3K/AKT Pathway
The PI3K/AKT pathway is a key regulator of cell growth and survival, and its dysregulation is commonly associated with cancer. FHIT negatively regulates this pathway by inhibiting the activity of PI3K, thereby reducing AKT activation. This inhibition of the PI3K/AKT

pathway by FHIT leads to decreased cell proliferation and increased apoptosis.

Loss of FHIT expression results in the unchecked activation of the PI3K/AKT pathway, promoting cell survival and proliferation, which contributes to tumorigenesis. This pathway represents a potential therapeutic target, as restoring FHIT expression or function could inhibit the PI3K/AKT pathway and suppress tumor growth.

FHIT and the Wnt/β-Catenin Pathway

The Wnt/β-catenin signaling pathway is involved in regulating cell proliferation, differentiation, and survival. Aberrant activation of this pathway is associated with various cancers. FHIT has been shown to interact with components of the Wnt/β-catenin pathway, inhibiting β-catenin-mediated transcriptional activity. By suppressing the Wnt/β-catenin pathway, FHIT reduces the expression of genes involved in cell proliferation and survival, thereby exerting its tumor suppressor effects.

FHIT in Cancer

FHIT Alterations in Cancer

Alterations in the FHIT gene are common in various cancer types, including lung, breast, esophageal, and gastric cancers. These alterations include deletions, rearrangements, and epigenetic silencing of the FHIT gene. The loss of FHIT expression is associated with poor prognosis and increased tumor aggressiveness.

- **Lung Cancer**: FHIT gene alterations are frequently observed in non-small cell lung cancer (NSCLC). These alterations are often associated with smoking and result in reduced FHIT expression, contributing to the development and progression of lung cancer.
- **Breast Cancer**: In breast cancer, FHIT gene deletions and promoter hypermethylation lead to decreased FHIT expression. The loss of FHIT function in breast cancer cells is linked to increased cell proliferation and resistance to apoptosis.

- **Gastrointestinal Cancers**: FHIT alterations are also common in esophageal and gastric cancers. In these cancers, the loss of FHIT expression is associated with increased genomic instability and tumor progression.

The FHIT gene is a crucial tumor suppressor gene that plays a significant role in regulating apoptosis, DNA damage response, and signal transduction pathways. Its loss or inactivation is associated with various cancer types, highlighting its importance in maintaining genomic stability and preventing tumorigenesis.

MUTYH

The MUTYH gene, known for encoding the DNA glycosylase enzyme MUTYH, plays a critical role in maintaining genomic integrity. This gene's primary function involves the prevention of mutations that can arise due to oxidative DNA damage. MUTYH-associated polyposis (MAP), a condition linked to mutations in the MUTYH gene, is characterized by an increased risk of colorectal cancer, among other cancers.

Function of the MUTYH Gene
DNA Repair and Oxidative Damage

MUTYH is integral to the base excision repair (BER) pathway, which is essential for correcting oxidative DNA damage. Oxidative stress can lead to the formation of 8-oxoguanine (8-oxoG), a highly mutagenic lesion that pairs erroneously with adenine during DNA replication. MUTYH encodes an adenine DNA glycosylase enzyme that recognizes and excises adenine that has been mispaired with 8-oxoG, thereby preventing G to T transversions, a common type of mutation caused by oxidative stress.

Prevention of Mutations and Cancer Suppression

By correcting the misincorporation of adenine opposite 8-oxoG, MUTYH plays a vital role in preventing mutations that could lead to carcinogenesis. The importance of this function is underscored by the association between biallelic mutations in the MUTYH gene and the development of colorectal adenomas and carcinomas, as seen in individuals with MAP.

Production of the MUTYH Protein
Gene Expression and Translation

The MUTYH gene is located on chromosome 1p34.1 and spans approximately 11 exons. The expression of the MUTYH gene is regulated by a complex interplay of transcription factors that respond to cellular signals, including those induced by oxidative stress. Once transcribed into mRNA, the MUTYH gene undergoes translation in the cytoplasm to produce the MUTYH protein, which is then imported into the nucleus and mitochondria, where it performs its DNA repair functions.

Post-Translational Modifications

Post-translational modifications (PTMs) are critical for the functionality of the MUTYH protein. These modifications include phosphorylation, acetylation, and ubiquitination, which regulate the protein's stability, localization, and interaction with other proteins involved in the BER pathway. Phosphorylation, for example, is essential for the activation and proper functioning of MUTYH in response to DNA damage.

Regulation of the MUTYH Gene
Transcriptional Regulation

The transcription of the MUTYH gene is tightly controlled by several transcription factors, including p53, which is activated in response to DNA damage. The p53 protein can bind to the promoter region of the MUTYH gene, enhancing its expression as part of the cellular response to oxidative stress . Other factors, such as NRF2, a key regulator of the antioxidant response, also play a role in upregulating MUTYH expression under conditions of oxidative stress.

Epigenetic Regulation

Epigenetic modifications, such as DNA methylation and histone acetylation, also influence MUTYH expression. Hypermethylation of the MUTYH promoter region has been observed in various cancers, leading to reduced expression of the gene and, consequently, impaired DNA repair capabilities . This epigenetic silencing of MUTYH is a significant factor in the development of tumors, particularly in individuals with a predisposition to cancer due to germline mutations in other DNA repair genes.

Post-Transcriptional Regulation

The stability and translation efficiency of MUTYH mRNA are regulated post-transcriptionally by microRNAs (miRNAs) and RNA-binding proteins. miRNAs can bind to the 3′ untranslated region (UTR) of MUTYH mRNA, leading to its degradation or the inhibition of translation. Dysregulation of miRNAs that target MUTYH has been implicated in various cancers, further highlighting the importance of precise regulatory mechanisms.

Pathways Involving MUTYH

Base Excision Repair (BER) Pathway

The MUTYH gene plays a pivotal role in the BER pathway, which is responsible for repairing small base lesions in DNA, such as those caused by oxidation, alkylation, or deamination. The BER pathway involves several key steps:

1. **Recognition of DNA Damage:** MUTYH identifies and binds to adenine residues that are mispaired with 8-oxoG.

2. **Excision of the Mispair:** The adenine base is excised by MU-TYH's glycosylase activity, creating an abasic site.

3. **Processing of the Abasic Site:** The abasic site is processed by an apurinic/apyrimidinic endonuclease (APE1), which cuts the DNA backbone.

4. **DNA Synthesis and Ligation:** DNA polymerase β fills in the gap with the correct nucleotide, and DNA ligase seals the nick, completing the repair process.

This pathway is crucial for preventing mutations that could lead to cancer, particularly in tissues exposed to high levels of oxidative stress, such as the colon.

Interaction with Other DNA Repair Proteins

MUTYH interacts with other proteins involved in DNA repair, such as OGG1 and MSH2. OGG1 is responsible for excising 8-oxoG from the DNA, while MSH2, part of the mismatch repair (MMR) system, helps recruit MUTYH to sites of oxidative damage. The coordination between these proteins ensures the accurate repair of oxidative lesions, preventing mutagenesis and tumorigenesis.

Wnt/β-catenin Pathway

The Wnt/β-catenin signaling pathway is involved in cell proliferation, differentiation, and survival. Dysregulation of this pathway is a common feature in colorectal cancer, particularly in patients with MAP. Studies have shown that mutations in MUTYH can lead to aberrant activation of the Wnt/β-catenin pathway, promoting tumorigenesis. This occurs because oxidative DNA damage, which is not properly repaired due to defective MUTYH, can result in mutations in key regulators of the Wnt pathway, such as APC (Adenomatous Polyposis Coli).

p53 Pathway

The tumor suppressor protein p53 plays a critical role in maintaining genomic stability by inducing cell cycle arrest, apoptosis, or DNA repair in response to DNA damage. MUTYH is involved in the p53 pathway as part of the cellular response to oxidative stress. When DNA damage occurs, p53 is activated and can upregulate the expression of DNA repair genes, including MUTYH. This ensures that oxidative lesions are repaired before they can lead to mutations and cancer.

Role in Colorectal Cancer

Colorectal cancer is one of the most well-studied cancers associated with MUTYH mutations. Individuals with biallelic MUTYH mutations have a significantly increased risk of developing colorectal adenomas, which can progress to carcinoma if left untreated. The cancer risk in these individuals is attributed to the accumulation of G to T transversions in key oncogenes and tumor suppressor genes, resulting from defective oxidative DNA damage repair.

Role in Other Cancers

In addition to colorectal cancer, mutations in the MUTYH gene have been implicated in other cancers, including gastric, breast, and endometrial cancers. The common thread among these cancers is the role of oxidative stress and the resulting DNA damage, which, if not repaired due to dysfunctional MUTYH, can lead to mutagenesis and cancer development.

Clinical Implications of MUTYH Dysfunction
MUTYH-Associated Polyposis (MAP)

MAP is an autosomal recessive disorder characterized by the development of multiple colorectal adenomas and an increased risk of colorectal cancer. The condition is caused by biallelic germline mutations in the MUTYH gene. Individuals with MAP typically develop polyps in their 40s or 50s, although the onset can be earlier. The clinical management of MAP includes regular surveillance colonoscopies and, in some cases, prophylactic colectomy to prevent the progression to colorectal cancer.

Genetic Testing and Counseling

Given the hereditary nature of MAP, genetic testing for MUTYH mutations is recommended for individuals with a family history of colorectal polyps or cancer, especially if they develop polyps at a young age.

Identifying biallelic MUTYH mutations in a patient can inform clinical management, including increased surveillance and consideration of risk-reducing surgery. Genetic counseling is also important for family members of affected individuals, as they may be carriers of MUTYH mutations and at risk of developing MAP.

The MUTYH gene is a critical component of the DNA repair machinery, specifically in the context of oxidative DNA damage. Its role in preventing mutations through the BER pathway underscores its importance as a tumor suppressor. Mutations in the MUTYH gene lead to a failure in repairing oxidative lesions, resulting in an increased risk of colorectal cancer and other malignancies.

CHEK2

The CHEK2 (Checkpoint kinase 2) gene is a crucial component of the cell cycle control machinery and a significant tumor suppressor gene. Mutations in this gene have been linked to various cancers, most notably breast cancer, prostate cancer, and colorectal cancer.

Function of the CHEK2 Gene

The CHEK2 gene encodes a protein kinase that is involved in the DNA damage response (DDR) pathway, particularly in the regulation of the cell cycle. This gene is a key player in maintaining genomic stability by ensuring that cells with damaged DNA do not progress through the cell cycle, thereby preventing the accumulation of mutations that could lead to cancer.

DNA Damage Response

The primary function of the CHEK2 protein is to act as a checkpoint in the cell cycle, particularly in response to DNA damage. Upon detecting DNA double-strand breaks (DSBs), the CHEK2 protein is activated by phosphorylation through the ATM (Ataxia Telangiectasia Mutated) kinase. Once activated, CHEK2 phosphorylates several downstream substrates, including the tumor suppressor protein p53, the BRCA1 protein, and the CDC25A phosphatase.

- **p53 Activation**: CHEK2 phosphorylates p53 on serine 20, stabilizing p53 by preventing its interaction with MDM2, an E3 ubiquitin ligase that tags p53 for degradation. The stabilization of p53 leads to the transcription of genes involved in cell cycle arrest, DNA repair, and apoptosis.
- **BRCA1 Phosphorylation**: CHEK2 also phosphorylates BRCA1, a gene involved in the repair of DNA DSBs through homologous recombination. This phosphorylation enhances the ability of BRCA1 to mediate DNA repair, further contributing to genomic stability.
- **CDC25A Inhibition**: By phosphorylating CDC25A, CHEK2 inhibits the activity of this phosphatase, preventing the activation of CDK2/cyclin E and CDK1/cyclin B complexes. This action results in cell cycle arrest at the G1/S and G2/M checkpoints, allowing time for DNA repair.

Apoptosis Induction

When DNA damage is irreparable, CHEK2 plays a role in inducing apoptosis, a programmed cell death process. This is crucial for eliminating cells that harbor potentially oncogenic mutations. CHEK2-mediated activation of p53 leads to the transcription of pro-apoptotic genes such as BAX, PUMA, and NOXA, which initiate the apoptotic cascade.

Production of the CHEK2 Protein

The CHEK2 gene is located on chromosome 22q12.1 and consists of 14 exons. The gene encodes a protein of 543 amino acids with a molecular weight of approximately 62 kDa. The production of CHEK2 protein involves the following processes:

Transcription

The transcription of the CHEK2 gene is regulated by various transcription factors, including p53, E2F1, and NF-κB. These factors bind to the promoter region of the CHEK2 gene, initiating the synthesis of mRNA.

- **p53**: As a master regulator of the DDR pathway, p53 can directly regulate the transcription of CHEK2. Under conditions of DNA damage, p53 binds to the p53 response elements in the CHEK2 promoter, upregulating its transcription.
- **E2F1**: E2F1, a transcription factor involved in cell cycle regulation, can also induce CHEK2 expression, particularly in response to DNA damage. This upregulation is part of the broader cellular response to ensure cell cycle arrest and repair.
- **NF-κB**: The NF-κB pathway, typically activated in response to stress signals, can also enhance CHEK2 transcription. This regulation links CHEK2 activity to inflammatory responses and stress signaling.

Translation

Once transcribed, the CHEK2 mRNA is translated into protein in the cytoplasm. The translation of CHEK2 mRNA is tightly regulated by ribosomal machinery, ensuring that sufficient levels of CHEK2 protein are produced in response to DNA damage.

Post-Translational Modifications

The activity and stability of the CHEK2 protein are regulated by various post-translational modifications (PTMs), including phosphorylation, ubiquitination, and acetylation.

- **Phosphorylation**: CHEK2 is phosphorylated on several residues, including threonine 68 (Thr68), by ATM kinase. This phosphorylation is essential for the activation of CHEK2 and its ability to phosphorylate downstream targets.

- **Ubiquitination**: CHEK2 is subject to ubiquitination, which can lead to its proteasomal degradation. This process is regulated by several E3 ubiquitin ligases, including MDM2 and CHIP, which ensure that CHEK2 levels are kept in check to prevent excessive cell cycle arrest.

- **Acetylation**: Acetylation of CHEK2 can modulate its activity and interactions with other proteins. This PTM is less understood but is believed to play a role in fine-tuning CHEK2's function in response to specific cellular contexts.

Regulation of the CHEK2 Gene

The regulation of CHEK2 involves multiple layers of control, including transcriptional regulation, post-translational modifications, and interactions with other proteins. These mechanisms ensure that CHEK2 activity is precisely controlled in response to DNA damage and other cellular stressors.

1. Transcriptional Regulation

As mentioned earlier, transcriptional regulation of CHEK2 is mediated by transcription factors such as p53, E2F1, and NF-κB. Additionally, the chromatin state around the CHEK2 promoter can influence its transcription. For example, histone modifications such as acetylation and methylation can make the CHEK2 promoter more or less accessible to transcription factors, thus modulating its expression.

2. Post-Translational Modifications

PTMs are crucial for regulating the activity of the CHEK2 protein. Phosphorylation, in particular, is a key regulatory mechanism that controls CHEK2 activation in response to DNA damage. ATM-mediated phosphorylation of CHEK2 at Thr68 is a critical step in its activation, allowing it to phosphorylate downstream targets such as p53 and BRCA1.

3. Protein-Protein Interactions

CHEK2 interacts with several proteins that modulate its activity and function. For example, CHEK2 forms complexes with BRCA1 and MDC1 (Mediator of DNA Damage Checkpoint 1), which are essential for its role in the DDR pathway. These interactions facilitate the recruitment of CHEK2 to sites of DNA damage and enhance its ability to phosphorylate target proteins.

4. Negative Regulation

To prevent excessive or inappropriate activation of CHEK2, several negative regulatory mechanisms are in place. For instance, the PP2A phosphatase can dephosphorylate CHEK2, reversing its activation and allowing cells to resume the cell cycle once DNA repair is complete. Additionally, ubiquitination by E3 ligases such as MDM2 targets CHEK2 for degradation, ensuring that its levels do not accumulate excessively.

Pathways Involving CHEK2

CHEK2 is a central player in several key cellular pathways, particularly those related to the DDR, cell cycle regulation, and apoptosis. Understanding these pathways provides insight into how CHEK2 functions as a tumor suppressor and how its dysregulation can lead to cancer.

1. DNA Damage Response Pathway

The DDR pathway is the primary pathway in which CHEK2 functions. This pathway is activated in response to DNA damage, particularly DSBs, which are one of the most lethal forms of DNA damage.

- **ATM Activation**: In response to DSBs, the ATM kinase is rapidly activated. ATM then phosphorylates CHEK2 at Thr68, initiating its activation.
- **CHEK2 Activation and Substrate Phosphorylation**: Once activated, CHEK2 phosphorylates several key substrates, including p53, BRCA1, and CDC25A. These phosphorylation events lead to cell cycle arrest, allowing time for DNA repair. If the dam-

age is too severe, CHEK2-mediated activation of p53 can lead to apoptosis.

- **Homologous Recombination Repair (HRR)**: CHEK2 plays a role in the HRR pathway by phosphorylating BRCA1. This phosphorylation enhances BRCA1's ability to mediate the repair of DSBs through HRR, a high-fidelity repair mechanism that uses a sister chromatid as a template.

2. Cell Cycle Regulation

CHEK2 is a critical regulator of the cell cycle, particularly at the G1/S and G2/M checkpoints. These checkpoints are crucial for maintaining genomic stability by preventing the progression of cells with damaged DNA.

- **G1/S Checkpoint**: At the G1/S checkpoint, CHEK2-mediated phosphorylation of CDC25A inhibits its activity, preventing the activation of CDK2/cyclin E complexes. This inhibition leads to cell cycle arrest, allowing time for DNA repair before the cell enters S phase.
- **G2/M Checkpoint**: Similarly, at the G2/M checkpoint, CHEK2 phosphorylates CDC25C, preventing the activation of CDK1/cyclin B complexes. This action results in cell cycle arrest at the G2/M transition, ensuring that cells do not enter mitosis with damaged DNA.

3. Apoptosis Pathway

In cases where DNA damage is irreparable, CHEK2 plays a pivotal role in inducing apoptosis to eliminate potentially oncogenic cells.

- **p53-Mediated Apoptosis**: CHEK2 activates p53 by phosphorylating it at serine 20. Activated p53 then transcribes pro-apoptotic genes such as BAX, PUMA, and NOXA, which initiate the mitochondrial apoptotic pathway. This leads to the release of cytochrome c from mitochondria, the activation of caspases, and ultimately, cell death.

- **CHEK2-Independent Apoptosis**: Although CHEK2 is primarily involved in p53-mediated apoptosis, it can also induce apoptosis through p53-independent mechanisms. For example, CHEK2 can phosphorylate the pro-apoptotic protein BAD, promoting its activation and leading to apoptosis.

Implications of CHEK2 Mutations

Mutations in the CHEK2 gene can lead to a loss of its tumor suppressor function, contributing to the development of cancer. The most common mutation associated with cancer is the CHEK2*1100delC variant, which results in a truncated, non-functional CHEK2 protein.

- **Breast Cancer**: Individuals with the CHEK2*1100delC mutation have an increased risk of developing breast cancer. This mutation impairs CHEK2's ability to activate p53 and BRCA1, leading to defects in DNA repair and cell cycle control.
- **Prostate Cancer**: CHEK2 mutations are also associated with an increased risk of prostate cancer. The loss of CHEK2 function can result in unchecked cell proliferation and the accumulation of genetic mutations, driving tumorigenesis.
- **Colorectal Cancer**: In colorectal cancer, CHEK2 mutations are linked to defects in the DDR pathway, leading to chromosomal instability and the progression of cancer.

The CHEK2 tumor suppressor gene is a critical component of the DNA damage response and plays a vital role in maintaining genomic stability. Through its regulation of the cell cycle, DNA repair, and apoptosis, CHEK2 prevents the accumulation of mutations that can lead to cancer. However, mutations in the CHEK2 gene can compromise its tumor suppressor function, increasing the risk of cancer development.

BAP1

The BRCA1-associated protein-1 (BAP1) is a deubiquitinating enzyme that plays a critical role in various cellular processes, including DNA damage response, cell cycle regulation, chromatin remodeling, and apoptosis. As a tumor suppressor gene, BAP1 has garnered significant attention in cancer research due to its involvement in several cancer types.

BAP1 is a nuclear protein encoded by the BAP1 gene, located on chromosome 3p21.1. It was first identified as a binding partner of the BRCA1 gene, a well-known tumor suppressor implicated in breast and ovarian cancers. The BAP1 protein contains a ubiquitin carboxyl-terminal hydrolase (UCH) domain, which confers its deubiquitinating enzyme activity. This activity is crucial for maintaining protein stability and regulating various cellular functions.

The loss or mutation of BAP1 has been linked to a predisposition to several cancers, including uveal melanoma, mesothelioma, renal cell carcinoma, and others. Germline mutations in BAP1 have also been associated with a hereditary cancer predisposition syndrome known as BAP1 tumor predisposition syndrome (BAP1-TPDS).

Function of BAP1

The BAP1 protein functions primarily as a deubiquitinating enzyme, meaning it removes ubiquitin moieties from target proteins, thereby regulating their degradation, localization, and activity. This activity places BAP1 at the center of multiple cellular pathways, many of which are directly linked to tumor suppression.

DNA Damage Response and Repair

One of the most critical functions of BAP1 is its role in the DNA damage response (DDR). BAP1 is recruited to sites of DNA damage, where it interacts with other DDR proteins to facilitate DNA repair. BAP1 has been shown to deubiquitinate histone H2A at DNA damage sites, which is a crucial step in the recruitment of other repair proteins, including BRCA1.

BAP1's involvement in homologous recombination (HR), a critical DNA repair mechanism, is of particular importance. HR is responsible for repairing double-strand breaks in DNA, a type of damage that, if not properly repaired, can lead to chromosomal instability and cancer development. By facilitating the recruitment of BRCA1 and other repair proteins to damage sites, BAP1 plays an essential role in maintaining genomic stability.

Chromatin Remodeling

BAP1 is also involved in chromatin remodeling, a process that regulates the accessibility of DNA to transcription factors and other proteins. By deubiquitinating histone H2A, BAP1 influences the structure of chromatin, making it more or less accessible for transcription.

Chromatin remodeling is essential for gene expression, and dysregulation of this process can lead to aberrant gene expression, a hallmark of cancer. BAP1's role in chromatin remodeling underscores its importance in maintaining normal cellular function and preventing oncogenesis.

Cell Cycle Regulation and Apoptosis

BAP1 has been implicated in the regulation of the cell cycle and apoptosis, two processes that are tightly controlled to prevent uncontrolled cell proliferation and tumor formation. BAP1 can deubiquitinate and stabilize proteins involved in cell cycle progression, such as

HCF-1 (Host Cell Factor-1). By regulating the stability and activity of these proteins, BAP1 helps control the transition between different phases of the cell cycle.

In addition to its role in cell cycle regulation, BAP1 is involved in apoptosis, the programmed cell death process that eliminates damaged or unwanted cells. BAP1 can deubiquitinate and stabilize proteins involved in apoptosis, thereby promoting cell death in response to cellular stress or damage. The loss of BAP1 function can lead to the evasion of apoptosis, a hallmark of cancer cells.

Production of BAP1

The production of the BAP1 protein begins with the transcription of the BAP1 gene, which is regulated by various transcription factors. The BAP1 mRNA is then translated into the BAP1 protein, which undergoes several post-translational modifications that regulate its activity, stability, and localization.

Transcriptional Regulation

The transcription of the BAP1 gene is controlled by several transcription factors, including E2F, a family of transcription factors that play a critical role in cell cycle regulation. E2F binding sites have been identified in the promoter region of the BAP1 gene, suggesting that E2F may positively regulate BAP1 transcription during the cell cycle.

Other transcription factors, such as SP1 and p53, have also been implicated in the regulation of BAP1 transcription. SP1 is a general transcription factor that binds to GC-rich regions of promoters, while p53 is a well-known tumor suppressor that regulates the expression of genes involved in the DNA damage response, cell cycle arrest, and apoptosis. The regulation of BAP1 transcription by these factors underscores its importance in maintaining cellular homeostasis.

Post-Translational Modifications

After translation, the BAP1 protein undergoes several post-translational modifications that regulate its activity and stability. These modifications include phosphorylation, ubiquitination, and acetylation.

Phosphorylation of BAP1 by kinases such as ATM (ataxia-telangiectasia mutated) and ATR (ataxia-telangiectasia and Rad3-related) in response to DNA damage enhances its activity and promotes its recruitment to DNA damage sites. Ubiquitination, on the other hand, can target BAP1 for degradation by the proteasome, thereby regulating its levels in the cell.

Acetylation of BAP1 by acetyltransferases can also regulate its activity and interactions with other proteins. These post-translational modifications provide a mechanism for the dynamic regulation of BAP1 activity in response to cellular signals.

Protein Interactions

BAP1 functions as part of a multi-protein complex that includes ASXL1 (Additional Sex Combs Like 1), ASXL2, and other proteins. The BAP1-ASXL complex is essential for the deubiquitination of histone H2A and the regulation of gene expression.

BAP1 also interacts with other proteins involved in the DNA damage response, chromatin remodeling, and apoptosis. These interactions are crucial for the recruitment of BAP1 to sites of DNA damage and its role in tumor suppression.

Regulation of BAP1

The regulation of BAP1 is complex and involves multiple layers of control, including transcriptional regulation, post-translational modifications, and interactions with other proteins. Dysregulation of BAP1 can lead to its loss of function, which is associated with tumorigenesis.

Genetic Mutations

Mutations in the BAP1 gene are a common mechanism of BAP1 inactivation in cancer. These mutations can be germline (inherited) or somatic (acquired). Germline mutations in BAP1 are associated with BAP1 tumor predisposition syndrome, which increases the risk of developing several types of cancer, including uveal melanoma, mesothelioma, and renal cell carcinoma.

Somatic mutations in BAP1 have been identified in various cancers, including lung cancer, breast cancer, and hepatocellular carcinoma. These mutations often result in the loss of BAP1 protein function, leading to dysregulation of the cellular processes it controls.

Epigenetic Regulation

Epigenetic modifications, such as DNA methylation and histone modifications, can also regulate BAP1 expression. Hypermethylation of the BAP1 promoter has been observed in some cancers, leading to decreased BAP1 expression. Histone modifications, such as methylation and acetylation, can also influence BAP1 expression by altering chromatin structure and accessibility.

Epigenetic regulation of BAP1 adds another layer of complexity to its control and highlights the importance of maintaining proper BAP1 expression for tumor suppression.

MicroRNAs

MicroRNAs (miRNAs) are small non-coding RNAs that regulate gene expression by binding to the 3' untranslated region (UTR) of target mRNAs, leading to their degradation or inhibition of translation. Several miRNAs have been identified that target BAP1 mRNA, including miR-31 and miR-203. These miRNAs can downregulate BAP1 expression, contributing to the loss of BAP1 function in cancer.

The regulation of BAP1 by miRNAs underscores the importance of post-transcriptional control in maintaining proper levels of this critical tumor suppressor.

Pathways Involving BAP1

BAP1 is involved in several key cellular pathways, including those related to DNA damage response, chromatin remodeling, cell cycle regulation, and apoptosis. The dysregulation of these pathways due to the loss of BAP1 function can lead to tumorigenesis.

DNA Damage Response Pathway

As mentioned earlier, BAP1 plays a crucial role in the DNA damage response (DDR) pathway. In response to DNA damage, BAP1 is recruited to the damage sites, where it deubiquitinates histone H2A. This deubiquitination is a critical step in the recruitment of other DDR proteins, including BRCA1, to the damage sites.

BAP1's role in the DDR pathway is essential for maintaining genomic stability. The loss of BAP1 function can impair DNA repair, leading to the accumulation of DNA damage and increased risk of cancer development.

Chromatin Remodeling Pathway

BAP1 is also involved in the regulation of chromatin structure through its deubiquitination of histone H2A. Chromatin remodeling is essential for regulating gene expression, and dysregulation of this process can lead to aberrant gene expression and cancer.

The BAP1-ASXL complex plays a key role in this pathway by removing ubiquitin from histone H2A, thereby altering chromatin structure and gene expression. The loss of BAP1 function can disrupt this process, leading to changes in gene expression that contribute to tumorigenesis.

Cell Cycle Regulation Pathway

BAP1 regulates the cell cycle by deubiquitinating and stabilizing proteins involved in cell cycle progression, such as HCF-1. By controlling the stability and activity of these proteins, BAP1 helps regulate the transition between different phases of the cell cycle.

The loss of BAP1 function can lead to uncontrolled cell proliferation, a hallmark of cancer. BAP1's role in cell cycle regulation highlights its importance in preventing tumorigenesis.

Apoptosis Pathway

BAP1 is involved in the regulation of apoptosis by deubiquitinating and stabilizing proteins involved in the apoptotic process. This activity promotes cell death in response to cellular stress or damage, helping to eliminate damaged or unwanted cells.

The loss of BAP1 function can impair apoptosis, allowing damaged cells to survive and proliferate, contributing to cancer development.

BAP1 and Cancer

The loss of BAP1 function has been linked to several types of cancer, including uveal melanoma, mesothelioma, renal cell carcinoma, and others. BAP1 mutations, both germline and somatic, are a common mechanism of BAP1 inactivation in these cancers.

Uveal Melanoma

Uveal melanoma is the most common primary intraocular malignancy in adults. Germline mutations in BAP1 have been identified in families with a predisposition to uveal melanoma, suggesting that BAP1 is a key tumor suppressor in this cancer. Somatic mutations in BAP1 are also common in sporadic cases of uveal melanoma.

The loss of BAP1 function in uveal melanoma is associated with a more aggressive disease and poorer prognosis. The mechanisms by which BAP1 loss contributes to uveal melanoma include impaired DNA repair, dysregulation of gene expression, and evasion of apoptosis.

Mesothelioma

Mesothelioma is an aggressive cancer that develops in the lining of the lungs, abdomen, or heart. Germline mutations in BAP1 have been linked to a predisposition to mesothelioma, and somatic mutations in BAP1 are common in sporadic cases of this cancer.

The loss of BAP1 function in mesothelioma is associated with increased tumor aggressiveness and resistance to therapy. The mechanisms by which BAP1 loss contributes to mesothelioma include impaired DNA repair, chromatin remodeling, and cell cycle regulation.

Renal Cell Carcinoma

Renal cell carcinoma (RCC) is the most common type of kidney cancer. Germline mutations in BAP1 have been identified in families with a predisposition to RCC, and somatic mutations in BAP1 are common in sporadic cases of this cancer.

The loss of BAP1 function in RCC is associated with a more aggressive disease and poorer prognosis. The mechanisms by which BAP1 loss contributes to RCC include impaired DNA repair, dysregulation of gene expression, and evasion of apoptosis.

Other Cancers

In addition to uveal melanoma, mesothelioma, and RCC, BAP1 mutations have been identified in other cancers, including lung cancer, breast cancer, and hepatocellular carcinoma. The loss of BAP1 function in these cancers is associated with increased tumor aggressiveness and resistance to therapy.

The BAP1 tumor suppressor gene plays a critical role in maintaining cellular homeostasis through its involvement in the DNA damage response, chromatin remodeling, cell cycle regulation, and apoptosis. The loss of BAP1 function, whether through genetic mutations or other mechanisms, is associated with an increased risk of cancer development.

BAP1's involvement in multiple cellular pathways underscores its importance as a tumor suppressor.

4

Types of Cancer

In this chapter, we will delve into some of the most prevalent and impactful types of cancers. While it is impossible to cover every type of cancer within the scope of this work, my focus will be on those that are most common and pose significant challenges to public health. The cancers discussed include those that affect various organs and tissues in the body, such as breast, colon, brain, prostate, and skin cancer, among others. Each of these cancers presents unique characteristics, but they also share common biological pathways that drive their development, progression, and, in some cases, response to treatment.

As you read through this chapter, you may notice that certain pathways, such as those involving cell cycle regulation, apoptosis, and DNA repair mechanisms, are mentioned repeatedly. This is intentional and necessary. Cancer, at its core, is a disease of the cellular machinery, where normal processes go awry due to genetic mutations, environmental factors, or a combination of both. Because these fundamental pathways are critical to the function and survival of all cells, their disruption is a common theme across many different types of cancers.

By exploring these pathways in the context of each specific cancer type, we aim to provide a comprehensive understanding of how these diseases operate at a molecular level. For example, the role of the p53 tumor suppressor gene is a recurring topic in cancer biology. This gene is often referred to as the "guardian of the genome" because of its role in preventing the accumulation of mutations. In cancers such as breast and colon cancer, mutations in p53 are frequently observed, leading to

unchecked cell division and tumor growth. However, the specific consequences of p53 malfunction can vary depending on the tissue type and
the presence of other mutations, which is why it is necessary to revisit
this pathway in different contexts.

Similarly, angiogenesis, the process by which tumors establish their
own blood supply, is a critical aspect of cancer progression that is relevant to many cancer types. By understanding how this process occurs in
different cancers, we can appreciate the nuances in how tumors adapt to
their environments.

While some pathways may seem redundant at first glance, their repeated discussion serves to highlight the universality and importance of
these mechanisms in cancer biology. It also underscores the complexity
of cancer as a disease, where similar processes can lead to vastly different
outcomes depending on the cellular and molecular context.

Ultimately, the goal of this chapter is to equip you with a deeper understanding of the commonalities and differences among various cancers. This knowledge is crucial not only for understanding the biology
of cancer but also for appreciating the rationale behind current and
emerging therapeutic strategies. As you progress through the chapter,
keep in mind that the repetition of certain pathways is not a sign of re-
dundancy but rather a reflection of the interconnected nature of cancer
biology. Each instance offers new insights and underscores the importance of these pathways in the development and treatment of cancer.

Bladder Cancer

Bladder cancer is one of the most common cancers, especially in industrialized nations, and primarily affects older adults. It arises from the tissues of the bladder, an organ in the pelvic area that stores urine before it is excreted from the body. The vast majority of bladder cancers begin in the urothelial cells, which line the inside of the bladder. Understanding the function, production, and regulation of bladder cancer, as well as the pathways involved, is crucial for developing effective treatments. Moreover, investigating the causes linked to animal products and exploring how a plant-based diet can aid in reversing bladder cancer offers valuable insights into prevention and management strategies.

Function and Structure of the Bladder

The bladder is a hollow, muscular organ located in the lower abdomen, primarily responsible for storing urine produced by the kidneys before it is excreted through the urethra. The bladder's wall consists of several layers, each playing a crucial role in its function:

1. **Mucosa**: The innermost layer, composed of urothelial cells, is the starting point for most bladder cancers. This layer provides a barrier that protects the underlying tissues from the toxic substances in urine.
2. **Lamina Propria**: Just beneath the mucosa is a layer of connective tissue that supports the mucosa and contains blood vessels, nerves, and lymphatics.
3. **Muscularis Propria**: The thick muscle layer responsible for the contraction of the bladder during urination.
4. **Perivesical Fat**: The outermost layer of fat and connective tissue surrounds the bladder and provides additional support and insulation.

Production and Development of Bladder Cancer

Bladder cancer primarily arises from genetic mutations in the urothelial cells. These mutations can lead to uncontrolled cell growth and tumor formation. The development of bladder cancer can be categorized into several stages:

1. **Initiation**: The initiation stage involves genetic mutations in urothelial cells, often triggered by exposure to carcinogens, such as those found in tobacco smoke or certain chemicals used in the dye industry. These mutations may affect genes that regulate cell growth and division, such as TP53 or FGFR3.
2. **Promotion**: During the promotion stage, the mutated cells begin to proliferate abnormally. This stage is often influenced by additional factors like chronic inflammation, which can be caused by infections or prolonged exposure to irritants like those found in certain animal products.
3. **Progression**: As the cancer progresses, the tumor grows and invades deeper layers of the bladder wall. Tumor cells may acquire additional mutations that allow them to evade apoptosis (programmed cell death) and suppress the immune response.
4. **Metastasis**: In advanced cases, bladder cancer cells can spread to other parts of the body, such as the lymph nodes, bones, liver, or lungs. This is a critical stage where the cancer becomes more difficult to treat and significantly reduces the patient's prognosis.

Regulation of Bladder Cancer Development

The body has several mechanisms in place to regulate cell growth and prevent cancer development. These regulatory pathways are crucial in maintaining normal cellular function and preventing uncontrolled cell proliferation:

1. **Tumor Suppressor Genes**: Genes like TP53 and RB1 play a critical role in controlling cell division and inducing apoptosis in cells with damaged DNA. Mutations in these genes can lead to a loss of regulatory control, contributing to cancer development.

2. **DNA Repair Mechanisms**: The body has several pathways, such as the mismatch repair pathway, that identify and correct DNA damage. Defects in these repair mechanisms can lead to the accumulation of genetic mutations, increasing the risk of cancer.

3. **Cell Cycle Regulation**: The cell cycle is tightly regulated by various proteins, including cyclins and cyclin-dependent kinases (CDKs). Disruptions in these regulatory proteins can lead to uncontrolled cell division and tumor formation.

4. **Immune Surveillance**: The immune system plays a vital role in identifying and destroying cancerous cells. However, some bladder cancer cells can evade the immune response by expressing immune checkpoint proteins, such as PD-L1, which inhibit the activity of T cells.

Pathways Involved in Bladder Cancer

Bladder cancer development and progression involve several key molecular pathways:

1. **RAS-MAPK Pathway**: The RAS-MAPK pathway is involved in cell proliferation, differentiation, and survival. Mutations in components of this pathway, such as FGFR3 or RAS, can lead to increased cell growth and contribute to bladder cancer development.

2. **PI3K-AKT Pathway**: The PI3K-AKT pathway plays a significant role in regulating cell survival and metabolism. Mutations or amplifications in this pathway can promote tumor growth and resistance to apoptosis.

3. **p53 Pathway**: The p53 protein is a crucial tumor suppressor that regulates the cell cycle and apoptosis. Mutations in the TP53 gene are common in bladder cancer and can lead to a loss of p53 function, allowing cancer cells to proliferate uncontrollably.

4. **Epigenetic Alterations**: In addition to genetic mutations, epigenetic changes, such as DNA methylation and histone modification, can also contribute to bladder cancer development. These changes can lead to the silencing of tumor suppressor genes or the activation of oncogenes.

Known Causes Related to Animal Products

Several dietary factors have been associated with an increased risk of bladder cancer, particularly those related to animal products:

1. **Red and Processed Meats**: Consumption of red and processed meats has been linked to an increased risk of bladder cancer. These meats contain high levels of nitrates and nitrites, which can be converted into carcinogenic N-nitroso compounds in the body. A study published in the *International Journal of Cancer* found that high intake of red and processed meats was associated with a significantly increased risk of bladder cancer, particularly among smokers .

2. **Dairy Products**: Some studies suggest a potential link between dairy consumption and bladder cancer risk. Dairy products contain hormones like estrogen, which may promote the growth of hormone-sensitive cancers, including bladder cancer. However, the evidence is mixed, and more research is needed to establish a clear connection.

3. **High-Fat Diets**: Diets high in saturated fats, often found in animal products, have been associated with an increased risk of bladder cancer. High-fat diets can lead to obesity and chronic in-

flammation, both of which are risk factors for cancer development.

4. **Heterocyclic Amines (HCAs) and Polycyclic Aromatic Hydrocarbons (PAHs)**: These carcinogenic compounds are formed when meat is cooked at high temperatures, such as grilling or frying. HCAs and PAHs can induce DNA mutations in urothelial cells, increasing the risk of bladder cancer.

How a Plant-Based Diet Can Help with Reversal

A plant-based diet, rich in fruits, vegetables, whole grains, legumes, and nuts, offers several protective factors against bladder cancer and may even help in its reversal:

1. **Antioxidants and Phytochemicals**: Plant-based foods are abundant in antioxidants and phytochemicals, which help neutralize free radicals and reduce oxidative stress, a key factor in cancer development. For example, cruciferous vegetables like broccoli and cauliflower contain sulforaphane, a compound that has been shown to inhibit the growth of bladder cancer cells .

2. **Anti-Inflammatory Properties**: Many plant-based foods have anti-inflammatory properties, which can reduce chronic inflammation, a known risk factor for cancer. Omega-3 fatty acids, found in flaxseeds and walnuts, are particularly effective in reducing inflammation.

3. **Fiber**: A high-fiber diet, characteristic of plant-based eating, helps promote regular bowel movements and the excretion of toxins, reducing the exposure of the bladder to carcinogens. Fiber also aids in maintaining a healthy weight, lowering the risk of obesity-related cancers.

4. **Isoflavones and Lignans**: These phytoestrogens, found in soy products, flaxseeds, and whole grains, may help regulate hormone

levels and reduce the risk of hormone-sensitive cancers like bladder cancer.

5. **Glucosinolates**: Found in cruciferous vegetables, glucosinolates are converted into bioactive compounds like indoles and isothiocyanates during digestion. These compounds have been shown to modulate detoxification enzymes and inhibit the growth of cancer cells.

6. **Lowering IGF-1 Levels**: Insulin-like Growth Factor 1 (IGF-1) is a hormone linked to cancer growth. Animal products tend to increase IGF-1 levels, while plant-based diets are associated with lower IGF-1 levels, which can reduce the risk of cancer proliferation.

7. **Detoxification Support**: Plant-based diets support the body's natural detoxification processes, particularly through the liver. Foods like garlic, onions, and cruciferous vegetables enhance the activity of detoxification enzymes, aiding in the elimination of carcinogens.

Bladder cancer is a complex disease influenced by genetic, environmental, and dietary factors. While the consumption of certain animal products has been associated with an increased risk of bladder cancer, a plant-based diet offers numerous protective benefits. The antioxidants, phytochemicals, and fiber in plant-based foods can help prevent the initiation and progression of bladder cancer. Additionally, the anti-inflammatory and detoxifying properties of a plant-based diet can support the body's natural defenses against cancer. By adopting a plant-based diet, individuals may not only reduce their risk of developing bladder cancer but also support the reversal of the disease.

Brain Cancer

Brain cancer, one of the most complex and challenging forms of cancer, arises when abnormal cells grow uncontrollably in the brain or the surrounding tissues. The intricate nature of the brain, with its delicate balance of neurons, glial cells, and other critical components, makes brain cancer a particularly formidable disease. This report delves into the function, production, and regulation of brain cancer, providing an in-depth analysis of the pathways involved in its development, the impact of animal products as potential causes, and the role of a plant-based diet in reversing this condition.

Function of Brain Cancer

Brain cancer disrupts the normal function of the brain by invading and destroying healthy brain tissue. The brain is the control center for the body, responsible for managing vital functions such as movement, sensation, memory, emotion, and cognition. Brain tumors, whether malignant or benign, can interfere with these functions depending on their location, size, and growth rate.

Malignant brain tumors, or brain cancer, are particularly aggressive because they tend to infiltrate surrounding brain tissue, making complete surgical removal difficult. These tumors can increase intracranial pressure, leading to symptoms like headaches, nausea, vomiting, and changes in mental status. Depending on the location of the tumor, patients may experience neurological deficits such as weakness, loss of vision, speech difficulties, and seizures.

The primary goal of brain cancer treatment is to remove or reduce the tumor's size to alleviate symptoms and improve the patient's quality of life. However, due to the brain's complexity, achieving this goal while preserving neurological function is a significant challenge.

Production of Brain Cancer

The production of brain cancer involves a series of genetic mutations and alterations in cellular pathways that lead to uncontrolled cell growth. Brain tumors can originate from various types of cells in the brain, including neurons, glial cells, and the meninges (the protective membranes surrounding the brain).

Genetic Mutations

Brain cancer often begins with genetic mutations in the DNA of brain cells. These mutations can occur spontaneously or be inherited. Key genes involved in the regulation of cell growth and division, such as tumor suppressor genes and oncogenes, may be affected by these mutations.

1. **Tumor Suppressor Genes**: These genes normally act as brakes on cell growth, ensuring that cells do not divide uncontrollably. Mutations in tumor suppressor genes, such as TP53, can lead to a loss of function, allowing cells to proliferate unchecked.
2. **Oncogenes**: Oncogenes are genes that promote cell growth and division. Mutations or overexpression of oncogenes, such as EGFR (epidermal growth factor receptor), can drive the uncontrolled growth of cells, contributing to tumor formation.

Cellular Pathways

Several key cellular pathways are implicated in the production of brain cancer. These pathways are responsible for regulating cell growth, division, and survival. Dysregulation of these pathways due to genetic mutations can lead to the development of brain tumors.

1. **PI3K/AKT/mTOR Pathway**: This pathway is crucial for cell growth and survival. Mutations in components of this pathway, such as PTEN (a tumor suppressor gene), can lead to its hyperactivation, promoting tumor growth.
2. **RAS/RAF/MEK/ERK Pathway**: This pathway is involved in cell proliferation and differentiation. Mutations in genes like

BRAF can activate this pathway, leading to uncontrolled cell growth.

3. **p53 Pathway**: The p53 protein is a critical regulator of the cell cycle and apoptosis (programmed cell death). Mutations in the TP53 gene can impair the function of p53, allowing cells with damaged DNA to survive and proliferate, leading to tumor formation.

4. **Wnt/β-catenin Pathway**: This pathway plays a role in cell proliferation and differentiation. Aberrant activation of the Wnt/β-catenin pathway has been implicated in various cancers, including brain cancer.

Regulation of Brain Cancer

The regulation of brain cancer involves complex interactions between genetic, epigenetic, and environmental factors. Understanding these regulatory mechanisms is essential for developing effective treatments.

Genetic Regulation

Genetic regulation of brain cancer involves the activation or suppression of specific genes that control cell growth, division, and survival. Mutations in these genes can disrupt normal regulatory processes, leading to tumor formation.

1. **Epigenetic Modifications**: Epigenetic changes, such as DNA methylation and histone modification, can alter gene expression without changing the DNA sequence. These modifications can silence tumor suppressor genes or activate oncogenes, contributing to brain cancer development.

2. **MicroRNAs (miRNAs)**: miRNAs are small non-coding RNAs that regulate gene expression by binding to messenger RNAs (mRNAs) and inhibiting their translation. Dysregulation of miRNAs has been implicated in brain cancer, as they can influ-

ence the expression of genes involved in cell proliferation and apoptosis.

Environmental Regulation

Environmental factors, such as exposure to radiation, chemicals, and certain dietary components, can influence the risk of developing brain cancer. These factors can cause DNA damage, leading to mutations that contribute to tumor formation.

1. **Radiation Exposure**: High doses of ionizing radiation, such as those used in radiation therapy, are a known risk factor for brain cancer. Radiation can cause DNA damage and increase the likelihood of mutations in brain cells.
2. **Chemical Exposure**: Certain chemicals, such as vinyl chloride and formaldehyde, have been linked to an increased risk of brain cancer. These chemicals can cause DNA damage and promote the development of tumors.
3. **Dietary Factors**: Diet can play a role in regulating the risk of brain cancer. For example, diets high in animal products have been associated with an increased risk of certain cancers, including brain cancer. Conversely, plant-based diets rich in antioxidants and anti-inflammatory compounds may help protect against brain cancer.

Detailed Pathways Involved in Brain Cancer

The development and progression of brain cancer involve multiple cellular pathways. Understanding these pathways is crucial for identifying potential targets for treatment and prevention.

PI3K/AKT/mTOR Pathway

The PI3K/AKT/mTOR pathway is one of the most commonly dysregulated pathways in brain cancer. This pathway is responsible for regulating cell growth, survival, and metabolism.

1. **Activation of PI3K**: Phosphoinositide 3-kinase (PI3K) is activated by growth factors and other signals. Once activated, PI3K generates phosphatidylinositol-3,4,5-trisphosphate (PIP3), which recruits and activates AKT.
2. **AKT Activation**: AKT is a serine/threonine kinase that promotes cell survival and growth. Activated AKT phosphorylates and inactivates several downstream targets, including the tumor suppressor protein p53.
3. **mTOR Activation**: The mammalian target of rapamycin (mTOR) is a key regulator of cell growth and metabolism. mTOR is activated by AKT and promotes protein synthesis, cell growth, and survival.
4. **Dysregulation in Brain Cancer**: In brain cancer, mutations in genes such as PTEN (a negative regulator of the PI3K/AKT/ mTOR pathway) can lead to hyperactivation of this pathway, promoting tumor growth and resistance to apoptosis.

RAS/RAF/MEK/ERK Pathway

The RAS/RAF/MEK/ERK pathway, also known as the MAPK pathway, is another critical pathway involved in brain cancer. This pathway regulates cell proliferation, differentiation, and survival.

1. **Activation of RAS**: RAS is a small GTPase that is activated by growth factors and other signals. Once activated, RAS recruits and activates RAF, a serine/threonine kinase.
2. **RAF Activation**: Activated RAF phosphorylates and activates MEK, which in turn phosphorylates and activates ERK.
3. **ERK Activation**: ERK is a kinase that translocates to the nucleus and regulates the expression of genes involved in cell proliferation and survival.
4. **Dysregulation in Brain Cancer**: Mutations in genes such as BRAF can lead to constitutive activation of the RAS/RAF/

MEK/ERK pathway, driving uncontrolled cell growth and tumor formation.

p53 Pathway

The p53 pathway is a critical regulator of the cell cycle and apoptosis. p53 is often referred to as the "guardian of the genome" due to its role in preventing the proliferation of cells with damaged DNA.

1. **Activation of p53**: In response to DNA damage or other stress signals, p53 is activated and functions as a transcription factor. p53 induces the expression of genes involved in cell cycle arrest, DNA repair, and apoptosis.
2. **Induction of Apoptosis**: If the damage is irreparable, p53 triggers apoptosis to eliminate the damaged cell. This prevents the propagation of potentially cancerous cells.
3. **Dysregulation in Brain Cancer**: Mutations in the TP53 gene are common in brain cancer. These mutations can lead to the loss of p53 function, allowing cells with damaged DNA to survive and proliferate, contributing to tumor formation.

Wnt/β-catenin Pathway

The Wnt/β-catenin pathway plays a role in cell proliferation, differentiation, and migration. Dysregulation of this pathway has been implicated in the development of various cancers, including brain cancer.

1. **Activation of Wnt Signaling**: Wnt proteins bind to Frizzled receptors on the cell surface, leading to the stabilization and accumulation of β-catenin in the cytoplasm.
2. **β-catenin Translocation**: β-catenin translocates to the nucleus, where it acts as a transcriptional co-activator for target genes involved in cell proliferation and survival.

3. **Dysregulation in Brain Cancer**: Aberrant activation of the Wnt/β-catenin pathway can lead to uncontrolled cell proliferation and tumor growth.

Known Causes Related to Animal Products

Dietary factors, particularly the consumption of animal products, have been associated with an increased risk of various cancers, including brain cancer. Several mechanisms may explain this association.

High Saturated Fat and Cholesterol

Animal products are often high in saturated fat and cholesterol, which have been linked to an increased risk of cancer. High levels of saturated fat and cholesterol can promote inflammation and oxidative stress, both of which contribute to cancer development.

1. **Inflammation**: Saturated fats can induce chronic inflammation by activating pro-inflammatory pathways, such as the NF-κB pathway. Chronic inflammation can create a microenvironment that supports tumor growth and progression.
2. **Oxidative Stress**: High levels of cholesterol can lead to the generation of reactive oxygen species (ROS), which can cause DNA damage and promote mutations that contribute to cancer.

Heme Iron

Heme iron, found in red meat and other animal products, has been implicated in the development of cancer. Heme iron can catalyze the formation of free radicals, leading to oxidative stress and DNA damage.

1. **Oxidative Stress**: Heme iron can promote the formation of ROS, which can damage DNA, proteins, and lipids, contributing to cancer development.
2. **N-nitroso Compounds (NOCs)**: Heme iron can also catalyze the formation of NOCs, which are potent carcinogens. NOCs

can induce mutations in DNA, promoting the development of cancer.

Hormones and Growth Factors

Animal products, particularly dairy products and meat, can contain hormones and growth factors that may promote cancer development.

1. **Insulin-like Growth Factor-1 (IGF-1)**: IGF-1 is a hormone that promotes cell growth and proliferation. Elevated levels of IGF-1, which can result from the consumption of animal products, have been linked to an increased risk of cancer.
2. **Estrogens**: Dairy products can contain estrogens, which are hormones that can promote the growth of hormone-sensitive tumors, such as certain types of brain cancer.

How a Plant-Based Diet Can Help with Reversal

A plant-based diet, rich in fruits, vegetables, whole grains, legumes, nuts, and seeds, offers numerous benefits for preventing and potentially reversing brain cancer. This diet is naturally low in harmful components found in animal products and high in beneficial compounds that protect against cancer.

Antioxidants

Plant-based foods are rich in antioxidants, such as vitamins C and E, beta-carotene, and flavonoids, which help neutralize free radicals and protect cells from oxidative stress.

1. **Neutralization of ROS**: Antioxidants in plant foods can neutralize ROS, reducing DNA damage and the risk of mutations that lead to cancer.
2. **DNA Repair**: Some antioxidants, such as vitamin C, play a role in DNA repair processes, helping to maintain the integrity of the genome and prevent cancer development.

Anti-Inflammatory Compounds

A plant-based diet is rich in anti-inflammatory compounds, such as omega-3 fatty acids, polyphenols, and phytochemicals, which can help reduce chronic inflammation.

1. **Reduction of Inflammation**: Anti-inflammatory compounds in plant foods can inhibit pro-inflammatory pathways, such as NF-κB, reducing the risk of tumor development and progression.
2. **Modulation of Immune Response**: A diet rich in anti-inflammatory foods can support a healthy immune response, enhancing the body's ability to recognize and eliminate cancer cells.

Fiber

Dietary fiber, abundant in plant-based foods, plays a crucial role in maintaining gut health and reducing the risk of cancer.

1. **Gut Microbiota Modulation**: Fiber supports the growth of beneficial gut bacteria, which produce short-chain fatty acids (SCFAs) with anti-inflammatory and anti-cancer properties.
2. **Estrogen Metabolism**: Fiber can bind to estrogens in the digestive tract, reducing their reabsorption and lowering the risk of hormone-sensitive cancers, including certain types of brain cancer.

Phytochemicals

Phytochemicals are bioactive compounds found in plants that have been shown to have anti-cancer properties.

1. **Apoptosis Induction**: Phytochemicals such as sulforaphane (found in cruciferous vegetables) can induce apoptosis in cancer cells, helping to eliminate them from the body.

2. **Cell Cycle Regulation**: Some phytochemicals, such as curcumin (found in turmeric), can modulate the cell cycle, preventing the uncontrolled proliferation of cancer cells.

3. **Inhibition of Angiogenesis**: Certain phytochemicals, such as resveratrol (found in grapes), can inhibit angiogenesis, the process by which tumors develop their own blood supply, thereby limiting tumor growth.

Brain cancer is a complex and challenging disease, characterized by the uncontrolled growth of abnormal cells in the brain. Its development involves a series of genetic mutations and dysregulated cellular pathways, influenced by both genetic and environmental factors. Dietary factors, particularly the consumption of animal products, have been associated with an increased risk of brain cancer due to their potential to promote inflammation, oxidative stress, and hormonal imbalances.

Conversely, a plant-based diet offers numerous protective benefits against brain cancer. Rich in antioxidants, anti-inflammatory compounds, fiber, and phytochemicals, a plant-based diet can help reduce the risk of cancer development and potentially aid in the reversal of the disease by promoting apoptosis, regulating the cell cycle, and inhibiting tumor growth.

Breast Cancer

Breast cancer is one of the most common cancers worldwide, affecting millions of women and a smaller percentage of men. This malignancy arises from the cells of the breast, particularly the milk ducts or lobules, and can spread to other parts of the body if not diagnosed and treated early. The development and progression of breast cancer involve complex interactions between genetic, hormonal, and environmental factors.

The Function of Breast Cancer Cells

Breast cancer cells, like all cancer cells, are characterized by uncontrolled growth and the ability to invade surrounding tissues. Unlike normal cells, which grow, divide, and die in an orderly manner, cancer cells continue to divide without the normal regulatory mechanisms, leading to the formation of tumors. The primary function of these cancerous cells is to proliferate and survive, often at the expense of the host's health.

The abnormal behavior of breast cancer cells is driven by mutations in genes that regulate cell growth and division, such as oncogenes and tumor suppressor genes. Oncogenes, when mutated, can cause cells to grow uncontrollably, while mutations in tumor suppressor genes can lead to a loss of control over cell division. For example, mutations in the BRCA1 and BRCA2 genes are well-known risk factors for the development of breast cancer, as these genes normally help repair DNA damage and prevent abnormal cell growth.

The Production of Breast Cancer

The production of breast cancer, also referred to as tumorigenesis or carcinogenesis, involves several stages:

Initiation

The initiation stage begins with genetic mutations in a single cell. These mutations can be caused by various factors, including exposure to carcinogens, radiation, hormonal influences, and inherited genetic predispositions. During initiation, the normal regulatory mechanisms of the cell are disrupted, leading to the potential for uncontrolled growth.

Promotion

In the promotion stage, the initiated cell undergoes clonal expansion. This means that the cell begins to divide and create more cells with the same mutations. Hormones such as estrogen can act as promoters by binding to estrogen receptors on breast cells, stimulating cell division, and increasing the likelihood of further genetic mutations.

Progression

Progression is the stage where the tumor becomes malignant. During this phase, the cancer cells acquire additional mutations that allow them to invade surrounding tissues, metastasize to distant organs, and resist cell death. The tumor may also recruit new blood vessels through angiogenesis, ensuring a continuous supply of nutrients to support its growth.

Metastasis

Metastasis is the spread of cancer cells from the primary tumor to other parts of the body. Breast cancer commonly metastasizes to the bones, liver, lungs, and brain. This process involves the detachment of cancer cells from the primary tumor, their invasion into the bloodstream or lymphatic system, and their colonization of new tissues.

The Regulation of Breast Cancer

The regulation of breast cancer involves a complex network of genetic, hormonal, and environmental factors. Understanding these regulatory mechanisms is essential for developing effective strategies for prevention, diagnosis, and treatment.

Genetic Regulation

Genetic regulation plays a central role in breast cancer development. Mutations in key genes such as BRCA1, BRCA2, TP53, and HER2 are closely associated with an increased risk of breast cancer. These genes are involved in DNA repair, cell cycle control, and apoptosis (programmed cell death).

- **BRCA1 and BRCA2**: These tumor suppressor genes are responsible for repairing damaged DNA. Mutations in these genes can lead to the accumulation of genetic damage and increase the risk of breast and ovarian cancer. Women with BRCA1 or

BRCA2 mutations have a significantly higher lifetime risk of developing breast cancer compared to the general population.

- **TP53**: The TP53 gene encodes the p53 protein, which acts as a guardian of the genome. It plays a critical role in regulating the cell cycle, DNA repair, and apoptosis. Mutations in TP53 are found in a significant proportion of breast cancers and are associated with more aggressive tumors and poor prognosis.
- **HER2**: HER2 (Human Epidermal growth factor Receptor 2) is an oncogene that promotes cell growth and division. Overexpression of HER2 is observed in approximately 20-30% of breast cancers and is associated with a more aggressive disease course.

Hormonal Regulation

Hormones, particularly estrogen and progesterone, play a crucial role in the regulation of breast cancer. Many breast cancers are hormone receptor-positive, meaning they have receptors for estrogen (ER) and/or progesterone (PR) on their surface. These hormones bind to their respective receptors, promoting cell division and tumor growth.

- **Estrogen**: Estrogen is a steroid hormone that regulates the growth and development of breast tissue. It binds to estrogen receptors (ER) in breast cells, activating signaling pathways that promote cell proliferation. Prolonged exposure to estrogen, whether due to early menarche, late menopause, hormone replacement therapy, or obesity, is associated with an increased risk of breast cancer.
- **Progesterone**: Like estrogen, progesterone also influences breast cancer development. Progesterone receptors (PR) are often co-expressed with estrogen receptors in breast cancer cells. The interaction between estrogen and progesterone receptors can modulate the growth of breast cancer cells and their response to hormonal therapies.

- **HER2 Regulation**: HER2 is another critical player in the hormonal regulation of breast cancer. HER2-positive breast cancers are characterized by the overexpression of the HER2 protein, which promotes cell growth and survival.

Environmental and Lifestyle Regulation

Environmental and lifestyle factors also play a significant role in the regulation of breast cancer. Diet, physical activity, alcohol consumption, and exposure to environmental toxins can influence breast cancer risk.

- **Diet**: Diet is a major modifiable risk factor for breast cancer. High-fat diets, particularly those rich in saturated fats and animal products, have been associated with an increased risk of breast cancer. In contrast, a diet rich in fruits, vegetables, whole grains, and plant-based foods is associated with a lower risk.
- **Physical Activity**: Regular physical activity has been shown to reduce the risk of breast cancer by regulating hormone levels, reducing inflammation, and improving immune function. Exercise can also help prevent obesity, which is a known risk factor for breast cancer.
- **Alcohol Consumption**: Alcohol consumption is a well-established risk factor for breast cancer. Alcohol can increase estrogen levels in the body and may also cause DNA damage, leading to the development of cancer. The risk of breast cancer increases with the amount of alcohol consumed.
- **Environmental Toxins**: Exposure to environmental toxins, such as endocrine-disrupting chemicals (EDCs), can interfere with hormone regulation and increase the risk of breast cancer. EDCs are found in various products, including plastics, pesticides, and personal care products.

Detailed Pathways Involved in Breast Cancer

Breast cancer development and progression are governed by several key signaling pathways. Understanding these pathways provides insight into the molecular mechanisms underlying breast cancer and highlights potential therapeutic targets.

Estrogen Receptor (ER) Pathway

The estrogen receptor (ER) pathway is a critical driver of breast cancer, particularly in hormone receptor-positive tumors. Estrogen binds to ERs in breast cells, activating the receptor and leading to the transcription of genes involved in cell proliferation, survival, and differentiation.

- **ER Activation**: Upon binding to estrogen, the ER undergoes a conformational change that allows it to bind to specific DNA sequences known as estrogen response elements (EREs). This binding promotes the transcription of target genes that drive cell proliferation.
- **Co-Regulators**: The activity of ER is modulated by co-regulators, including co-activators and co-repressors. Co-activators enhance ER-mediated gene transcription, while co-repressors inhibit it. The balance between co-activators and co-repressors influences the response of breast cancer cells to estrogen and hormonal therapies.

HER2 Pathway

The HER2 pathway is activated in HER2-positive breast cancers, where the HER2 protein is overexpressed. HER2 is a receptor tyrosine kinase that, when activated, triggers downstream signaling cascades that promote cell proliferation, survival, and migration.

- **HER2 Dimerization**: HER2 can dimerize with itself (homodimerization) or with other members of the HER family (heterodimerization), such as HER3. Dimerization activates the intrinsic kinase activity of HER2, leading to the phosphorylation of tyrosine residues in the intracellular domain.

- **Downstream Signaling**: The activated HER2 receptor initiates multiple downstream signaling pathways, including the PI3K/Akt/mTOR and MAPK/ERK pathways. These pathways promote cell growth, survival, and resistance to apoptosis.

PI3K/Akt/mTOR Pathway

The PI3K/Akt/mTOR pathway is a key regulator of cell growth, survival, and metabolism in breast cancer. This pathway is frequently activated in breast cancer due to mutations in genes such as PIK3CA (which encodes the p110α subunit of PI3K) and PTEN (a tumor suppressor that negatively regulates PI3K).

- **PI3K Activation**: The PI3K enzyme is activated by receptor tyrosine kinases (RTKs), such as HER2, or by G-protein-coupled receptors (GPCRs). Activated PI3K converts PIP2 to PIP3, leading to the recruitment and activation of Akt.
- **Akt Signaling**: Akt is a serine/threonine kinase that promotes cell survival by inhibiting pro-apoptotic proteins and activating survival pathways. Akt also activates mTOR, a key regulator of cell growth and metabolism.

MAPK/ERK Pathway

The MAPK/ERK pathway is another critical signaling pathway involved in breast cancer. This pathway is activated by growth factors, cytokines, and other extracellular signals that bind to receptor tyrosine kinases.

- **MAPK Cascade**: The activation of receptor tyrosine kinases leads to the activation of the MAPK kinase cascade, which involves the sequential phosphorylation and activation of MAP-

KKKs (e.g., Raf), MAPKKs (e.g., MEK), and MAPKs (e.g., ERK).

- **ERK Activation**: Activated ERK translocates to the nucleus, where it phosphorylates and activates transcription factors that regulate the expression of genes involved in cell proliferation, differentiation, and survival.

Known Causes of Breast Cancer Related to Animal Products

There is growing evidence that certain animal products are associated with an increased risk of breast cancer. These associations are thought to be mediated by various mechanisms, including the promotion of inflammation, hormone disruption, and the presence of carcinogenic compounds.

Red and Processed Meats

Red and processed meats have been linked to an increased risk of breast cancer. These meats contain high levels of saturated fats, heme iron, and carcinogens formed during cooking, such as heterocyclic amines (HCAs) and polycyclic aromatic hydrocarbons (PAHs).

- **Saturated Fats**: Diets high in saturated fats, commonly found in red and processed meats, can lead to increased levels of circulating estrogen, which may promote the development of hormone receptor-positive breast cancers.
- **Heme Iron**: Heme iron, found in red meat, can catalyze the formation of reactive oxygen species (ROS), leading to oxidative stress and DNA damage. This oxidative stress may contribute to the initiation and progression of breast cancer.
- **Carcinogens**: Cooking methods that involve high temperatures, such as grilling or frying, can produce HCAs and PAHs, which are known to be mutagenic and carcinogenic. These compounds can damage DNA and promote the development of breast cancer.

Dairy Products

Dairy products have also been implicated in breast cancer risk due to their content of hormones, growth factors, and saturated fats.

- **Hormones and Growth Factors**: Dairy products, especially those derived from pregnant cows, contain hormones such as estrogen and insulin-like growth factor 1 (IGF-1). These hormones can promote cell proliferation and inhibit apoptosis, potentially contributing to breast cancer development.
- **Saturated Fats**: Like red meat, dairy products are high in saturated fats, which can increase estrogen levels and inflammation, both of which are risk factors for breast cancer.
- **Casein Protein**: Casein, the primary protein in milk, has been shown to promote the growth of cancer cells in some studies. The consumption of casein may stimulate the production of IGF-1, further increasing the risk of breast cancer.

Animal Fats and Cholesterol

Animal fats, particularly those high in cholesterol, have been associated with an increased risk of breast cancer. Cholesterol is a precursor for the synthesis of steroid hormones, including estrogen, which can promote the growth of hormone receptor-positive breast cancers.

- **Cholesterol Metabolites**: Cholesterol can be metabolized into 27-hydroxycholesterol (27-HC), a compound that mimics the effects of estrogen and can promote the growth of ER-positive breast cancer cells.
- **Inflammation**: High levels of dietary cholesterol can lead to chronic inflammation, which is a known risk factor for cancer development, including breast cancer.

The Role of a Plant-Based Diet in Breast Cancer Reversal

A plant-based diet, rich in fruits, vegetables, whole grains, legumes, nuts, and seeds, offers numerous benefits for the prevention and reversal of breast cancer. Such a diet is low in saturated fats and free of cholesterol, while being high in fiber, antioxidants, and phytochemicals that can protect against cancer.

Antioxidants and Phytochemicals

Plant-based foods are abundant in antioxidants and phytochemicals, which play a crucial role in neutralizing free radicals, reducing oxidative stress, and preventing DNA damage that can lead to cancer.

- **Flavonoids**: Flavonoids, found in fruits, vegetables, and tea, have been shown to inhibit the growth of breast cancer cells and induce apoptosis. They also have anti-inflammatory and antioxidant properties that can protect against cancer development.
- **Carotenoids**: Carotenoids, such as beta-carotene and lycopene, are pigments found in colorful fruits and vegetables. These compounds have been linked to a reduced risk of breast cancer due to their ability to scavenge free radicals and enhance immune function.
- **Sulforaphane**: Sulforaphane, a compound found in cruciferous vegetables like broccoli and Brussels sprouts, has potent anti-cancer properties. It can inhibit the growth of breast cancer cells by inducing phase II detoxification enzymes, promoting apoptosis, and inhibiting angiogenesis.

Fiber and Gut Health

A plant-based diet is high in dietary fiber, which is beneficial for gut health and may play a role in reducing breast cancer risk.

- **Estrogen Metabolism**: Fiber can bind to estrogen in the digestive tract and promote its excretion, reducing the levels of

circulating estrogen and thereby lowering the risk of hormone receptor-positive breast cancer.

- **Gut Microbiome**: The gut microbiome plays a crucial role in metabolizing and regulating hormones, including estrogen. A diet rich in fiber promotes a healthy gut microbiome, which may help in the prevention and reversal of breast cancer.

Anti-Inflammatory Effects

Chronic inflammation is a key contributor to cancer development. A plant-based diet has strong anti-inflammatory effects, which can help prevent the initiation and progression of breast cancer.

- **Omega-3 Fatty Acids**: While plant-based diets are typically low in omega-6 fatty acids, which can promote inflammation, they are rich in omega-3 fatty acids found in flaxseeds, chia seeds, and walnuts. Omega-3 fatty acids have anti-inflammatory properties and may help protect against breast cancer.
- **Polyphenols**: Polyphenols, found in a variety of plant foods, have anti-inflammatory and antioxidant effects. They can inhibit the production of inflammatory cytokines and reduce the risk of cancer development.

Hormonal Regulation

A plant-based diet can help regulate hormone levels and reduce the risk of hormone-dependent cancers such as breast cancer.

- **Lignans**: Lignans, found in flaxseeds and other plant foods, are phytoestrogens that can modulate estrogen metabolism. They may reduce the risk of breast cancer by binding to estrogen receptors and exerting a weaker estrogenic effect compared to endogenous estrogen.
- **Isoflavones**: Isoflavones, found in soy products, are another class of phytoestrogens. They have been shown to reduce the risk of

breast cancer, particularly in premenopausal women, by modulating estrogen receptors and inhibiting the growth of cancer cells.

Breast cancer is a complex disease influenced by genetic, hormonal, and environmental factors. The pathways involved in its development and progression are intricately regulated, and various risk factors, including the consumption of animal products, can contribute to its onset. However, a plant-based diet offers a powerful strategy for both the prevention and reversal of breast cancer. By providing a rich source of antioxidants, phytochemicals, fiber, and anti-inflammatory compounds, a plant-based diet can reduce the risk of breast cancer and support the body's natural defenses against this malignancy.

Triple Negative Breast Cancer

Triple Negative Breast Cancer (TNBC) is a subtype of breast cancer characterized by the absence of three common receptors known to fuel most breast cancers: estrogen receptors (ER), progesterone receptors (PR), and human epidermal growth factor receptor 2 (HER2). This absence makes TNBC more challenging to treat compared to other breast cancer types. TNBC accounts for about 10-15% of all breast cancers and is more likely to affect younger women, women of African American descent, and those with a BRCA1 gene mutation.

Molecular Pathways Involved in Triple Negative Breast Cancer

1. **PI3K/AKT/mTOR Pathway**
   The phosphatidylinositol 3-kinase (PI3K)/AKT/mammalian target of rapamycin (mTOR) pathway is frequently activated in

TNBC. This pathway plays a critical role in cell growth, survival, and metabolism. Dysregulation of this pathway, often due to mutations or amplification of PIK3CA (the gene encoding the catalytic subunit of PI3K), leads to uncontrolled cell proliferation and survival, contributing to the aggressive nature of TNBC.

2. **EGFR Pathway**

Epidermal growth factor receptor (EGFR) is overexpressed in a significant percentage of TNBC cases. The EGFR pathway is involved in cell proliferation, differentiation, and survival. Overactivation of EGFR can result in increased tumor cell proliferation and resistance to apoptosis (programmed cell death), making it a potential therapeutic target in TNBC.

3. **JAK/STAT Pathway**

The Janus kinase (JAK)/signal transducer and activator of transcription (STAT) pathway is another critical pathway in TNBC. It is involved in promoting cell proliferation and survival, particularly in response to cytokines and growth factors. Aberrant activation of the JAK/STAT pathway has been associated with poor prognosis in TNBC patients.

4. **NOTCH Signaling Pathway**

NOTCH signaling is implicated in cell fate determination, stem cell maintenance, and differentiation. In TNBC, NOTCH signaling is often dysregulated, contributing to the maintenance of cancer stem cells, which are thought to drive tumor recurrence and resistance to conventional therapies.

5. **Wnt/β-Catenin Pathway**

The Wnt/β-catenin pathway is involved in regulating cell proliferation and differentiation. Aberrant activation of this pathway in TNBC leads to increased cell proliferation, invasion, and metastasis. The pathway's role in maintaining cancer stem cells also contributes to the aggressive behavior of TNBC.

6. **Immune Checkpoint Pathways**

TNBC is known to have a higher level of tumor-infiltrating lymphocytes (TILs) compared to other breast cancer subtypes. However, the immune environment in TNBC can be immunosuppressive, often involving the upregulation of immune checkpoint molecules like PD-1/PD-L1. These molecules inhibit the immune system's ability to attack the cancer, making immune checkpoint inhibitors a promising area of research for TNBC treatment.

Known Causes Related to Animal Products

1. **High Saturated Fat Intake**
   Several studies have linked the consumption of animal products, particularly those high in saturated fats, with an increased risk of developing TNBC. Saturated fats, primarily found in red and processed meats, can promote inflammation and oxidative stress, which contribute to cancer development. In particular, high-fat diets have been shown to activate the PI3K/AKT/mTOR pathway, leading to enhanced cell proliferation and survival in TNBC.

2. **Heme Iron**
   Heme iron, found in animal products like red meat, has been associated with an increased risk of breast cancer. Heme iron can catalyze the formation of free radicals, leading to oxidative DNA damage, which is a precursor to cancer development. Additionally, high levels of iron can promote the growth of cancer cells by providing essential nutrients for their rapid proliferation.

3. **Hormones in Dairy Products**
   Dairy products, especially those derived from cows treated with hormones, contain estrogen and other growth factors that may influence breast cancer risk. Even though TNBC is defined by the lack of hormone receptors, exposure to exogenous estrogens and growth factors may still promote cancer development through al-

ternative pathways, such as the IGF (Insulin-like Growth Factor) signaling pathway.

4. **Carcinogenic Compounds in Processed Meats**

   Processed meats, such as bacon, sausages, and hot dogs, contain carcinogenic compounds like N-nitroso compounds and polycyclic aromatic hydrocarbons (PAHs). These compounds can induce mutations in DNA, leading to the initiation and progression of cancer. TNBC, which lacks effective receptor-targeted therapies, might be particularly susceptible to the mutagenic effects of these compounds.

5. **High Protein Diets**

   Diets high in animal proteins, particularly from red and processed meats, have been linked to an increased risk of cancer, including TNBC. High protein intake can lead to increased levels of insulin-like growth factor 1 (IGF-1), which promotes cell proliferation and inhibits apoptosis. The IGF-1 pathway is known to be involved in the development and progression of various cancers, including TNBC.

Reversing TNBC Through a Plant-Based Diet

1. **Rich in Antioxidants**

   A plant-based diet is naturally rich in antioxidants, which help neutralize free radicals and reduce oxidative stress, a key contributor to cancer development. Foods such as berries, leafy greens, and nuts are high in antioxidants like vitamin C, vitamin E, and polyphenols, which have been shown to inhibit the growth of cancer cells and promote apoptosis.

2. **Low in Saturated Fats**

   Plant-based diets are typically low in saturated fats, which can reduce the risk of cancer progression. Replacing animal fats with healthy plant-based fats from sources like avocados, nuts, and seeds can help decrease inflammation and improve overall metabolic health, which is beneficial for preventing and managing TNBC.

3. **Rich in Phytochemicals**

   Phytochemicals are bioactive compounds found in plants that have been shown to have anti-cancer properties. Cruciferous vegetables like broccoli, cauliflower, and Brussels sprouts contain sulforaphane, a compound that can inhibit the growth of cancer cells and enhance detoxification pathways. Similarly, soy products contain isoflavones, which have been shown to reduce the risk of breast cancer recurrence.

4. **High in Fiber**

   A plant-based diet is high in dietary fiber, which has been associated with a reduced risk of breast cancer. Fiber helps regulate hormone levels, including estrogen, by promoting the excretion of excess hormones through the digestive tract. This is particularly important in reducing the risk of hormone-related cancers, but it also benefits overall gut health and immune function, which are crucial in managing TNBC.

5. **Anti-inflammatory Properties**

   Chronic inflammation is a known contributor to cancer development and progression. A plant-based diet, rich in fruits, vegetables, whole grains, and legumes, has potent anti-inflammatory effects. Foods like turmeric, ginger, and garlic contain anti-inflammatory compounds that can help reduce the inflammation associated with cancer progression.

6. **Modulation of Immune Function**

   The immune system plays a critical role in recognizing and destroying cancer cells. A plant-based diet can enhance immune function by providing essential vitamins, minerals, and phytonutrients that support the body's natural defense mechanisms. For example, mushrooms contain beta-glucans, which have been shown to modulate the immune system and enhance its ability to target and destroy cancer cells.

7. **Reduction in IGF-1 Levels**

Plant-based diets are typically lower in protein, particularly animal protein, which leads to lower levels of IGF-1. As mentioned earlier, high levels of IGF-1 are associated with increased cancer risk. By reducing IGF-1 levels, a plant-based diet can help slow the progression of TNBC and reduce the risk of recurrence.

8. **Detoxification Support**

Many plant-based foods support the body's natural detoxification processes. For example, cruciferous vegetables are known to enhance the activity of detoxification enzymes in the liver, which help to remove carcinogens from the body. This can be particularly beneficial for individuals with TNBC, as it reduces the overall toxic burden on the body and helps prevent cancer progression.

Triple Negative Breast Cancer is a complex and aggressive subtype of breast cancer that lacks the common receptors targeted by many therapies. The molecular pathways involved in TNBC, such as the PI3K/AKT/mTOR, EGFR, JAK/STAT, NOTCH, and Wnt/β-catenin pathways, contribute to its aggressive nature and poor prognosis. However, lifestyle factors, particularly diet, play a crucial role in both the development and management of TNBC.

The consumption of animal products, particularly those high in saturated fats, heme iron, and carcinogenic compounds, has been linked to an increased risk of TNBC. In contrast, a plant-based diet offers numerous benefits, including reduced inflammation, enhanced immune function, and improved detoxification, all of which contribute to a reduced risk of cancer progression and recurrence.

By adopting a plant-based diet, individuals with TNBC can potentially improve their prognosis and overall health outcomes. The anti-cancer properties of plant-based foods, coupled with their ability to modulate key pathways involved in cancer development, make this dietary approach a promising strategy for the prevention and management of Triple Negative Breast Cancer.

Cervical Cancer

Cervical cancer is one of the most common cancers affecting women globally, particularly in low- and middle-income countries. It originates in the cervix, the lower part of the uterus that connects to the vagina. Despite advancements in screening, cervical cancer remains a significant health issue due to its complex etiology and the involvement of multiple risk factors, including viral infections, genetic predisposition, and lifestyle choices.

Function of Cervical Cancer

Cervical cancer primarily arises from the epithelial cells of the cervix. It can be classified into two main types:

- **Squamous cell carcinoma**: The most common form, originating from the squamous cells lining the outer part of the cervix.
- **Adenocarcinoma**: Arising from the glandular cells of the cervix, which produce mucus.

Cervical cancer progresses slowly over time, beginning with pre-cancerous changes, known as cervical intraepithelial neoplasia (CIN) or dysplasia. These changes can be detected through regular Pap smear tests and treated before they develop into invasive cancer.

Immune Response and Cancer Development

The immune system plays a crucial role in the regulation of cervical cancer. Typically, the body can clear infections within a few months. However, in some cases, the virus persists and integrates its DNA into the host cells, leading to uncontrolled cell proliferation and, eventually, cancer. Factors such as immune suppression, chronic inflammation, and genetic susceptibility can hinder the immune system's ability to eliminate the virus, allowing cancer to develop.

Production of Cervical Cancer
1. Cellular Transformation

The production of cervical cancer involves a series of cellular transformations driven by cellular machinery.

2. Dysregulation of Cellular Pathways

The inactivation of p53 and Rb disrupts normal cell cycle control, leading to the accumulation of DNA damage and the eventual transformation of normal cervical cells into malignant cells. This dysregulation also promotes angiogenesis (the formation of new blood vessels) and metastasis (the spread of cancer to other parts of the body).

3. Progression to Invasive Cancer

The progression from pre-cancerous lesions to invasive cervical cancer is a multi-step process. It often takes several years or even decades for these changes to occur. The rate of progression can be influenced by various factors, smoking, co-infection with other sexually transmitted infections, and hormonal influences such as long-term use of oral contraceptives.

Regulation of Cervical Cancer
1. Genetic and Epigenetic Regulation

The regulation of cervical cancer involves both genetic and epigenetic mechanisms. Genetic mutations in oncogenes (genes that promote cancer) and tumor suppressor genes (genes that prevent cancer) play a pivotal role in cancer development. Epigenetic changes, such as DNA methylation and histone modification, also contribute to the silencing of tumor suppressor genes and the activation of oncogenes.

2. Role of the Microenvironment

The tumor microenvironment, which includes immune cells, blood vessels, and extracellular matrix, plays a significant role in the regulation of cervical cancer. Chronic inflammation within the cervix creates a favorable environment for cancer development. Cytokines and growth factors released by immune cells can promote tumor growth and invasion.

3. Hormonal Influences

Hormonal factors, particularly estrogen, can influence the regulation of cervical cancer. Estrogen receptors are present in cervical cells, and estrogen exposure has been linked to an increased risk of cervical cancer.

Detailed Pathways in Cervical Cancer Development

1. P53 Inactivation

P53 is a critical tumor suppressor that regulates cell cycle arrest and apoptosis in response to DNA damage. The inactivation of p53 allows cells with damaged DNA to continue dividing, leading to the accumulation of mutations and the development of cancer.

2. Rb Pathway Disruption

Rb normally controls the transition from the G1 phase to the S phase of the cell cycle by inhibiting the activity of E2F transcription factors.

3. Angiogenesis and Metastasis

As cervical cancer progresses, it acquires the ability to promote angiogenesis through the secretion of vascular endothelial growth factor (VEGF) and other pro-angiogenic factors. The formation of new blood vessels provides the growing tumor with nutrients and oxygen, facilitating its growth and the potential for metastasis. Cancer cells can invade surrounding tissues and spread to distant organs through the lymphatic system or bloodstream.

Known Causes Related to Animal Products
1. High Consumption of Animal Fats
Several studies have suggested a link between the consumption of animal fats and an increased risk of cervical cancer. Animal fats are rich in saturated fats, which can promote chronic inflammation and oxidative stress, both of which are risk factors for cancer. Additionally, animal products, particularly red and processed meats, have been associated with the production of carcinogenic compounds, such as heterocyclic amines and polycyclic aromatic hydrocarbons, during cooking.

2. Dairy Products and Hormonal Influence
Dairy products contain hormones such as estrogen and insulin-like growth factor 1 (IGF-1), which have been implicated in the development of hormone-related cancers, including cervical cancer. Estrogen can promote the growth of estrogen receptor-positive cervical cells, while IGF-1 can stimulate cell proliferation and inhibit apoptosis.

3. Processed Meats and Nitrosamines
Processed meats, such as sausages, bacon, and hot dogs, often contain nitrites and nitrates as preservatives. These compounds can be converted into nitrosamines, which are potent carcinogens. Nitrosamines have been shown to induce DNA mutations and promote the development of various cancers, including cervical cancer.

The Role of a Plant-Based Diet in Reversing Cervical Cancer
1. Antioxidant-Rich Foods and DNA Protection
A plant-based diet rich in fruits, vegetables, and whole grains provides an abundance of antioxidants, such as vitamins C and E, carotenoids, and polyphenols. These antioxidants protect cells from ox-

idative damage by neutralizing free radicals, thereby reducing the risk of DNA mutations that can lead to cancer. Foods like berries, leafy greens, and cruciferous vegetables are particularly high in these protective compounds.

2. Anti-Inflammatory Effects of Plant Foods

Chronic inflammation is a known risk factor for cancer development, including cervical cancer. A plant-based diet, particularly one high in anti-inflammatory foods like turmeric, ginger, flaxseeds, and walnuts, can help reduce inflammation in the body. The omega-3 fatty acids found in flaxseeds and walnuts are particularly effective in modulating inflammatory pathways.

3. Fiber and Gut Health

Dietary fiber, abundant in plant-based foods, plays a crucial role in maintaining gut health and regulating the immune system. Fiber promotes a healthy gut microbiome, which is essential for immune function and the prevention of chronic inflammation. A healthy gut can also enhance the body's ability to clear infections, reducing the risk of cervical cancer development.

4. Phytochemicals and Cancer Cell Inhibition

Phytochemicals, which are naturally occurring compounds found in plants, have been shown to inhibit cancer cell growth and induce apoptosis in cancer cells. For example, sulforaphane, found in cruciferous vegetables like broccoli and Brussels sprouts, has potent anti-cancer properties. Curcumin, the active compound in turmeric, has also been shown to inhibit the growth of cervical cancer cells and enhance the effectiveness of conventional treatments.

5. Immune System Support

A plant-based diet supports the immune system by providing essential vitamins and minerals, such as vitamin C, vitamin E, zinc, and selenium. These nutrients are vital for the proper functioning of immune cells and the body's ability to fight infections. A strong immune system is crucial for preventing the progression of cervical dysplasia to invasive cancer.

6. Hormonal Balance through Plant-Based Foods

Phytoestrogens, found in foods like soy, flaxseeds, and legumes, can help balance hormone levels in the body. Unlike the estrogen found in animal products, phytoestrogens have a weaker effect and can compete with endogenous estrogen for receptor binding, potentially reducing the risk of hormone-driven cancers like cervical cancer.

7. Detoxification Pathways and Cancer Prevention

A plant-based diet supports the body's natural detoxification processes, particularly in the liver, where harmful toxins and carcinogens are metabolized and excreted. Cruciferous vegetables, such as broccoli, cauliflower, and kale, contain compounds that activate detoxification enzymes, helping to eliminate potential cancer-causing agents from the body.

8. Reducing Exposure to Carcinogens

By eliminating or reducing the intake of animal products, individuals can lower their exposure to dietary carcinogens, such as nitrosamines, heterocyclic amines, and polycyclic aromatic hydrocarbons. A plant-based diet minimizes the consumption of these harmful compounds and reduces the overall carcinogenic burden on the body.

9. Weight Management and Cancer Risk

Obesity is a known risk factor for many cancers, including cervical cancer. A plant-based diet, which is typically lower in calories and higher in fiber, can help with weight management and reduce the risk of obesity-related cancers. Maintaining a healthy weight is crucial for hormone balance and reducing the risk of cancer recurrence.

10. Enhancing the Effectiveness of Conventional Treatments

Research suggests that a plant-based diet may enhance the effectiveness of conventional cancer treatments, such as chemotherapy and radiation. The anti-inflammatory and antioxidant properties of plant foods can help reduce treatment-related side effects and improve overall outcomes. For example, curcumin has been shown to sensitize cancer cells to chemotherapy, making them more susceptible to treatment.

Cervical cancer is a complex disease with a multifaceted etiology involving genetic, environmental, and lifestyle factors. The interplay between immune system regulation, and lifestyle choices, particularly diet, plays a crucial role in the development and progression of cervical cancer. While animal products, particularly those high in saturated fats, hormones, and carcinogens, have been linked to an increased risk of cervical cancer, a plant-based diet offers a protective and potentially therapeutic effect.

By providing a rich source of antioxidants, anti-inflammatory compounds, fiber, and phytochemicals, a plant-based diet can support the body's natural defenses against cancer, promote hormonal balance, and enhance the effectiveness of conventional treatments. The evidence suggests that adopting a plant-based diet may not only reduce the risk of developing cervical cancer but also aid in the reversal of pre-cancerous lesions and improve outcomes for those diagnosed with the disease.

Colon Cancer

Colon cancer, also known as colorectal cancer, is a malignant tumor arising from the inner lining of the colon or rectum. It is one of the most common types of cancer globally, with significant morbidity and mortality rates. Understanding the function, production, and regulation of colon cancer is essential for devising preventive strategies and effective treatments. This report explores the intricate pathways involved in colon cancer development, the known causes linked to animal products, and how a plant-based diet can aid in its reversal.

Function of Colon Cancer

Colon cancer originates from the epithelial cells lining the colon, which undergo a series of mutations leading to uncontrolled cell growth and tumor formation. The colon's primary function is to absorb water and nutrients from food, forming and storing feces for excretion. When cancer develops, it disrupts these functions, leading to symptoms such as altered bowel habits, abdominal pain, and rectal bleeding.

The progression of colon cancer involves multiple stages:

1. **Hyperplasia**: This initial stage involves the abnormal proliferation of cells in the colon lining, forming benign polyps.
2. **Adenoma Formation**: Some polyps develop into adenomas, which are precancerous growths.
3. **Carcinoma in situ**: Adenomas can further progress to carcinoma in situ, where cancerous cells remain confined within the colon lining.
4. **Invasive Carcinoma**: At this stage, cancer cells invade deeper layers of the colon wall and can spread to nearby lymph nodes and distant organs (metastasis).

Production of Colon Cancer

The production of colon cancer is a complex process involving genetic, environmental, and lifestyle factors. The key steps in colon cancer production include:

1. **Genetic Mutations**: Colon cancer often arises from genetic mutations in specific genes that regulate cell growth and apoptosis (programmed cell death). The most common mutations occur in the APC gene, which controls the Wnt signaling pathway, crucial for cell proliferation and differentiation. Other genes frequently mutated include KRAS, TP53, and SMAD4.

2. **Epigenetic Changes**: In addition to genetic mutations, epigenetic changes, such as DNA methylation and histone modification, can silence tumor suppressor genes, leading to unchecked cell growth.

3. **Inflammation**: Chronic inflammation in the colon, often due to conditions like inflammatory bowel disease (IBD), can promote cancer development. Inflammatory cytokines and reactive oxygen species (ROS) can cause DNA damage and stimulate tumor growth.

4. **Dietary Factors**: Diet plays a crucial role in colon cancer production. Diets high in red and processed meats, animal fats, and low in fiber are associated with an increased risk of colon cancer. These foods can lead to the production of carcinogenic compounds, such as N-nitroso compounds and heterocyclic amines, which can damage the colon lining and initiate cancerous changes.

5. **Gut Microbiota**: The gut microbiota, consisting of trillions of microorganisms, also influences colon cancer production. Dysbiosis, or an imbalance in gut bacteria, can promote inflammation, alter bile acid metabolism, and produce metabolites that induce carcinogenesis.

Regulation of Colon Cancer

The regulation of colon cancer involves a complex interplay of genetic, molecular, and environmental factors. Key regulatory pathways include:

1. **Wnt/β-catenin Pathway**: This pathway is critical for regulating cell proliferation and differentiation in the colon. Mutations in the APC gene lead to the activation of the Wnt pathway, resulting in the accumulation of β-catenin in the nucleus, where it drives

the expression of genes promoting cell growth and survival. This pathway is frequently dysregulated in colon cancer.

2. **p53 Pathway**: The p53 tumor suppressor protein plays a crucial role in regulating the cell cycle and apoptosis. Mutations in the TP53 gene, which encodes p53, are common in colon cancer. Loss of p53 function allows cells with damaged DNA to evade apoptosis, leading to tumor progression.

3. **TGF-β Pathway**: The TGF-β signaling pathway is involved in regulating cell proliferation, differentiation, and immune response. In colon cancer, mutations in genes like SMAD4 disrupt this pathway, promoting tumor growth and metastasis.

4. **EGFR Pathway**: The epidermal growth factor receptor (EGFR) pathway is involved in regulating cell growth and survival. Overexpression of EGFR and mutations in downstream effectors like KRAS are common in colon cancer, leading to uncontrolled cell proliferation.

5. **MicroRNAs**: MicroRNAs (miRNAs) are small non-coding RNAs that regulate gene expression post-transcriptionally. Dysregulation of miRNAs has been implicated in colon cancer, where they can act as oncogenes or tumor suppressors by targeting key regulatory genes.

Detailed Pathways Involved in Colon Cancer

The development of colon cancer involves several intricate pathways, each contributing to different aspects of tumor initiation, progression, and metastasis. Some of the most significant pathways include:

1. **Wnt/β-catenin Pathway**:
   - **Initiation**: Mutations in the APC gene lead to the activation of the Wnt pathway, allowing β-catenin to accumulate in the nucleus.

- **Progression**: β-catenin forms a complex with TCF/LEF transcription factors, driving the expression of genes like MYC and CCND1, which promote cell proliferation.
- **Metastasis**: Dysregulation of the Wnt pathway can also enhance cell motility and invasiveness, contributing to metastasis.

2. **PI3K/AKT/mTOR Pathway**:
   - **Initiation**: Activation of the PI3K/AKT pathway occurs through mutations in PIK3CA or loss of PTEN, leading to increased cell survival and growth.
   - **Progression**: The AKT protein activates the mTOR pathway, promoting protein synthesis and cell proliferation.
   - **Metastasis**: This pathway also regulates cell metabolism and angiogenesis, facilitating tumor growth and metastasis.

3. **p53 Pathway**:
   - **Initiation**: Mutations in TP53 lead to the loss of p53 function, allowing cells with DNA damage to survive and proliferate.
   - **Progression**: Loss of p53 also impairs the cell's ability to respond to stress signals, leading to unchecked cell growth.
   - **Metastasis**: The dysregulation of p53 can enhance the ability of cancer cells to invade surrounding tissues and spread to distant organs.

4. **TGF-β Pathway**:
   - **Initiation**: Mutations in SMAD4 or other components of the TGF-β pathway disrupt its tumor-suppressive effects, allowing cells to proliferate.
   - **Progression**: The loss of TGF-β signaling promotes epithelial-mesenchymal transition (EMT), a process by which cancer cells gain migratory and invasive properties.
   - **Metastasis**: EMT is a key step in metastasis, enabling cancer cells to break away from the primary tumor and colonize distant organs.

5. **Mismatch Repair (MMR) Pathway**:
- **Initiation**: Defects in the MMR pathway, often due to mutations in genes like MLH1, MSH2, and MSH6, lead to microsatellite instability (MSI), a hallmark of certain types of colon cancer.
- **Progression**: MSI results in the accumulation of mutations in other genes, driving tumor progression.
- **Metastasis**: Tumors with MSI may have different metastatic behaviors and responses to treatment compared to microsatellite-stable tumors.

Known Causes of Colon Cancer Linked to Animal Products

Numerous studies have established a strong link between the consumption of animal products and an increased risk of colon cancer. Some of the key factors include:

1. **Red and Processed Meats**:
- **Carcinogens**: Red and processed meats are known to contain carcinogenic compounds, such as heterocyclic amines (HCAs) and polycyclic aromatic hydrocarbons (PAHs), which form during cooking at high temperatures. These compounds can damage the DNA in colon cells, initiating carcinogenesis.
- **N-nitroso Compounds**: Processed meats often contain nitrates and nitrites, which can form N-nitroso compounds (NOCs) in the gut. NOCs are potent carcinogens that can induce DNA mutations and promote tumor growth.
- **Saturated Fats**: High intake of saturated fats from animal products can lead to the production of secondary bile acids in the colon, which have been shown to have carcinogenic effects.

2. **Dairy Products**:
   - **Growth Factors**: Dairy products contain insulin-like growth factor 1 (IGF-1), a hormone that can promote cell proliferation and inhibit apoptosis. Elevated levels of IGF-1 have been linked to an increased risk of colon cancer.
   - **Calcium**: While calcium is essential for health, excessive intake from dairy products may have a dual effect. While it may protect against colorectal cancer by binding to secondary bile acids and free fatty acids, high calcium levels can also inhibit the absorption of other beneficial nutrients, potentially increasing cancer risk.

3. **Eggs**:
   - **Choline and TMAO**: Eggs are rich in choline, which is metabolized by gut bacteria into trimethylamine-N-oxide (TMAO). High levels of TMAO have been associated with an increased risk of colon cancer, possibly due to its pro-inflammatory effects and ability to promote tumor growth.

The Role of a Plant-Based Diet in Reversing Colon Cancer

A plant-based diet, rich in fruits, vegetables, whole grains, legumes, nuts, and seeds, has been shown to have numerous protective effects against colon cancer. The mechanisms by which a plant-based diet can help in reversing colon cancer include:

1. **High Fiber Intake**:
   - **Gut Health**: A diet high in fiber promotes a healthy gut microbiota, which can produce short-chain fatty acids (SCFAs) like butyrate. Butyrate has anti-inflammatory and anti-carcinogenic properties, protecting the colon lining from damage and reducing cancer risk.
   - **Bile Acid Metabolism**: Fiber binds to bile acids, reducing their conversion into secondary bile acids, which are car-

cinogenic. This decreases the exposure of the colon lining to harmful substances.

2. **Phytochemicals**:
   - **Antioxidants**: Plant-based foods are rich in antioxidants, such as flavonoids, carotenoids, and polyphenols, which protect cells from oxidative stress and DNA damage.
   - **Anti-inflammatory Effects**: Many phytochemicals have anti-inflammatory properties, which can reduce chronic inflammation, a key driver of colon cancer.
   - **Apoptosis Induction**: Certain compounds in plants, like sulforaphane (found in cruciferous vegetables) and curcumin (found in turmeric), can induce apoptosis in cancer cells, helping to eliminate them from the body.

3. **Lower Intake of Carcinogens**:
   - **Absence of HCAs and PAHs**: A plant-based diet naturally avoids the carcinogens found in cooked meats, such as HCAs and PAHs, reducing the risk of DNA damage and cancer initiation.
   - **Reduced NOC Formation**: Plant-based diets are low in nitrates and nitrites, minimizing the formation of NOCs in the gut.

4. **Improved Insulin Sensitivity**:
   - **Lower IGF-1 Levels**: A plant-based diet can lead to lower levels of IGF-1, reducing the promotion of cell proliferation and the inhibition of apoptosis in the colon.
   - **Blood Sugar Regulation**: Plant-based diets have been shown to improve insulin sensitivity and reduce blood sugar levels, which may lower cancer risk by reducing the insulin/IGF-1 signaling pathway that promotes tumor growth.

5. **Healthy Weight Maintenance**:
   - **Obesity and Cancer**: Obesity is a significant risk factor for colon cancer. A plant-based diet is generally lower in calo-

ries and higher in nutrients, which can help in maintaining a healthy weight and reducing cancer risk.
- **Hormonal Regulation**: By maintaining a healthy weight, a plant-based diet also helps regulate hormones like insulin and leptin, which are involved in cancer progression.

Colon cancer is a multifactorial disease influenced by genetic, environmental, and dietary factors. The function, production, and regulation of colon cancer involve complex pathways that drive tumor initiation, progression, and metastasis. The consumption of animal products, particularly red and processed meats, dairy, and eggs, has been strongly linked to an increased risk of colon cancer due to the presence of carcinogens, growth factors, and pro-inflammatory compounds.

Conversely, a plant-based diet offers a protective effect against colon cancer through multiple mechanisms. High fiber intake, the presence of phytochemicals, lower intake of carcinogens, improved insulin sensitivity, and healthy weight maintenance all contribute to reducing cancer risk and potentially reversing the disease. By adopting a plant-based diet, individuals can take proactive steps towards reducing their risk of colon cancer and supporting overall health and well-being.

Endometrial Cancer

Endometrial cancer is one of the most common gynecological cancers, primarily affecting the lining of the uterus, known as the endometrium. It is a complex disease with multifactorial origins, including genetic, environmental, and lifestyle factors. Understanding the function, production, and regulation of endometrial cancer is essential for developing effective prevention and treatment strategies.

The Endometrium: Function and Structure

The endometrium is the inner lining of the uterus, playing a critical role in the menstrual cycle and pregnancy. It undergoes cyclic changes in response to hormonal fluctuations, particularly estrogen and progesterone. The endometrium thickens during the menstrual cycle to prepare for potential embryo implantation. If fertilization does not occur, the endometrial lining is shed during menstruation.

Hormonal Regulation of the Endometrium

The menstrual cycle is regulated by a complex interplay of hormones:

- **Estrogen**: Produced primarily by the ovaries, estrogen stimulates the growth of the endometrial lining during the proliferative phase of the menstrual cycle.
- **Progesterone**: Following ovulation, the corpus luteum produces progesterone, which stabilizes the endometrium and prepares it for possible implantation.
- **Luteinizing Hormone (LH) and Follicle-Stimulating Hormone (FSH)**: These pituitary hormones regulate the production of estrogen and progesterone.

Pathogenesis of Endometrial Cancer

Endometrial cancer arises when the normal regulatory mechanisms of the endometrium are disrupted, leading to uncontrolled cell growth. There are two primary types of endometrial cancer: Type I (endometrioid adenocarcinoma) and Type II (non-endometrioid cancers, including serous and clear cell carcinomas). Type I is more common and is often associated with estrogen exposure, while Type II is more aggressive and less hormonally driven.

Molecular Pathways Involved in Endometrial Cancer

Several key molecular pathways are implicated in the development and progression of endometrial cancer:

- **PI3K/AKT/mTOR Pathway**: This pathway is frequently altered in endometrial cancer, particularly in Type I tumors. Mutations in PTEN, PIK3CA, and AKT genes lead to increased signaling through this pathway, promoting cell growth and survival.
- **Wnt/β-catenin Pathway**: Dysregulation of the Wnt signaling pathway, often due to mutations in the CTNNB1 gene (which encodes β-catenin), can lead to uncontrolled cell proliferation.
- **p53 Pathway**: Mutations in the TP53 gene, which encodes the tumor suppressor protein p53, are common in Type II endometrial cancers. Loss of p53 function allows cells with DNA damage to proliferate, contributing to cancer development.
- **Estrogen Receptor Signaling**: Estrogen plays a significant role in Type I endometrial cancer. Overexpression of estrogen receptors (ERα) can lead to excessive proliferation of endometrial cells.

Role of Estrogen in Endometrial Cancer

Unopposed estrogen exposure is a well-established risk factor for endometrial cancer. Estrogen promotes the proliferation of endometrial cells, and in the absence of counteracting progesterone, this can lead to hyperplasia and, eventually, cancer. Conditions such as obesity, polycystic ovary syndrome (PCOS), and hormone replacement therapy (HRT) with estrogen alone increase estrogen levels and, consequently, the risk of endometrial cancer.

Known Causes Related to Animal Products

The consumption of animal products has been linked to an increased risk of endometrial cancer. This is primarily due to the presence of exogenous hormones, high levels of saturated fats, and the potential for increased estrogen production.

Dietary Fats and Endometrial Cancer

Diets high in saturated fats, particularly from animal sources, have been associated with a higher risk of endometrial cancer. Saturated fats can increase estrogen production by promoting the conversion of androgens to estrogens in adipose tissue. Furthermore, high-fat diets may contribute to obesity, a significant risk factor for endometrial cancer.

Meat Consumption and Endometrial Cancer

Red and processed meats have been implicated in the development of various cancers, including endometrial cancer. These meats contain heme iron, which can promote oxidative stress and DNA damage, leading to cancerous changes. Additionally, cooking meat at high temperatures can produce carcinogenic compounds like heterocyclic amines (HCAs) and polycyclic aromatic hydrocarbons (PAHs).

Dairy Products and Endometrial Cancer

Dairy products, particularly those high in fat, have also been linked to an increased risk of endometrial cancer. The hormones present in dairy, including estrogen and insulin-like growth factor-1 (IGF-1), may contribute to cancer development. IGF-1 is known to promote cell proliferation and inhibit apoptosis, creating an environment conducive to cancer growth.

Plant-Based Diet Role in Reversing Endometrial Cancer

A plant-based diet, rich in fruits, vegetables, whole grains, legumes, nuts, and seeds, has been shown to reduce the risk of various cancers, including endometrial cancer. This diet provides a plethora of nutrients and phytochemicals that can inhibit cancer development and promote overall health.

Antioxidants and Phytochemicals

Plant-based foods are abundant in antioxidants and phytochemicals, which can neutralize free radicals, reduce oxidative stress, and prevent DNA damage. Key antioxidants include vitamins C and E, carotenoids, and flavonoids. These compounds can inhibit the growth of cancer cells and induce apoptosis.

- **Carotenoids**: Found in carrots, sweet potatoes, and leafy greens, carotenoids like beta-carotene have been shown to inhibit the proliferation of endometrial cancer cells.
- **Flavonoids**: Present in berries, citrus fruits, and onions, flavonoids like quercetin have anti-inflammatory and anti-cancer properties.

Fiber and Gut Health

A diet rich in fiber supports a healthy gut microbiome, which plays a crucial role in regulating estrogen levels. Fiber binds to estrogen in the intestines, facilitating its excretion and reducing circulating estrogen levels. This is particularly important in reducing the risk of estrogen-dependent cancers like endometrial cancer.

- **Whole Grains**: Foods like oats, brown rice, and quinoa are excellent sources of fiber that can help regulate estrogen levels.
- **Legumes**: Beans, lentils, and peas provide both fiber and phytoestrogens, which can have a protective effect against endometrial cancer.

Anti-Inflammatory Effects

Chronic inflammation is a known contributor to cancer development. A plant-based diet is naturally anti-inflammatory, reducing the risk of chronic diseases, including cancer. Omega-3 fatty acids, found in flaxseeds, chia seeds, and walnuts, are particularly effective in reducing inflammation.

- **Curcumin**: The active compound in turmeric, curcumin, has potent anti-inflammatory and anti-cancer properties.

- **Ginger**: Ginger contains gingerol, which has been shown to reduce inflammation and inhibit cancer cell growth.

Impact on Obesity

Obesity is a significant risk factor for endometrial cancer, primarily due to its role in increasing estrogen production. A plant-based diet, which is typically lower in calories and higher in nutrients, can aid in weight management and reduce the risk of obesity-related cancers.

- **Low-Calorie Density**: Plant-based foods tend to have a lower calorie density, allowing individuals to consume larger portions without excessive calorie intake, promoting weight loss and maintenance.
- **Metabolic Health**: A diet rich in plant-based foods improves insulin sensitivity and reduces the risk of metabolic syndrome, further decreasing the risk of endometrial cancer.

Detailed Pathways in Endometrial Cancer
Estrogen-Driven Pathways

The estrogen-driven pathway is one of the most significant mechanisms in the development of Type I endometrial cancer. Estrogen binds to estrogen receptors (ERα) in the endometrial cells, leading to the activation of various genes involved in cell proliferation and survival.

- **ERα Signaling**: Upon binding to estrogen, ERα translocates to the nucleus, where it acts as a transcription factor, promoting the expression of genes like c-myc, cyclin D1, and Bcl-2, which are involved in cell cycle progression and inhibition of apoptosis.
- **PI3K/AKT/mTOR Pathway**: Estrogen signaling can activate the PI3K/AKT/mTOR pathway, leading to increased cell growth and survival. Mutations in PTEN, a tumor suppressor gene that

negatively regulates this pathway, are common in endometrial cancer, leading to unchecked activation of mTOR signaling.

Inflammation-Related Pathways

Chronic inflammation can contribute to the development of endometrial cancer by promoting an environment conducive to DNA damage and cell proliferation. Key inflammatory pathways include:

- **NF-κB Pathway**: NF-κB is a transcription factor that regulates the expression of pro-inflammatory cytokines and chemokines. In endometrial cancer, NF-κB can be activated by various stimuli, including cytokines like TNF-α, leading to increased inflammation and cancer progression.
- **COX-2 Pathway**: Cyclooxygenase-2 (COX-2) is an enzyme involved in the production of prostaglandins, which are mediators of inflammation. Overexpression of COX-2 has been observed in endometrial cancer, promoting angiogenesis, cell proliferation, and resistance to apoptosis.

Insulin and IGF-1 Pathways

Insulin resistance and elevated levels of insulin and insulin-like growth factor-1 (IGF-1) are associated with an increased risk of endometrial cancer. These factors can promote cell proliferation and inhibit apoptosis through several pathways:

- **Insulin Receptor Signaling**: Insulin binds to its receptor on the cell surface, activating the PI3K/AKT pathway, similar to estrogen signaling. This leads to increased cell growth and survival, contributing to cancer development.
- **IGF-1 Signaling**: IGF-1 binds to its receptor (IGF-1R), triggering signaling cascades that promote cell proliferation and inhibit apoptosis. High levels of IGF-1 are associated with a higher risk of endometrial cancer, particularly in obese individuals.

A Plant-Based Diet Can Help Reverse Endometrial Cancer

A plant-based diet can play a significant role in reversing endometrial cancer by targeting the underlying mechanisms involved in cancer development and progression.

Modulation of Estrogen Levels

As mentioned earlier, a diet rich in fiber can reduce circulating estrogen levels by promoting its excretion. Additionally, phytoestrogens found in soy products, flaxseeds, and other plant foods can have a protective effect by competing with endogenous estrogen for binding to estrogen receptors, thereby reducing estrogenic stimulation of the endometrium.

- **Soy Isoflavones**: Isoflavones, such as genistein and daidzein, found in soy, are weak estrogen agonists. They can bind to ERα with lower affinity than endogenous estrogen, leading to reduced estrogenic effects and a lower risk of endometrial cancer.
- **Lignans**: Found in flaxseeds, lignans are converted by gut bacteria into enterolactone and enterodiol, which have weak estrogenic activity. These compounds can help balance estrogen levels and reduce cancer risk.

Reduction of Inflammation

A plant-based diet's anti-inflammatory properties can help reduce the chronic inflammation associated with endometrial cancer. Foods rich in omega-3 fatty acids, curcumin, ginger, and other anti-inflammatory compounds can inhibit inflammatory pathways, reducing the risk of cancer progression.

- **Omega-3 Fatty Acids**: These fatty acids, found in flaxseeds, chia seeds, and walnuts, can inhibit the NF-κB pathway, reducing the production of pro-inflammatory cytokines and chemokines.

- **Curcumin**: Curcumin can inhibit the COX-2 pathway, reducing prostaglandin production and inflammation. It also has direct anti-cancer effects by inducing apoptosis and inhibiting cell proliferation.

Improvement of Insulin Sensitivity

A plant-based diet is effective in improving insulin sensitivity and reducing the risk of insulin resistance, a significant risk factor for endometrial cancer. Whole grains, legumes, and vegetables have a low glycemic index, leading to more stable blood sugar levels and reduced insulin demand.

- **Low Glycemic Index Foods**: Foods like oats, quinoa, and legumes have a low glycemic index, leading to slower digestion and absorption, which helps maintain stable blood glucose levels and improves insulin sensitivity.
- **Polyphenols**: Found in fruits, vegetables, and whole grains, polyphenols like quercetin and resveratrol have been shown to improve insulin sensitivity and reduce the risk of insulin resistance-related cancers.

Weight Management and Obesity Reduction

A plant-based diet, with its emphasis on low-calorie, nutrient-dense foods, is highly effective for weight management. Reducing body fat lowers estrogen production in adipose tissue, decreasing the risk of estrogen-dependent cancers like endometrial cancer.

- **Caloric Density**: Foods like fruits, vegetables, and whole grains have a low caloric density, allowing for larger portions with fewer calories, which aids in weight loss and management.
- **Thermogenesis**: Plant-based diets may increase thermogenesis (the process of heat production in organisms), leading to greater energy expenditure and further aiding in weight management.

Enhanced Detoxification and Elimination

A plant-based diet supports the body's natural detoxification processes, aiding in the elimination of carcinogens and excess hormones that may contribute to cancer development. Cruciferous vegetables like broccoli, kale, and Brussels sprouts are particularly beneficial in this regard.

- **Glucosinolates**: Found in cruciferous vegetables, glucosinolates are compounds that, when broken down, form bioactive compounds like indoles and isothiocyanates. These compounds enhance the activity of detoxification enzymes, helping to eliminate potential carcinogens.
- **Chlorophyll**: The green pigment in leafy vegetables, chlorophyll, binds to carcinogenic molecules and facilitates their excretion from the body.

Endometrial cancer is a complex disease with multiple contributing factors, including hormonal imbalances, chronic inflammation, insulin resistance, and dietary influences. Animal products, particularly those high in fat and hormones, have been linked to an increased risk of endometrial cancer, highlighting the importance of dietary choices in cancer prevention.

A plant-based diet offers numerous protective benefits, from modulating estrogen levels and reducing inflammation to improving insulin sensitivity and aiding in weight management. By targeting the underlying mechanisms of endometrial cancer, a plant-based diet not only reduces the risk of developing the disease but also offers potential for reversing its progression.

Esophageal Cancer

Esophageal cancer is a malignancy that arises in the tissues of the esophagus, the muscular tube responsible for moving food and liquids from the throat to the stomach. This type of cancer is notorious for its aggressive nature and poor prognosis, often diagnosed in advanced stages due to the absence of early symptoms. Understanding the function, production, and regulation of esophageal cancer at a cellular level is critical for developing effective prevention and treatment strategies. Additionally, the role of diet—particularly the impact of animal products and the potential benefits of a plant-based diet—has garnered significant attention in recent years.

Function of Esophageal Cancer

The esophagus plays a vital role in the digestive system by transporting food and liquids from the mouth to the stomach. Esophageal cancer disrupts this function, leading to symptoms such as difficulty swallowing (dysphagia), weight loss, chest pain, and regurgitation. As the cancer progresses, it can obstruct the esophagus, making it increasingly difficult for patients to consume solid foods and even liquids. This obstruction not only impairs nutrition but also severely affects the quality of life.

The biological function of esophageal cancer cells is similar to that of other cancerous cells: they divide uncontrollably, evade apoptosis (programmed cell death), sustain angiogenesis (the formation of new blood vessels), and invade surrounding tissues. These malignant cells have the potential to metastasize, spreading to distant organs such as the liver, lungs, and bones. The aggressive nature of esophageal cancer is partly due to its ability to rapidly invade surrounding tissues and metastasize to other parts of the body.

Production of Esophageal Cancer

The production of esophageal cancer involves a series of genetic and epigenetic alterations that transform normal esophageal epithelial cells into malignant ones. These alterations can be triggered by various factors, including environmental exposures, dietary habits, and underlying medical conditions.

Genetic Mutations and Pathways

Several key genetic mutations have been identified in esophageal cancer. These mutations often affect genes involved in cell cycle regulation, DNA repair, and apoptosis. Some of the most commonly mutated genes in esophageal cancer include:

- **TP53**: This tumor suppressor gene is frequently mutated in esophageal cancer. TP53 encodes the p53 protein, which plays a crucial role in regulating the cell cycle and inducing apoptosis in response to DNA damage. Mutations in TP53 lead to the loss of its tumor-suppressive function, allowing cells with damaged DNA to continue dividing.
- **CDKN2A**: This gene encodes the p16 protein, a cyclin-dependent kinase inhibitor that regulates the cell cycle by inhibiting the activity of cyclin-dependent kinases (CDKs). Loss of CDKN2A function leads to unchecked cell cycle progression and contributes to the development of cancer.
- **NOTCH1**: This gene is involved in cell differentiation, proliferation, and apoptosis. Mutations in NOTCH1 have been associated with both squamous cell carcinoma and adenocarcinoma of the esophagus.
- **EGFR**: The epidermal growth factor receptor (EGFR) gene is involved in cell proliferation and survival. Overexpression or amplification of EGFR is common in esophageal cancer and is associated with poor prognosis.

These genetic alterations disrupt normal cellular processes, leading to uncontrolled cell growth, evasion of apoptosis, and the potential for metastasis. In addition to these genetic mutations, epigenetic changes such as DNA methylation and histone modifications also play a role in the development and progression of esophageal cancer.

Histological Subtypes

Esophageal cancer can be classified into two main histological subtypes: esophageal squamous cell carcinoma (ESCC) and esophageal adenocarcinoma (EAC).

- **Esophageal Squamous Cell Carcinoma (ESCC)**: This subtype arises from the squamous cells that line the upper and middle portions of the esophagus. ESCC is more common in regions with high rates of tobacco and alcohol consumption. It is also associated with dietary factors such as the consumption of hot beverages, which can cause thermal injury to the esophageal lining.
- **Esophageal Adenocarcinoma (EAC)**: This subtype originates from glandular cells that are typically found in the lower part of the esophagus. EAC is strongly associated with gastroesophageal reflux disease (GERD) and Barrett's esophagus, a condition in which the normal squamous epithelium of the esophagus is replaced with columnar epithelium due to chronic acid exposure.

Regulation of Esophageal Cancer

The regulation of esophageal cancer involves a complex interplay of genetic, epigenetic, and environmental factors. Key signaling pathways and molecular mechanisms play critical roles in the regulation of cell growth, survival, and apoptosis in esophageal cancer.

Signaling Pathways

Several signaling pathways are dysregulated in esophageal cancer, contributing to its initiation and progression:

- **PI3K/AKT/mTOR Pathway**: This pathway is involved in regulating cell growth, survival, and metabolism. Activation of the PI3K/AKT/mTOR pathway is common in esophageal cancer and is associated with resistance to apoptosis and increased cell proliferation.

- **Wnt/β-catenin Pathway**: The Wnt/β-catenin pathway plays a key role in cell proliferation and differentiation. Dysregulation of this pathway, often due to mutations in the APC gene, leads to the accumulation of β-catenin in the nucleus, where it promotes the transcription of target genes involved in cell proliferation.
- **NF-κB Pathway**: The NF-κB pathway is involved in regulating the immune response, inflammation, and cell survival. Chronic activation of NF-κB in esophageal cancer cells promotes inflammation and resistance to apoptosis, contributing to tumor growth and metastasis.
- **Hedgehog Signaling Pathway**: The Hedgehog pathway is involved in regulating cell differentiation and tissue patterning during development. Aberrant activation of this pathway has been implicated in the development of esophageal adenocarcinoma.

Epigenetic Regulation

Epigenetic changes, such as DNA methylation and histone modifications, play a significant role in the regulation of gene expression in esophageal cancer. Hypermethylation of tumor suppressor genes, such as CDKN2A and RASSF1A, leads to their silencing and contributes to the development of cancer. Additionally, global hypomethylation can result in genomic instability and the activation of oncogenes.

Tumor Microenvironment

The tumor microenvironment (TME) in esophageal cancer consists of various cell types, including cancer-associated fibroblasts, immune cells, and endothelial cells. The TME plays a critical role in promoting tumor growth, angiogenesis, and metastasis. Cancer-associated fibroblasts secrete growth factors and cytokines that support cancer cell survival and invasion. Additionally, the immune cells within the TME can be co-opted by cancer cells to suppress anti-tumor immune responses.

Detailed Pathways Involved in Esophageal Cancer

Esophageal cancer development and progression involve multiple molecular pathways that regulate cell proliferation, survival, apoptosis, and metastasis. These pathways are often dysregulated due to genetic mutations and epigenetic alterations. Some of the key pathways involved in esophageal cancer are outlined below.

TP53 Pathway

The TP53 pathway is one of the most critical tumor suppressor pathways in esophageal cancer. The p53 protein, encoded by the TP53 gene, acts as a "guardian of the genome" by regulating the cell cycle, DNA repair, and apoptosis in response to cellular stress and DNA damage. In normal cells, p53 activation leads to cell cycle arrest, allowing for DNA repair or the initiation of apoptosis if the damage is irreparable.

In esophageal cancer, mutations in TP53 are common and result in the loss of p53 function. This allows cells with damaged DNA to continue proliferating, leading to the accumulation of additional genetic mutations and the development of cancer. Loss of p53 function is associated with poor prognosis and resistance to chemotherapy in esophageal cancer.

PI3K/AKT/mTOR Pathway

The PI3K/AKT/mTOR pathway is a key regulator of cell growth, survival, and metabolism. In esophageal cancer, this pathway is often hyperactivated due to mutations in PIK3CA (the gene encoding the catalytic subunit of PI3K) or loss of function of PTEN (a tumor suppressor that negatively regulates the pathway).

Activation of the PI3K/AKT/mTOR pathway promotes cell proliferation, inhibits apoptosis, and enhances resistance to chemotherapy. This pathway also plays a role in promoting angiogenesis, which is essential for tumor growth and metastasis. Targeting this pathway with inhibitors has shown promise in preclinical models of esophageal cancer.

Wnt/β-catenin Pathway

The Wnt/β-catenin pathway is involved in regulating cell proliferation, differentiation, and migration. In normal cells, β-catenin is kept at low levels through degradation by the destruction complex, which includes the APC protein. However, mutations in the APC gene or other components of the pathway can lead to the accumulation of β-catenin in the nucleus, where it activates the transcription of target genes involved in cell proliferation and survival.

In esophageal cancer, dysregulation of the Wnt/β-catenin pathway contributes to uncontrolled cell growth and resistance to apoptosis. This pathway is particularly important in the development of esophageal adenocarcinoma, where it plays a role in the progression from Barrett's esophagus to malignancy.

NF-κB Pathway

The NF-κB pathway is a key regulator of inflammation and immune responses. In esophageal cancer, chronic activation of the NF-κB pathway promotes inflammation, cell survival, and resistance to apoptosis. This pathway is often activated by inflammatory cytokines, such as TNF-α, which are present in the tumor microenvironment.

The NF-κB pathway also plays a role in the epithelial-mesenchymal transition (EMT), a process by which cancer cells acquire invasive and metastatic properties. Inhibition of the NF-κB pathway has been shown to reduce tumor growth and metastasis in preclinical models of esophageal cancer.

Hedgehog Signaling Pathway

The Hedgehog signaling pathway is involved in regulating cell differentiation and tissue patterning during embryonic development. Aberrant activation of this pathway has been implicated in the development of several cancers, including esophageal adenocarcinoma.

In esophageal cancer, the Hedgehog pathway promotes cell proliferation, survival, and invasion. This pathway is activated by the binding of Hedgehog ligands to the Patched receptor, leading to the activation of the Smoothened protein and the subsequent transcription of target genes. Inhibition of the Hedgehog pathway has shown promise as a therapeutic strategy in esophageal adenocarcinoma.

Known Causes Related to Animal Products

Dietary habits, particularly the consumption of certain animal products, have been implicated in the development of esophageal cancer. Several studies have identified specific components of animal-based diets that increase the risk of this malignancy.

1. Processed Meats

Processed meats, such as bacon, sausages, and hot dogs, have been classified as Group 1 carcinogens by the International Agency for Research on Cancer (IARC). The consumption of processed meats has been linked to an increased risk of esophageal cancer, particularly esophageal adenocarcinoma. The carcinogenicity of processed meats is attributed to the presence of nitrosamines, which are formed during the processing and cooking of these products. Nitrosamines are known to cause DNA damage and promote the development of cancer.

2. Red Meat

Red meat, including beef, pork, and lamb, has also been associated with an increased risk of esophageal cancer. The cooking of red meat at high temperatures, such as grilling or barbecuing, can lead to the formation of heterocyclic amines (HCAs) and polycyclic aromatic hydrocarbons (PAHs), both of which are carcinogenic. These compounds can induce genetic mutations and contribute to the development of esophageal cancer.

3. Animal Fats

High consumption of animal fats, particularly saturated fats found in meat and dairy products, has been linked to an increased risk of esophageal cancer. Diets rich in saturated fats can promote obesity, which is a known risk factor for esophageal adenocarcinoma. Obesity contributes to the development of gastroesophageal reflux disease

(GERD), a major risk factor for Barrett's esophagus and esophageal adenocarcinoma.

4. Dairy Products

The consumption of dairy products, particularly those high in fat, has been associated with an increased risk of esophageal cancer. The exact mechanisms are not fully understood, but it is hypothesized that the high-fat content in dairy products may contribute to the development of obesity and GERD, both of which are risk factors for esophageal adenocarcinoma.

The Role of a Plant-Based Diet in Reversal and Prevention

A growing body of evidence suggests that a plant-based diet can play a significant role in the prevention and even reversal of esophageal cancer. Plant-based diets are rich in fruits, vegetables, whole grains, legumes, nuts, and seeds, which provide a wide range of nutrients, antioxidants, and phytochemicals that have anti-cancer properties.

1. Antioxidants and Phytochemicals

Fruits and vegetables are rich in antioxidants, such as vitamins C and E, beta-carotene, and flavonoids, which help neutralize free radicals and reduce oxidative stress, a key factor in cancer development. Additionally, phytochemicals such as sulforaphane (found in cruciferous vegetables like broccoli) and lycopene (found in tomatoes) have been shown to inhibit the growth of cancer cells and promote apoptosis. A "Randomized Phase II Trial of Lyophilized Strawberries in Patients with Dysplastic Precancerous Lesions of the Esophagus" found that strawberries have the ability to reverse esophageal cancer in 80.6% of people in the study, with 60 grams of strawberry powder daily. At the end of the study over 50% of people in the study had a total reversal of their esophageal cancer.

2. Fiber

A plant-based diet is typically high in dietary fiber, which has been shown to reduce the risk of esophageal cancer. Fiber aids in digestion and helps prevent constipation, which can reduce the risk of GERD and, consequently, esophageal adenocarcinoma. Additionally, fiber binds to potential carcinogens in the digestive tract and facilitates their excretion, reducing their contact with the esophageal lining.

3. Anti-inflammatory Effects

Chronic inflammation is a key factor in the development and progression of esophageal cancer. A plant-based diet, rich in anti-inflammatory foods such as leafy greens, berries, and nuts, can help reduce inflammation and lower the risk of cancer. Omega-3 fatty acids, found in flaxseeds and walnuts, are particularly effective in reducing inflammation and may help prevent the development of esophageal cancer.

4. Weight Management

Obesity is a significant risk factor for esophageal adenocarcinoma. A plant-based diet, which is typically lower in calories and fat than an animal-based diet, can help with weight management and reduce the risk of obesity-related cancers. Studies have shown that individuals who follow a plant-based diet tend to have lower body mass indices (BMIs) and lower rates of obesity.

5. Protection Against GERD

Gastroesophageal reflux disease (GERD) is a major risk factor for esophageal adenocarcinoma. A plant-based diet, particularly one that is low in fat and high in fiber, can help reduce the incidence of GERD. Foods that are known to trigger GERD, such as high-fat dairy products, red meat, and processed foods, are often excluded from a plant-based diet.

6. Reversal Potential

There is evidence to suggest that a plant-based diet may not only prevent but also help reverse esophageal cancer. The consumption of whole, plant-based foods has been associated with the regression of precancerous lesions and early-stage cancers in some studies. This is likely due to the combined effects of the diet's anti-inflammatory, antioxidant, and immune-boosting properties.

For example, a study published in the *Journal of the American College of Nutrition* found that a diet rich in fruits and vegetables was associated with a lower risk of esophageal cancer and that high consumption of plant-based foods could potentially reverse the progression of precancerous conditions such as Barrett's esophagus.

Esophageal cancer is a complex disease with multifactorial causes, including genetic mutations, epigenetic changes, and environmental factors such as diet. The consumption of certain animal products, particularly processed meats, red meats, and high-fat dairy products, has been associated with an increased risk of esophageal cancer. These dietary factors contribute to carcinogenesis through the formation of carcinogenic compounds, promotion of obesity, and exacerbation of gastroesophageal reflux disease.

Conversely, a plant-based diet, rich in fruits, vegetables, whole grains, legumes, and nuts, offers protective effects against esophageal cancer. The antioxidants, phytochemicals, and fiber found in plant-based foods help reduce oxidative stress, inflammation, and carcinogen exposure, while also promoting healthy weight management and reducing the risk of GERD. Additionally, there is evidence to suggest that a plant-based diet may have the potential to reverse precancerous lesions and early-stage esophageal cancers.

Gallbladder Cancer

Gallbladder cancer is a relatively rare but aggressive form of cancer that begins in the gallbladder, a small organ located beneath the liver. The gallbladder's primary function is to store bile, a digestive fluid produced by the liver that helps break down fats in the small intestine. Gallbladder cancer often goes undetected until it has reached an advanced stage due to its asymptomatic nature in the early phases, leading to poor prognosis.

Function of Gallbladder Cancer

The gallbladder, though small, plays a critical role in the digestive system. Gallbladder cancer occurs when malignant cells grow uncontrollably in the gallbladder tissue. The primary function of gallbladder cancer, like all cancers, is to proliferate and invade surrounding tissues. This proliferation disrupts normal cell function and can metastasize to other organs.

The malignant cells in gallbladder cancer originate from the epithelial cells lining the gallbladder. These cells can transform due to genetic mutations that alter their normal regulatory mechanisms. Gallbladder cancer can impair the organ's ability to function, causing symptoms such as abdominal pain, jaundice, and digestive issues. As the disease progresses, it may also affect the liver, bile ducts, and other nearby organs.

Production of Gallbladder Cancer

The production of gallbladder cancer begins with genetic mutations that cause normal gallbladder cells to become malignant. These mutations can occur due to various factors, including chronic inflammation, exposure to carcinogens, and genetic predispositions. The process of gallbladder cancer production involves several stages:

Initiation

The initiation stage involves genetic mutations in the DNA of gallbladder epithelial cells. These mutations can be caused by various factors, including chronic inflammation due to gallstones, infection with bacteria such as *Helicobacter pylori* or *Salmonella typhi*, and exposure to toxic substances in the bile.

Mutations often occur in genes responsible for cell growth and division, such as tumor suppressor genes (e.g., TP53) and oncogenes (e.g., KRAS). These mutations cause the cells to lose their normal regulatory mechanisms, leading to uncontrolled growth.

Promotion

During the promotion stage, the mutated cells begin to multiply rapidly. The presence of bile acids and chronic inflammation can create a microenvironment that promotes the proliferation of these mutated cells. This stage is characterized by the formation of pre-cancerous lesions, such as dysplasia or carcinoma in situ, which can eventually progress to invasive cancer.

Progression

In the progression stage, the pre-cancerous lesions evolve into invasive cancer. The malignant cells acquire additional mutations that enable them to invade surrounding tissues and spread to other parts of the body through the lymphatic system and bloodstream. This stage is marked by the development of a tumor that can obstruct the bile ducts, leading to symptoms such as jaundice and abdominal pain.

Regulation of Gallbladder Cancer

The regulation of gallbladder cancer involves various molecular pathways that control cell growth, division, and apoptosis. Dysregulation of these pathways is a hallmark of cancer, and understanding these mechanisms is crucial for developing targeted therapies. Key regulatory pathways involved in gallbladder cancer include:

The TP53 Pathway

The TP53 gene encodes the p53 protein, which is a critical tumor suppressor involved in regulating the cell cycle and inducing apoptosis in response to DNA damage. In many cases of gallbladder cancer, the TP53 gene is mutated, leading to a loss of p53 function. This loss allows cells with damaged DNA to continue dividing, contributing to tumor development.

The KRAS Pathway

KRAS is an oncogene that encodes a protein involved in the RAS/MAPK signaling pathway, which regulates cell proliferation and survival. Mutations in the KRAS gene can lead to constant activation of this pathway, driving uncontrolled cell growth. KRAS mutations are found in a significant proportion of gallbladder cancer cases and are associated with poor prognosis.

The Wnt/β-Catenin Pathway

The Wnt/β-catenin signaling pathway plays a role in regulating cell proliferation and differentiation. Aberrant activation of this pathway has been implicated in various cancers, including gallbladder cancer. Mutations or dysregulation of components of this pathway can lead to the accumulation of β-catenin in the nucleus, promoting the expression of genes that drive tumor growth.

The Notch Pathway

The Notch signaling pathway is involved in cell fate determination and differentiation. In gallbladder cancer, alterations in Notch signaling have been observed, contributing to the maintenance of cancer stem cells and resistance to chemotherapy. Dysregulation of this pathway can enhance the aggressiveness of gallbladder cancer.

The PI3K/AKT/mTOR Pathway

The PI3K/AKT/mTOR pathway is crucial for regulating cell growth, metabolism, and survival. In gallbladder cancer, mutations or overactivation of components of this pathway, such as PI3K or AKT, can lead to increased cell proliferation and resistance to apoptosis. Targeting this pathway is a potential therapeutic strategy for gallbladder cancer.

Detailed Pathways Involved in Gallbladder Cancer

Understanding the detailed pathways involved in gallbladder cancer provides insight into the disease's complexity and potential therapeutic targets. Several key pathways are implicated in the development and progression of gallbladder cancer:

The RAS/MAPK Pathway

The RAS/MAPK pathway is a critical regulator of cell proliferation and survival. In gallbladder cancer, mutations in the KRAS gene can lead to constitutive activation of this pathway, resulting in uncontrolled cell growth. The pathway involves the activation of RAS proteins, which then activate a cascade of kinases, including RAF, MEK, and ERK. Activated ERK translocates to the nucleus, where it promotes the expression of genes involved in cell cycle progression and survival.

The Wnt/β-Catenin Pathway

The Wnt/β-catenin pathway is involved in the regulation of cell proliferation and differentiation. In gallbladder cancer, aberrant activation of this pathway can occur due to mutations in components such as APC or β-catenin itself. This leads to the accumulation of β-catenin in the nucleus, where it interacts with transcription factors to promote the expression of oncogenes, driving tumor growth.

The Notch Pathway

The Notch pathway is involved in cell fate determination and maintenance of stem cell populations. In gallbladder cancer, dysregulation of Notch signaling can contribute to the maintenance of cancer stem cells, which are resistant to conventional therapies and can lead to tumor recurrence. Activation of Notch signaling involves the binding of ligands to Notch receptors, leading to the cleavage of the receptor and release of the Notch intracellular domain (NICD). The NICD translocates to the nucleus and regulates the expression of target genes involved in cell survival and proliferation.

The PI3K/AKT/mTOR Pathway

The PI3K/AKT/mTOR pathway is a key regulator of cell growth, metabolism, and survival. In gallbladder cancer, mutations or overactivation of this pathway can lead to increased cell proliferation and resistance to apoptosis. Activation of the pathway begins with the binding of growth factors to receptor tyrosine kinases (RTKs), leading to the activation of PI3K. PI3K generates PIP3, which recruits and activates AKT. Activated AKT phosphorylates downstream targets, including mTOR, promoting cell growth and survival.

The TGF-β Pathway

The TGF-β pathway is involved in the regulation of cell growth and differentiation. In gallbladder cancer, TGF-β signaling can have both tumor-suppressive and tumor-promoting effects, depending on the context. In the early stages of cancer, TGF-β acts as a tumor suppressor by inhibiting cell proliferation and inducing apoptosis. However, in later stages, cancer cells can become resistant to TGF-β's suppressive effects and instead exploit the pathway to promote invasion and metastasis.

Known Causes Related to Animal Products

Dietary factors, particularly the consumption of animal products, have been implicated in the development of gallbladder cancer. Several mechanisms by which animal products contribute to gallbladder cancer include:

High Saturated Fat Intake

Diets high in saturated fats, commonly found in red and processed meats, have been linked to an increased risk of gallbladder cancer. Saturated fats can lead to the formation of gallstones, which are a major risk factor for gallbladder cancer. Gallstones cause chronic inflammation of the gallbladder, creating an environment conducive to cancer development.

Heme Iron

Heme iron, found in animal products such as red meat, has been associated with an increased risk of gallbladder cancer. Heme iron can promote oxidative stress and the formation of reactive oxygen species (ROS), which can cause DNA damage and contribute to carcinogenesis. Additionally, heme iron can enhance the formation of N-nitroso compounds, which are potent carcinogens.

Cholesterol

High dietary intake of cholesterol, predominantly found in animal products, is another risk factor for gallbladder cancer. Cholesterol can promote the formation of gallstones and increase bile acid production, both of which contribute to chronic inflammation and cancer development. Moreover, cholesterol metabolites, such as oxysterols, can have pro-carcinogenic effects by promoting cell proliferation and survival.

Processed Meats

Processed meats, such as sausages, bacon, and ham, are classified as Group 1 carcinogens by the World Health Organization (WHO). The consumption of processed meats has been linked to an increased risk of various cancers, including gallbladder cancer. Processed meats often contain nitrates and nitrites, which can form N-nitroso compounds in the body, contributing to carcinogenesis.

Plant-Based Diet and Gallbladder Cancer Reversal

A plant-based diet, rich in fruits, vegetables, whole grains, and legumes, offers numerous health benefits, including a reduced risk of gallbladder cancer. Several mechanisms by which a plant-based diet can help reverse gallbladder cancer include:

Anti-Inflammatory Properties

Chronic inflammation is a key factor in the development of gallbladder cancer. A plant-based diet is rich in anti-inflammatory compounds, such as polyphenols, flavonoids, and carotenoids, which can help reduce inflammation and inhibit cancer progression. Foods like turmeric, ginger, and leafy greens are particularly potent in their anti-inflammatory effects.

Antioxidant Activity

A plant-based diet is abundant in antioxidants, such as vitamins C and E, and phytochemicals like quercetin and resveratrol. These antioxidants can neutralize ROS, reducing oxidative stress and DNA damage, which are critical steps in the prevention and reversal of cancer. Berries, citrus fruits, and cruciferous vegetables are excellent sources of antioxidants.

Fiber Content

Dietary fiber, found in fruits, vegetables, and whole grains, plays a significant role in reducing the risk of gallbladder cancer. Fiber helps in the regulation of bile acid metabolism and reduces the formation of gallstones. Additionally, fiber promotes the excretion of carcinogens and enhances gut health, which is crucial for overall cancer prevention.

Phytochemicals and Cancer Inhibition

Phytochemicals, naturally occurring compounds in plants, have been shown to have anti-cancer properties. For example, sulforaphane in cruciferous vegetables, lycopene in tomatoes, and catechins in green tea have all demonstrated the ability to inhibit cancer cell growth and induce apoptosis. A diet rich in these phytochemicals can help in the reversal of gallbladder cancer by targeting multiple pathways involved in cancer progression.

Regulation of Hormonal Balance

Certain cancers, including gallbladder cancer, are influenced by hormonal imbalances. A plant-based diet can help regulate hormone levels, particularly insulin and estrogen, which are known to play roles in cancer development. The consumption of phytoestrogens, found in soy products, can help modulate estrogen levels and reduce cancer risk.

Weight Management

Obesity is a known risk factor for gallbladder cancer, and a plant-based diet can aid in weight management. Plant-based foods are generally lower in calories and higher in nutrients, making them effective for maintaining a healthy weight. Weight loss can reduce the risk of gallstone formation and decrease the likelihood of developing gallbladder cancer.

Gallbladder cancer is a complex disease involving multiple genetic mutations and dysregulated pathways. The consumption of animal products, particularly those high in saturated fats, heme iron, and cholesterol, has been linked to an increased risk of gallbladder cancer. In contrast, a plant-based diet offers protective effects through its anti-inflammatory, antioxidant, and cancer-inhibitory properties.

By adopting a plant-based diet, individuals can reduce their risk of developing gallbladder cancer and potentially reverse the disease by targeting the underlying mechanisms of cancer progression. This diet not only supports overall health but also addresses specific risk factors associated with gallbladder cancer, such as chronic inflammation, oxidative stress, and hormonal imbalances.

Head and Neck Cancer

Head and neck cancers (HNCs) comprise a diverse group of malignant tumors that develop in or around the throat, larynx, nose, sinuses, and mouth. These cancers are categorized based on the specific location in the head or neck region where they originate. The most common types include cancers of the oral cavity, pharynx, and larynx. While HNCs can develop due to various factors, including genetic predispositions, lifestyle choices, and environmental exposures, increasing evidence suggests that dietary factors, particularly the consumption of animal products, play a significant role in their etiology. Conversely, a plant-based diet has been shown to offer protective benefits and may even aid in the reversal of these cancers.

Function and Types of Head and Neck Cancer
Function and Anatomy Involved

Head and neck cancers affect regions critical to basic human functions, such as breathing, eating, speaking, and sensory processes like smell and taste. These cancers typically originate from squamous cells, the thin, flat cells that line the mucosal surfaces of the head and neck.

- **Oral Cavity Cancer:** This type of cancer begins in the mouth, including the lips, tongue, gums, and the inner lining of the cheeks.
- **Pharyngeal Cancer:** It affects the pharynx, which includes the nasopharynx (upper part of the throat behind the nose), orophar-

ynx (middle part of the throat), and hypopharynx (lower part of the throat).

- **Laryngeal Cancer:** This cancer originates in the larynx (voice box), which houses the vocal cords.
- **Nasal Cavity and Paranasal Sinus Cancer:** These cancers develop in the space behind the nose and the sinus cavities.
- **Salivary Gland Cancer:** This type involves the salivary glands, which produce saliva to aid in digestion and keep the mouth moist.

Production and Development of Head and Neck Cancer

Head and neck cancers arise from the uncontrolled growth of cells within the mucosal surfaces of the head and neck. The production and development of these cancers follow a multi-step process that involves genetic mutations, environmental exposures, and lifestyle factors.

Carcinogenesis: The Initiation Phase

The first step in the production of HNCs is the initiation phase, during which the DNA of cells within the mucosal surfaces becomes damaged or mutated. These mutations can occur due to various factors:

- **Tobacco Use:** Smoking and chewing tobacco are the primary risk factors for HNCs. The carcinogens in tobacco cause direct DNA damage to the cells lining the oral cavity, pharynx, and larynx.
- **Alcohol Consumption:** Alcohol acts as a solvent, enhancing the penetration of carcinogens from tobacco into the mucosal cells. It also metabolizes into acetaldehyde, a toxic compound that can cause DNA damage.

Promotion Phase

During the promotion phase, the initiated cells are exposed to continuous stimuli, such as carcinogens or inflammatory agents, leading to their proliferation. Factors contributing to this phase include:

- **Chronic Inflammation:** Persistent inflammation in the mucosal surfaces, often caused by irritants like tobacco or alcohol, promotes the growth and division of mutated cells.
- **Nutrient Deficiencies:** Deficiencies in essential nutrients, such as vitamins A, C, and E, and minerals like selenium, can impair the body's ability to repair DNA damage and maintain normal cell function.

Progression Phase

The progression phase involves the accumulation of additional genetic mutations and alterations, leading to the malignant transformation of cells. During this phase, the cancer cells acquire the ability to invade surrounding tissues, metastasize to distant organs, and evade the body's immune system.

- **Genetic Alterations:** Mutations in tumor suppressor genes (e.g., TP53) and oncogenes (e.g., EGFR) drive the progression of HNCs by promoting uncontrolled cell growth and division.
- **Angiogenesis:** The formation of new blood vessels is essential for supplying nutrients and oxygen to the growing tumor. Tumor cells release growth factors, such as VEGF (vascular endothelial growth factor), to stimulate angiogenesis.

Regulation of Head and Neck Cancer

The regulation of head and neck cancer involves various molecular pathways that control cell proliferation, differentiation, and apoptosis (programmed cell death). Disruptions in these regulatory pathways can lead to the development and progression of cancer.

Cell Cycle Regulation

The cell cycle is tightly regulated by a network of proteins and signaling pathways that ensure cells divide only when necessary. Key regulators include:

- **Cyclins and Cyclin-Dependent Kinases (CDKs):** These proteins control the progression of cells through the different phases of the cell cycle. Overexpression of cyclins and CDKs has been observed in HNCs, leading to uncontrolled cell proliferation.
- **p53 Tumor Suppressor Protein:** p53 plays a crucial role in regulating the cell cycle and inducing apoptosis in response to DNA damage. Mutations in the TP53 gene are common in HNCs, resulting in the loss of this regulatory function.

Apoptosis Pathways

Apoptosis is a form of programmed cell death that eliminates damaged or unwanted cells. The regulation of apoptosis involves:

- **Intrinsic Pathway:** This pathway is triggered by internal signals, such as DNA damage or oxidative stress. Mitochondria release cytochrome c, which activates caspases, leading to cell death.
- **Extrinsic Pathway:** This pathway is activated by external signals, such as the binding of death ligands (e.g., FasL) to their receptors (e.g., Fas). This binding activates caspases, initiating apoptosis.
- **Inhibition of Apoptosis:** In HNCs, the intrinsic and extrinsic pathways are often disrupted, leading to the survival of cancer cells. For example, overexpression of anti-apoptotic proteins like Bcl-2 and IAPs (inhibitors of apoptosis proteins) has been observed in HNCs.

Signaling Pathways

Several signaling pathways are involved in the regulation of cell growth, differentiation, and survival in HNCs. Key pathways include:

- **EGFR Pathway:** The epidermal growth factor receptor (EGFR) is frequently overexpressed in HNCs. EGFR activation leads to the activation of downstream signaling pathways, such as the MAPK and PI3K/AKT pathways, which promote cell proliferation and survival.

- **NF-κB Pathway:** NF-κB is a transcription factor that regulates the expression of genes involved in inflammation, cell survival, and immune responses. In HNCs, NF-κB is often constitutively active, leading to the promotion of cancer cell survival and resistance to apoptosis.
- **Wnt/β-Catenin Pathway:** The Wnt/β-catenin pathway is involved in regulating cell proliferation and differentiation. Aberrant activation of this pathway has been implicated in the development and progression of HNCs.

Known Causes Related to Animal Products

The consumption of animal products has been linked to an increased risk of developing head and neck cancers. Several mechanisms explain this association, including the presence of carcinogens in animal products, the role of animal fats in promoting inflammation, and the potential for nutrient imbalances.

Carcinogens in Animal Products

Animal products can contain carcinogens, such as polycyclic aromatic hydrocarbons (PAHs), heterocyclic amines (HCAs), and nitrosamines, which are formed during the cooking process, particularly when meat is grilled, smoked, or processed.

- **Polycyclic Aromatic Hydrocarbons (PAHs):** PAHs are formed when meat is cooked at high temperatures, such as during grilling or barbecuing. These compounds can bind to DNA, causing mutations that initiate carcinogenesis.
- **Heterocyclic Amines (HCAs):** HCAs are formed when amino acids, sugars, and creatine in meat react at high temperatures.

HCAs are potent mutagens that can induce DNA damage, leading to the development of cancer.

- **Nitrosamines:** Nitrosamines are carcinogenic compounds that can form in processed meats, such as bacon, sausages, and hot dogs, due to the presence of nitrites and nitrates. Nitrosamines can cause DNA damage and contribute to the initiation of cancer.

Role of Animal Fats in Promoting Inflammation

Diets high in animal fats have been associated with chronic inflammation, a known risk factor for the development of HNCs. The mechanisms by which animal fats promote inflammation include:

- **Production of Pro-inflammatory Cytokines:** Consumption of saturated fats, commonly found in animal products, can lead to the production of pro-inflammatory cytokines, such as TNF-α and IL-6. These cytokines promote chronic inflammation, which can damage DNA and support cancer development.
- **Oxidative Stress:** Animal fats can increase oxidative stress by generating reactive oxygen species (ROS). ROS can cause DNA damage, lipid peroxidation, and protein oxidation, all of which contribute to the initiation and progression of cancer.
- **Activation of the NF-κB Pathway:** Saturated fats can activate the NF-κB pathway, which regulates the expression of genes involved in inflammation and cell survival. Chronic activation of this pathway can lead to the promotion of cancer cell survival and resistance to apoptosis.

Nutrient Imbalances and Deficiencies

Diets rich in animal products are often deficient in essential nutrients, such as fiber, vitamins, and antioxidants, which are critical for maintaining DNA integrity and regulating cell function.

- **Fiber Deficiency:** A lack of dietary fiber, which is abundant in plant-based foods, can lead to alterations in gut microbiota and the production of harmful metabolites, such as secondary bile acids. These metabolites can increase the risk of developing HNCs by promoting inflammation and DNA damage.
- **Vitamin Deficiencies:** Animal-based diets may lack sufficient vitamins A, C, and E, which are potent antioxidants that protect cells from oxidative damage. Deficiencies in these vitamins can impair the body's ability to repair DNA and regulate cell proliferation, increasing the risk of cancer.
- **Mineral Deficiencies:** Diets low in plant-based foods may be deficient in essential minerals, such as selenium and magnesium, which play a role in DNA repair and antioxidant defense. A lack of these minerals can contribute to the development of HNCs.

How a Plant-Based Diet Can Help with Reversal

A plant-based diet has been shown to offer numerous benefits in the prevention and reversal of head and neck cancers. This diet is rich in fruits, vegetables, whole grains, legumes, nuts, and seeds, which provide essential nutrients, antioxidants, and phytochemicals that support the body's natural defenses against cancer.

Antioxidant Protection

Plant-based foods are rich in antioxidants, such as vitamins A, C, and E, flavonoids, and polyphenols, which protect cells from oxidative damage and reduce inflammation.

- **Vitamin A:** Found in foods like carrots, sweet potatoes, and leafy greens, vitamin A plays a crucial role in maintaining the integrity of epithelial tissues and supporting the immune system. It also regulates cell differentiation and proliferation, helping to prevent the development of cancerous cells.

- **Vitamin C:** Abundant in citrus fruits, berries, and cruciferous vegetables, vitamin C is a potent antioxidant that neutralizes free radicals and supports the immune system. It also plays a role in collagen synthesis, which is essential for maintaining the structural integrity of tissues.
- **Vitamin E:** Found in nuts, seeds, and leafy greens, vitamin E protects cell membranes from oxidative damage and supports the immune response. It also regulates cell signaling pathways that control cell growth and differentiation.
- **Flavonoids and Polyphenols:** These phytochemicals, found in a variety of fruits, vegetables, and teas, have anti-inflammatory, antioxidant, and anti-cancer properties. They help to reduce the production of pro-inflammatory cytokines, inhibit angiogenesis, and promote apoptosis in cancer cells.

Anti-inflammatory Effects

A plant-based diet is naturally anti-inflammatory due to its high content of fiber, antioxidants, and omega-3 fatty acids.

- **Dietary Fiber:** Fiber, found in whole grains, fruits, vegetables, and legumes, promotes a healthy gut microbiota, which plays a role in regulating the immune response and reducing inflammation. Fiber also binds to carcinogens in the digestive tract, aiding in their elimination from the body.
- **Omega-3 Fatty Acids:** While plant-based sources of omega-3s, such as flaxseeds, chia seeds, and walnuts, are not as concentrated as those found in fish, they still provide essential anti-inflammatory benefits. Omega-3s inhibit the production of pro-inflammatory eicosanoids and reduce the activation of the NF-κB pathway.

Regulation of Cell Growth and Apoptosis

Plant-based foods contain compounds that regulate cell growth and promote apoptosis in cancer cells.

- **Indole-3-Carbinol (I3C):** Found in cruciferous vegetables like broccoli, cabbage, and kale, I3C modulates the expression of genes involved in cell cycle regulation and apoptosis. It also inhibits the activation of estrogen receptors, reducing the risk of hormone-related cancers.
- **Sulforaphane:** Another compound found in cruciferous vegetables, sulforaphane activates detoxification enzymes, promotes apoptosis, and inhibits angiogenesis. It also enhances the body's ability to repair DNA damage.
- **Resveratrol:** Found in grapes, berries, and peanuts, resveratrol has anti-cancer properties due to its ability to inhibit the proliferation of cancer cells, induce apoptosis, and reduce inflammation. It also modulates the expression of genes involved in cell cycle regulation and DNA repair.

Immune System Support

A plant-based diet supports the immune system by providing essential nutrients and phytochemicals that enhance immune function.

- **Beta-Glucans:** Found in mushrooms, oats, and barley, beta-glucans stimulate the activity of immune cells, such as macrophages, natural killer cells, and T-cells, which play a crucial role in identifying and destroying cancer cells.
- **Vitamin D:** While not exclusively found in plant-based foods, vitamin D can be obtained from fortified plant milks and supplements. It plays a critical role in regulating the immune response and enhancing the body's ability to fight off infections and cancer.

• **Zinc:** Found in nuts, seeds, and legumes, zinc is essential for the proper functioning of immune cells and the production of antibodies. It also plays a role in DNA repair and the regulation of apoptosis.

Mechanisms of Cancer Reversal

The potential for a plant-based diet to reverse head and neck cancer lies in its ability to target multiple pathways involved in cancer development and progression. These mechanisms include:

DNA Repair and Protection

Plant-based foods provide essential nutrients and antioxidants that support DNA repair and protect against further damage.

• **Folate:** Found in leafy greens, legumes, and fortified grains, folate is essential for DNA synthesis and repair. Adequate intake of folate has been associated with a reduced risk of developing HNCs.

• **Antioxidants:** As mentioned earlier, antioxidants neutralize free radicals, reducing oxidative stress and preventing DNA damage. This reduces the likelihood of mutations that could lead to cancer progression.

Epigenetic Modulation

Epigenetic changes, such as DNA methylation and histone modification, play a role in the regulation of gene expression. Certain plant-based compounds have been shown to modulate epigenetic changes, potentially reversing abnormal gene expression patterns associated with cancer.

• **Curcumin:** Found in turmeric, curcumin has been shown to modulate DNA methylation and histone acetylation, leading to the reactivation of tumor suppressor genes and the inhibition of oncogenes.

- **Green Tea Polyphenols:** Epigallocatechin gallate (EGCG), a polyphenol found in green tea, has been shown to modulate epigenetic changes, inhibiting the expression of genes involved in cancer cell proliferation and survival.

Inhibition of Angiogenesis

The inhibition of angiogenesis, the process of new blood vessel formation, is crucial for restricting the growth and spread of cancer. Plant-based compounds that inhibit angiogenesis include:

- **Lycopene:** Found in tomatoes and other red fruits, lycopene has been shown to inhibit angiogenesis by reducing the expression of VEGF and other pro-angiogenic factors.
- **Genistein:** A phytoestrogen found in soy products, genistein inhibits angiogenesis by modulating the expression of genes involved in the VEGF pathway.

Promotion of Apoptosis

The promotion of apoptosis in cancer cells is a key mechanism by which a plant-based diet can contribute to cancer reversal.

- **Quercetin:** Found in apples, onions, and berries, quercetin induces apoptosis in cancer cells by activating caspases and inhibiting anti-apoptotic proteins.
- **Apigenin:** Found in parsley, celery, and chamomile, apigenin promotes apoptosis by modulating the expression of pro-apoptotic and anti-apoptotic genes.

Head and neck cancers are a diverse group of malignancies with significant morbidity and mortality. While various factors contribute to their development, including genetic predispositions, lifestyle choices, and environmental exposures, diet plays a crucial role. The consump-

tion of animal products has been linked to an increased risk of developing these cancers due to the presence of carcinogens, the promotion of
inflammation, and nutrient imbalances.

Conversely, a plant-based diet offers protective benefits and may
even aid in the reversal of head and neck cancers. This diet provides
essential nutrients, antioxidants, and phytochemicals that support the
body's natural defenses against cancer, including DNA repair, immune
system support, and the regulation of cell growth and apoptosis. By targeting multiple pathways involved in cancer development and progression, a plant-based diet can play a vital role in both the prevention and
management of head and neck cancers.

Kidney Cancer

Kidney cancer, also known as renal cell carcinoma (RCC), originates
in the kidneys, which are responsible for filtering blood, removing
waste, and balancing electrolytes in the body. The kidneys play a critical
role in homeostasis, and their impairment can lead to and their impairment can lead to severe health consequences.

Function of Kidney Cancer

Kidney cancer typically develops in the renal tubules, the small tubes
in the kidney where the blood is filtered. The primary function of kidney cancer cells, like all cancer cells, is abnormal growth and proliferation. Unlike normal cells that undergo a regulated cycle of growth,
division, and death (apoptosis), cancer cells evade these controls, allowing them to grow unchecked. This uncontrolled growth can lead to the
formation of tumors, which can impair the kidney's ability to perform

its normal functions, such as filtering blood, balancing fluids, and regulating blood pressure.

As kidney cancer progresses, it can invade surrounding tissues and spread (metastasize) to other parts of the body, such as the lungs, bones, and brain. This metastatic spread is a key factor in the severity and prognosis of kidney cancer, as it complicates treatment and reduces the likelihood of a full recovery.

Production of Kidney Cancer

The production of kidney cancer involves a complex interplay of genetic, environmental, and lifestyle factors. The process begins at the cellular level, where mutations in specific genes lead to the abnormal behavior of kidney cells. These mutations can be inherited (germline mutations) or acquired during a person's lifetime (somatic mutations).

Genetic Mutations

Several key genes are implicated in the development of kidney cancer. The most well-known is the Von Hippel-Lindau (VHL) gene, which is mutated in approximately 90% of clear cell renal cell carcinomas (ccRCC), the most common subtype of kidney cancer. The VHL gene plays a crucial role in regulating cellular responses to hypoxia (low oxygen levels). When functioning normally, the VHL protein helps degrade hypoxia-inducible factors (HIFs) that promote angiogenesis (the formation of new blood vessels). However, when the VHL gene is mutated, HIFs accumulate, leading to increased angiogenesis, cell proliferation, and tumor growth.

Other genetic mutations associated with kidney cancer include alterations in the PBRM1, SETD2, BAP1, and TP53 genes. These mutations contribute to various aspects of tumor biology, including chromatin remodeling, DNA repair, and cell cycle regulation.

Environmental and Lifestyle Factors

Environmental and lifestyle factors also play a significant role in the production of kidney cancer. Smoking is a major risk factor, with studies showing that smokers are twice as likely to develop kidney cancer as non-smokers. Tobacco smoke contains carcinogenic compounds that can cause mutations in kidney cells, leading to cancer development.

Obesity is another important risk factor, as excess body weight is associated with chronic inflammation, insulin resistance, and increased levels of growth factors such as insulin-like growth factor (IGF-1), all of which can promote cancer development. Hypertension, often associated with obesity, is also linked to an increased risk of kidney cancer, possibly due to the damaging effects of high blood pressure on the kidney's blood vessels.

Dietary factors, particularly the consumption of animal products, have also been implicated in the production of kidney cancer. High intake of red and processed meats has been associated with an increased risk of RCC. This risk is thought to be related to the presence of carcinogenic compounds such as heterocyclic amines (HCAs) and polycyclic aromatic hydrocarbons (PAHs) that form during the cooking of meat at high temperatures.

Regulation of Kidney Cancer

The regulation of kidney cancer involves a network of signaling pathways that control cell growth, survival, and differentiation. In normal cells, these pathways maintain a balance between cell proliferation and apoptosis. However, in cancer cells, this balance is disrupted, leading to uncontrolled growth and tumor formation.

Hypoxia-Inducible Factor (HIF) Pathway

The HIF pathway is central to the regulation of kidney cancer, particularly in cases where the VHL gene is mutated. Under normal oxygen conditions, the VHL protein targets HIFs for degradation, preventing them from activating pro-angiogenic and pro-proliferative genes. However, in the absence of functional VHL, HIFs accumulate and activate genes that promote angiogenesis, cell proliferation, and glucose metabolism, all of which contribute to tumor growth.

Mammalian Target of Rapamycin (mTOR) Pathway

The mTOR pathway is another critical regulator of kidney cancer. mTOR is a kinase that integrates signals from growth factors, nutrients, and energy status to regulate cell growth and metabolism. In kidney cancer, the mTOR pathway is often hyperactivated, leading to increased cell growth and survival. This pathway is a key target for therapeutic intervention, with several mTOR inhibitors, such as everolimus and temsirolimus, approved for the treatment of advanced RCC.

Vascular Endothelial Growth Factor (VEGF) Pathway

The VEGF pathway is involved in the formation of new blood vessels (angiogenesis), which is essential for tumor growth and metastasis. In kidney cancer, the upregulation of VEGF, often due to HIF activation, leads to increased angiogenesis, allowing the tumor to obtain the nutrients and oxygen it needs to grow. VEGF inhibitors, such as bevacizumab and sunitinib, are used to block this pathway and inhibit tumor growth.

Cell Cycle Regulation

The cell cycle is tightly regulated by a series of checkpoints that ensure cells only divide when it is safe and necessary. In kidney cancer, mutations in genes such as TP53 and CDKN2A disrupt these checkpoints, allowing cells to proliferate unchecked. Therapeutic strategies that target cell cycle regulators are being explored as potential treatments for kidney cancer.

Pathways Involved in Kidney Cancer

Several key pathways are involved in the development and progression of kidney cancer. These pathways interact in complex ways to drive the growth and spread of tumors.

1. PI3K/AKT/mTOR Pathway

The PI3K/AKT/mTOR pathway is a critical regulator of cell growth, metabolism, and survival. In kidney cancer, this pathway is often hyperactivated due to mutations in genes such as PTEN and PIK3CA. Activation of this pathway promotes cell proliferation and survival while inhibiting apoptosis. The mTOR inhibitors mentioned earlier target this pathway to inhibit tumor growth.

2. HIF/VEGF Pathway

The HIF/VEGF pathway is central to the angiogenesis process in kidney cancer. As discussed earlier, mutations in the VHL gene lead to the accumulation of HIFs, which in turn activate the expression of VEGF and other pro-angiogenic factors. This pathway is a major target for anti-angiogenic therapies in kidney cancer.

3. WNT/β-Catenin Pathway

The WNT/β-catenin pathway is involved in regulating cell fate, proliferation, and migration. In kidney cancer, aberrant activation of this pathway can lead to increased cell proliferation and tumor growth. Mutations in genes such as CTNNB1 (which encodes β-catenin) have been found in some cases of RCC, contributing to tumor development.

4. p53 Pathway

The p53 pathway is a crucial regulator of the cell cycle and apoptosis. The TP53 gene, which encodes the p53 protein, is often mutated in various cancers, including kidney cancer. When functional, p53 acts as a tumor suppressor, triggering cell cycle arrest or apoptosis in response to DNA damage. However, mutations in TP53 can lead to the loss of this protective function, allowing cells to accumulate further mutations and become cancerous.

5. MET Pathway

The MET pathway is involved in cell growth, survival, and motility. Mutations in the MET gene, which encodes the hepatocyte growth factor receptor (HGFR), are found in a subset of kidney cancers, particularly in papillary RCC. Activation of the MET pathway promotes cell proliferation and metastasis, making it an important target for therapy.

6. NF-κB Pathway

The NF-κB pathway is a key regulator of inflammation and immune responses. In kidney cancer, chronic inflammation can activate the NF-κB pathway, leading to increased cell survival, proliferation, and resistance to apoptosis. This pathway is also involved in the tumor microenvironment, promoting angiogenesis and immune evasion.

Known Causes Related to Animal Products

The link between diet and cancer has been the subject of extensive research, with strong evidence pointing to the role of certain animal products in increasing the risk of various cancers, including kidney cancer.

Red and Processed Meats

Red and processed meats have been identified as significant risk factors for kidney cancer. Studies have shown that the consumption of these meats is associated with an increased risk of RCC. The carcinogenic potential of red and processed meats is thought to be due to several factors:

1. Heterocyclic Amines (HCAs) and Polycyclic Aromatic Hydrocarbons (PAHs): These compounds are formed during the cooking of meat at high temperatures, such as grilling, frying, or barbecuing. HCAs and PAHs are known to cause DNA damage, leading to mutations that can initiate cancer development.

2. Nitrites and Nitrates: These compounds are commonly used as preservatives in processed meats. In the body, nitrites and nitrates can be converted into nitrosamines, which are potent carcinogens. Nitrosamines can induce mutations in kidney cells, increasing the risk of cancer.

3. Saturated Fat: High intake of saturated fat, which is abundant in red and processed meats, has been linked to an increased risk of kidney cancer. Saturated fat can contribute to obesity, insulin resistance, and chronic inflammation, all of which are risk factors for cancer.

Dairy Products

Dairy products have also been implicated in the risk of kidney cancer. Some studies suggest that high consumption of dairy products, particularly those high in fat, may be associated with an increased risk of RCC. The potential mechanisms include:

1. Insulin-Like Growth Factor (IGF-1): Dairy products are a significant source of IGF-1, a hormone that promotes cell growth and proliferation. Elevated levels of IGF-1 have been linked to an increased risk of several cancers, including kidney cancer.

2. Calcium: While calcium is essential for bone health, excessive intake, particularly from dairy products, has been associated with an increased risk of kidney stones and possibly kidney cancer. High calcium intake can lead to hypercalciuria (excessive calcium in the urine), which may contribute to the development of RCC.

3. Hormones: Dairy products contain hormones such as estrogen and progesterone, which can influence cancer risk. The presence of these hormones in dairy products may promote the growth of hormone-sensitive tumors, including kidney cancer.

Eggs

The consumption of eggs has been associated with an increased risk of kidney cancer in some studies. The potential mechanisms include:

1. Choline: Eggs are a rich source of choline, a nutrient that can be converted into trimethylamine N-oxide (TMAO) in the body. High levels of TMAO have been linked to an increased risk of cancer, including kidney cancer.

2. Arachidonic Acid: Eggs contain arachidonic acid, an omega-6 fatty acid that can promote inflammation. Chronic inflammation is a known risk factor for cancer, including kidney cancer.

How a Plant-Based Diet Can Help with Reversal

A plant-based diet, which emphasizes fruits, vegetables, whole grains, legumes, nuts, and seeds, has been shown to offer numerous health benefits, including the potential to reduce the risk of cancer and even aid in the reversal of certain cancers, including kidney cancer.

Antioxidants and Phytochemicals

Plant-based foods are rich in antioxidants and phytochemicals, which have powerful anti-cancer properties. Antioxidants, such as vitamins C and E, beta-carotene, and selenium, help neutralize free radicals, which can cause DNA damage and lead to cancer. Phytochemicals, such as flavonoids, carotenoids, and polyphenols, have been shown to inhibit tumor growth, induce apoptosis, and block angiogenesis.

1. Flavonoids: Found in fruits, vegetables, and legumes, flavonoids have been shown to reduce the risk of kidney cancer. They work by inhibiting the proliferation of cancer cells, inducing apoptosis, and reducing inflammation.

2. Carotenoids: These pigments, found in colorful fruits and vegetables, have antioxidant properties that protect cells from damage. Carotenoids, such as lycopene and beta-carotene, have been linked to a reduced risk of several cancers, including kidney cancer.

3. Polyphenols: Present in foods like tea, coffee, berries, and dark chocolate, polyphenols have anti-inflammatory and anti-cancer effects. They can inhibit the growth of cancer cells, reduce angiogenesis, and enhance the body's immune response to cancer.

Fiber and Gut Health

A plant-based diet is naturally high in dietary fiber, which promotes gut health and may reduce the risk of kidney cancer. Fiber helps maintain a healthy gut microbiome, which plays a crucial role in modulating the immune system and protecting against cancer. A healthy gut microbiome can metabolize dietary fiber into short-chain fatty acids (SCFAs), such as butyrate, which have anti-inflammatory and anti-cancer properties.

Alkaline Diet

A plant-based diet is generally more alkaline than a diet rich in animal products. An alkaline diet helps maintain the body's pH balance, reducing the risk of chronic diseases, including cancer. Cancer cells thrive in an acidic environment, which can be promoted by the consumption of animal products. By contrast, a plant-based diet helps create a more alkaline internal environment, which is less conducive to cancer growth.

Reduced Exposure to Carcinogens

A plant-based diet reduces exposure to carcinogens commonly found in animal products, such as HCAs, PAHs, nitrosamines, and hormones. By avoiding these harmful substances, individuals can reduce their risk of developing kidney cancer and other cancers.

Weight Management

Obesity is a significant risk factor for kidney cancer, and a plant-based diet can help with weight management. Plant-based diets are typically lower in calories and higher in nutrients than diets rich in animal products, making it easier to maintain a healthy weight. Weight loss and maintenance reduce the risk of kidney cancer by lowering levels of insulin, IGF-1, and other growth factors that can promote cancer development.

Improved Insulin Sensitivity

A plant-based diet can improve insulin sensitivity, reducing the risk of kidney cancer. High insulin levels are associated with an increased risk of cancer, as insulin promotes cell proliferation and inhibits apoptosis. Plant-based diets, particularly those rich in whole grains, legumes, and vegetables, help regulate blood sugar levels and improve insulin sensitivity, reducing cancer risk.

Anti-Inflammatory Effects

Chronic inflammation is a known risk factor for cancer, and a plant-based diet has potent anti-inflammatory effects. Foods such as leafy greens, berries, nuts, seeds, and fatty fish contain anti-inflammatory compounds that can reduce the risk of cancer. By reducing inflammation, a plant-based diet can help prevent the initiation and progression of kidney cancer.

Epigenetic Modulation

Epigenetics refers to changes in gene expression that do not involve alterations in the DNA sequence. Diet can influence epigenetic modifications, which can impact cancer risk. A plant-based diet rich in folate, vitamin B12, and other nutrients can promote healthy epigenetic changes, reducing the risk of kidney cancer. For example, folate plays a crucial role in DNA methylation, a process that can silence oncogenes and protect against cancer.

Immune System Support

A plant-based diet supports the immune system, which is essential for preventing and fighting cancer. Foods such as mushrooms, garlic, ginger, and turmeric have immune-boosting properties that can enhance the body's ability to detect and destroy cancer cells. A strong immune system is crucial for the prevention and reversal of kidney cancer.

Kidney cancer is a complex disease influenced by genetic, environmental, and lifestyle factors. The production and regulation of kidney cancer involve various pathways, including the HIF/VEGF, mTOR, and p53 pathways. Known causes related to animal products, such as red and processed meats, dairy products, and eggs, contribute to the risk of kidney cancer through mechanisms involving carcinogens, hormones, and inflammation.

A plant-based diet offers a promising approach to reducing the risk of kidney cancer and aiding in its reversal. The rich array of antioxidants, phytochemicals, fiber, and other nutrients in plant-based foods supports the body's natural defenses against cancer. By reducing exposure to carcinogens, improving weight management, enhancing insulin sensitivity, and modulating epigenetics, a plant-based diet can play a crucial role in preventing and reversing kidney cancer.

Leukemia

Leukemia is a type of cancer that affects the blood and bone marrow, characterized by the overproduction of abnormal white blood cells. These cells, unlike normal white blood cells, do not function properly and can interfere with the production and function of normal blood cells, leading to a range of serious health issues. Understanding the function, production, regulation, and causes of leukemia, including its connection to diet, is crucial for developing effective strategies for prevention and treatment.

Function and Production of Leukemia Cells

Leukemia originates in the bone marrow, the soft tissue inside bones where blood cells are produced. Under normal conditions, the bone marrow produces three main types of blood cells: red blood cells (which carry oxygen), white blood cells (which fight infection), and platelets (which help with blood clotting). The production of these cells is tightly regulated by the body to ensure that the right amounts are produced at the right times.

In leukemia, this regulation is disrupted, leading to the overproduction of abnormal white blood cells. These cells, called leukemia cells, do not function properly and do not die when they should. Instead, they accumulate in the bone marrow, crowding out normal cells and preventing them from functioning correctly. Over time, these leukemia cells can spill into the bloodstream and spread to other parts of the body, including the lymph nodes, spleen, liver, central nervous system, and other organs.

Leukemia is classified into several types, based on the type of white blood cell affected and the speed at which the disease progresses. The main types include:

- **Acute Lymphoblastic Leukemia (ALL):** A fast-growing type of leukemia that affects lymphocytes, a type of white blood cell involved in the immune response.
- **Acute Myeloid Leukemia (AML):** A fast-growing leukemia that affects myeloid cells, which are precursors to various types of blood cells, including white blood cells, red blood cells, and platelets.

- **Chronic Lymphocytic Leukemia (CLL):** A slow-growing leukemia that affects lymphocytes and typically progresses over many years.
- **Chronic Myeloid Leukemia (CML):** A slow-growing leukemia that affects myeloid cells and can transition into a more aggressive phase over time.

Regulation of Leukemia Cells

The regulation of blood cell production in the bone marrow is a complex process that involves a variety of signaling pathways and regulatory proteins. Under normal circumstances, hematopoietic stem cells (HSCs) in the bone marrow differentiate into various types of blood cells in a highly controlled manner. This process is regulated by a network of growth factors, cytokines, and transcription factors that ensure the proper balance of cell proliferation, differentiation, and apoptosis (programmed cell death).

In leukemia, this regulatory network is disrupted, often due to genetic mutations that affect key regulatory proteins. These mutations can lead to uncontrolled cell proliferation, impaired differentiation, and resistance to apoptosis, all of which contribute to the accumulation of leukemia cells in the bone marrow and other tissues.

Several key pathways are involved in the regulation of blood cell production and are frequently altered in leukemia:

- **Notch Signaling Pathway:** This pathway plays a critical role in the regulation of hematopoietic stem cells and their differentiation into various blood cell lineages. Mutations or dysregulation of Notch signaling can lead to the development of leukemia by promoting the survival and proliferation of abnormal cells.
- **Wnt/β-catenin Pathway:** The Wnt/β-catenin pathway is involved in the regulation of stem cell self-renewal and differentiation. Dysregulation of this pathway can contribute to leukemia

by promoting the expansion of leukemic stem cells and inhibiting their differentiation.

- **JAK/STAT Pathway:** The JAK/STAT pathway is involved in the transmission of signals from growth factors and cytokines to the cell nucleus, where they regulate gene expression. Mutations in components of this pathway, such as the JAK2 gene, are commonly found in leukemia and can lead to uncontrolled cell proliferation.

- **PI3K/AKT/mTOR Pathway:** This pathway is involved in cell survival, growth, and metabolism. Dysregulation of the PI3K/AKT/mTOR pathway is frequently observed in leukemia and contributes to the resistance of leukemia cells to apoptosis.

- **p53 Pathway:** The p53 protein is a key regulator of the cell cycle and apoptosis. Mutations in the TP53 gene, which encodes p53, are common in many types of cancer, including leukemia, and can lead to the survival of cells with damaged DNA, contributing to the development and progression of the disease.

Detailed Pathways Involved in Leukemia

Leukemia is a multifactorial disease, with its development and progression influenced by a variety of genetic, environmental, and lifestyle factors. The following are some of the key molecular pathways involved in the pathogenesis of leukemia:

1. Genetic Mutations and Chromosomal Abnormalities

Genetic mutations and chromosomal abnormalities are common in leukemia and play a central role in its development. Some of the most well-known genetic alterations include:

- **Philadelphia Chromosome:** This chromosomal abnormality, resulting from a translocation between chromosomes 9 and 22, is found in the majority of cases of chronic myeloid leukemia (CML). It leads to the formation of the BCR-ABL fusion gene, which encodes an abnormal tyrosine kinase protein that drives uncontrolled cell proliferation.

- **FLT3 Mutations:** Mutations in the FLT3 gene, which encodes a receptor tyrosine kinase, are common in acute myeloid leukemia (AML) and are associated with a poor prognosis. These mutations lead to the constitutive activation of the FLT3 receptor, promoting cell survival and proliferation.
- **NPM1 Mutations:** Mutations in the NPM1 gene, which encodes a nucleophosmin protein involved in ribosome biogenesis and cellular stress responses, are found in a significant proportion of AML cases. These mutations are associated with increased survival and proliferation of leukemia cells.
- **IDH1/IDH2 Mutations:** Mutations in the IDH1 and IDH2 genes, which encode isocitrate dehydrogenase enzymes, are found in some cases of AML and are associated with altered cellular metabolism and epigenetic changes that contribute to leukemogenesis.

2. Epigenetic Alterations

Epigenetic changes, which involve modifications to DNA and histones that affect gene expression without altering the underlying DNA sequence, are also important in leukemia. These changes can lead to the silencing of tumor suppressor genes or the activation of oncogenes, contributing to the development and progression of the disease. Some key epigenetic alterations in leukemia include:

- **DNA Methylation:** Hypermethylation of CpG islands in the promoter regions of tumor suppressor genes can lead to their silencing, contributing to leukemogenesis. Hypomethylating agents, such as azacitidine and decitabine, are used in the treatment of some types of leukemia to reverse these changes.
- **Histone Modifications:** Alterations in histone acetylation and methylation can affect chromatin structure and gene expression

in leukemia cells. Inhibitors of histone deacetylases (HDACs) are being explored as potential therapies for leukemia.

- **MicroRNAs:** MicroRNAs (miRNAs) are small non-coding RNAs that regulate gene expression by binding to messenger RNAs (mRNAs) and preventing their translation. Dysregulation of miRNAs is common in leukemia and can contribute to the disease by affecting the expression of key regulatory genes.

3. Immune Evasion

Leukemia cells can evade the immune system through a variety of mechanisms, allowing them to survive and proliferate. Some of these mechanisms include:

- **PD-1/PD-L1 Pathway:** The interaction between the pro-grammed cell death protein 1 (PD-1) on T cells and its ligand PD-L1 on leukemia cells can inhibit the immune response, allowing the leukemia cells to evade detection and destruction. Immune checkpoint inhibitors that block this interaction are being inves-tigated as potential treatments for leukemia.
- **Cytokine Secretion:** Leukemia cells can secrete cytokines that suppress the immune response or promote the survival of leukemia cells. For example, interleukin-10 (IL-10) and trans-forming growth factor-beta (TGF-β) are cytokines that can in-hibit the activity of T cells and natural killer (NK) cells, allowing leukemia cells to escape immune surveillance.

Known Causes of Leukemia Related to Animal Products

While the exact causes of leukemia are not fully understood, research has identified several risk factors that can increase the likelihood of de-veloping the disease. Among these risk factors, diet, particularly the con-sumption of animal products, has been implicated in the development of certain types of leukemia.

1. Processed Meats and Leukemia

Processed meats, such as bacon, sausages, and hot dogs, have been classified as carcinogenic to humans by the International Agency for Research on Cancer (IARC), a part of the World Health Organization (WHO). These meats are often high in nitrates and nitrites, which can be converted into carcinogenic N-nitroso compounds (NOCs) in the body. Studies have shown that high consumption of processed meats is associated with an increased risk of several types of cancer, including leukemia.

The mechanisms by which processed meats contribute to leukemogenesis may involve:

- **DNA Damage:** NOCs and other carcinogens found in processed meats can cause DNA damage in hematopoietic stem cells, leading to mutations that contribute to the development of leukemia.
- **Oxidative Stress:** Processed meats are also high in saturated fats and cholesterol, which can increase oxidative stress in the body. Oxidative stress can lead to DNA damage and the activation of oncogenes, promoting the development of leukemia.

2. Red Meat and Leukemia

Red meat consumption has also been linked to an increased risk of leukemia, particularly in individuals who consume large amounts of well-done or charred meat. Cooking meat at high temperatures can produce carcinogenic compounds, such as heterocyclic amines (HCAs) and polycyclic aromatic hydrocarbons (PAHs), which can damage DNA and contribute to cancer development.

The potential mechanisms by which red meat contributes to leukemogenesis include:

- **HCAs and PAHs:** These carcinogenic compounds are formed when meat is cooked at high temperatures, such as grilling or frying. They can cause DNA mutations in hematopoietic stem cells, increasing the risk of leukemia.
- **Heme Iron:** Red meat is a rich source of heme iron, which can promote the formation of free radicals and oxidative stress in the body. Oxidative stress can damage DNA and contribute to the development of leukemia.

3. Dairy Products and Leukemia

The consumption of dairy products has been linked to an increased risk of certain cancers, including leukemia. Dairy products are high in saturated fats, hormones, and growth factors, which can promote the growth and proliferation of cancer cells.

The potential mechanisms by which dairy products contribute to leukemogenesis include:

- **Insulin-like Growth Factor-1 (IGF-1):** Dairy products are a significant source of IGF-1, a hormone that promotes cell growth and proliferation. Elevated levels of IGF-1 have been associated with an increased risk of several cancers, including leukemia.
- **Hormones:** Dairy products contain various hormones, including estrogen and progesterone, which can promote the growth of hormone-sensitive cancers. These hormones may also play a role in the development of leukemia by promoting the proliferation of abnormal cells.

How a Plant-Based Diet Can Help with Leukemia Reversal

A plant-based diet, rich in fruits, vegetables, whole grains, legumes, nuts, and seeds, has been shown to have numerous health benefits, including a reduced risk of cancer. For individuals with leukemia, a plant-based diet may offer several advantages that can help with the reversal of the disease and improve overall health.

1. Antioxidant and Anti-Inflammatory Properties

Plant-based foods are rich in antioxidants and anti-inflammatory compounds, which can help protect against DNA damage and reduce inflammation, both of which are important in the prevention and treatment of leukemia.

- **Fruits and Vegetables:** These foods are high in vitamins, minerals, and phytochemicals that have potent antioxidant and anti-inflammatory effects. For example, flavonoids found in fruits and vegetables can scavenge free radicals and reduce oxidative stress, protecting against DNA damage and the development of leukemia.
- **Whole Grains and Legumes:** Whole grains and legumes are rich in fiber, which has been shown to reduce inflammation and improve gut health. A healthy gut microbiome can support the immune system and reduce the risk of cancer, including leukemia.

2. Immune System Support

A plant-based diet can support the immune system by providing essential nutrients that are important for immune function, such as vitamins A, C, and E, as well as zinc and selenium.

- **Vitamin C:** This vitamin, found in high amounts in fruits and vegetables, is essential for the production and function of white blood cells, which are crucial for fighting infections and cancer cells. Vitamin C also has antioxidant properties that can protect against DNA damage.
- **Zinc:** Zinc is important for the development and function of immune cells, including T cells and natural killer (NK) cells. Plant-based sources of zinc include legumes, nuts, seeds, and whole grains.

3. Reduction of Carcinogenic Exposures

A plant-based diet eliminates or significantly reduces the consumption of processed meats, red meats, and dairy products, all of which have been linked to an increased risk of leukemia. By avoiding these foods, individuals can reduce their exposure to carcinogens and other harmful compounds that contribute to the development of leukemia.

4. Detoxification and Elimination of Toxins

Plant-based foods are rich in fiber, which supports healthy digestion and the elimination of toxins from the body. A diet high in fiber can help reduce the levels of carcinogens and other harmful compounds in the body, lowering the risk of leukemia and other cancers.

- **Cruciferous Vegetables:** Foods like broccoli, cauliflower, and Brussels sprouts contain compounds that support the body's detoxification processes, helping to eliminate carcinogens and protect against cancer.
- **Dark Leafy Greens:** These vegetables are high in chlorophyll, which can bind to carcinogens and support their elimination from the body.

5. Regulation of Blood Sugar and Insulin Levels

A plant-based diet can help regulate blood sugar and insulin levels, which is important for reducing the risk of cancer, including leukemia. High insulin levels have been associated with an increased risk of cancer, as insulin can promote cell growth and proliferation.

- **Low Glycemic Index Foods:** Plant-based foods, such as whole grains, legumes, and non-starchy vegetables, have a low glycemic index and can help maintain stable blood sugar levels.
- **Healthy Fats:** Nuts, seeds, and avocados are sources of healthy fats that can help regulate blood sugar levels and reduce inflammation.

6. Promotion of Apoptosis in Cancer Cells

Certain plant-based foods have been shown to promote apoptosis (programmed cell death) in cancer cells, which is a key mechanism for preventing the growth and spread of cancer.

- **Curcumin:** This compound, found in turmeric, has been shown to induce apoptosis in leukemia cells by activating various signaling pathways involved in cell death.
- **Green Tea:** Green tea contains polyphenols, such as epigallocatechin gallate (EGCG), which have been shown to induce apoptosis in leukemia cells and inhibit their proliferation.

7. Epigenetic Modulation

A plant-based diet can influence gene expression through epigenetic mechanisms, which may help in the prevention and treatment of leukemia. Phytochemicals found in plant-based foods can modulate the expression of genes involved in cell proliferation, apoptosis, and immune function.

- **Sulforaphane:** Found in cruciferous vegetables, sulforaphane has been shown to modulate gene expression and inhibit the growth of cancer cells, including leukemia cells.
- **Resveratrol:** This compound, found in grapes and berries, has been shown to affect gene expression and inhibit the proliferation of leukemia cells.

Leukemia is a complex and multifactorial disease that involves the dysregulation of normal blood cell production and function. While genetic mutations and chromosomal abnormalities are central to its development, environmental and lifestyle factors, including diet, also play a significant role. The consumption of animal products, particularly processed meats, red meats, and dairy, has been linked to an increased risk of leukemia due to the presence of carcinogenic compounds, hormones, and growth factors.

A plant-based diet offers numerous benefits that can help with the prevention and reversal of leukemia. By providing a rich source of antioxidants, anti-inflammatory compounds, and essential nutrients, a plant-based diet supports immune function, reduces inflammation, and promotes the elimination of toxins. Additionally, certain plant-based foods have been shown to induce apoptosis in leukemia cells and modulate gene expression, further contributing to the prevention and treatment of the disease.

Liver Cancer

Liver cancer, also known as hepatocellular carcinoma (HCC), is one of the most common types of cancer worldwide. Understanding the function, production, and regulation of liver cancer, as well as the detailed pathways involved in its development, is crucial for developing effective strategies for prevention and treatment.

Function of the Liver and Liver Cancer

The liver is one of the largest and most vital organs in the human body, responsible for numerous essential functions. It plays a key role in detoxification, protein synthesis, and the production of biochemicals necessary for digestion. The liver also regulates various metabolic processes, including the metabolism of carbohydrates, fats, and proteins. It stores glycogen, vitamins, and minerals, synthesizes plasma proteins such as albumin, and produces bile, which is crucial for the digestion and absorption of dietary fats.

Liver cancer typically arises from the hepatocytes, the main type of liver cells, leading to hepatocellular carcinoma. This form of cancer disrupts the liver's normal functions, leading to symptoms such as jaundice, abdominal pain, weight loss, and fatigue. As liver cancer progresses, it can impair the liver's ability to detoxify the blood, produce essential proteins, and manage glucose and fat metabolism, leading to severe systemic effects.

Production of Liver Cancer

The production of liver cancer is a multistep process involving genetic mutations, epigenetic alterations, and changes in cellular signaling pathways. Chronic liver inflammation, often due to viral hepatitis infections (hepatitis B and C), alcohol abuse, and non-alcoholic fatty liver disease (NAFLD), is a major risk factor for liver cancer. These conditions lead to repeated cycles of liver cell injury, death, and regeneration, creating an environment conducive to genetic mutations and the eventual development of cancer.

1. **Genetic Mutations and Alterations**: Liver cancer is driven by genetic mutations in key oncogenes and tumor suppressor genes. Mutations in the TERT promoter (telomerase reverse transcriptase), TP53, CTNNB1 (beta-catenin), and AXIN1 are commonly observed in HCC. These mutations lead to uncontrolled cell proliferation, resistance to apoptosis (programmed cell death), and increased survival of malignant cells.

2. **Epigenetic Changes**: In addition to genetic mutations, liver cancer involves epigenetic changes such as DNA methylation, histone modifications, and changes in non-coding RNA expression. These epigenetic alterations can silence tumor suppressor genes or activate oncogenes, further promoting cancer development.

3. **Cellular Signaling Pathways**: Several signaling pathways are implicated in the pathogenesis of liver cancer, including the Wnt/β-catenin pathway, PI3K/AKT/mTOR pathway, MAPK pathway, and TGF-β signaling pathway. These pathways regulate var-

ious cellular processes such as proliferation, differentiation, and survival, and their dysregulation can lead to cancer.

Regulation of Liver Cancer

The regulation of liver cancer involves both intrinsic cellular mechanisms and extrinsic factors such as the immune system and the tumor microenvironment.

1. **Tumor Suppressor Genes and Oncogenes**: The balance between tumor suppressor genes and oncogenes is crucial for the regulation of cell growth and division. In liver cancer, the inactivation of tumor suppressor genes such as TP53 and the activation of oncogenes such as MYC disrupt this balance, leading to uncontrolled cell proliferation.

2. **Immune System**: The immune system plays a dual role in liver cancer regulation. On one hand, it can recognize and destroy cancer cells through mechanisms such as cytotoxic T lymphocytes and natural killer cells. On the other hand, chronic inflammation, often driven by infections or liver damage, can create an immunosuppressive environment that promotes cancer development. Tumor-associated macrophages (TAMs) and regulatory T cells (Tregs) are often recruited to the tumor microenvironment, where they suppress anti-tumor immune responses and facilitate tumor growth.

3. **Tumor Microenvironment**: The tumor microenvironment, consisting of various cell types, extracellular matrix components, and signaling molecules, plays a critical role in liver cancer progression. Cancer-associated fibroblasts (CAFs), endothelial cells, and immune cells within the microenvironment interact with cancer cells to promote tumor growth, angiogenesis (formation of new blood vessels), and metastasis.

Detailed Pathways Involved in Liver Cancer Development

Several molecular pathways are involved in the development and progression of liver cancer. Understanding these pathways provides insights into potential therapeutic targets.

1. **Wnt/β-Catenin Pathway**: The Wnt/β-catenin signaling pathway is frequently activated in liver cancer, particularly in cases associated with hepatitis B and C infections. Mutations in the CTNNB1 gene, which encodes β-catenin, lead to the accumulation of β-catenin in the nucleus, where it activates the transcription of target genes involved in cell proliferation and survival. The dysregulation of this pathway contributes to the development and progression of liver cancer.

2. **PI3K/AKT/mTOR Pathway**: The PI3K/AKT/mTOR pathway is a key regulator of cell growth, metabolism, and survival. In liver cancer, this pathway is often activated due to mutations in genes such as PIK3CA, PTEN, and AKT. Activation of this pathway promotes cell proliferation, inhibits apoptosis, and enhances tumor growth. The mTOR inhibitor everolimus has shown some efficacy in treating liver cancer, highlighting the therapeutic potential of targeting this pathway.

3. **MAPK Pathway**: The MAPK (mitogen-activated protein kinase) pathway is another critical signaling pathway involved in liver cancer. It is activated by various growth factors and cytokines, leading to the phosphorylation and activation of downstream kinases such as ERK, JNK, and p38. These kinases regulate gene expression, cell proliferation, and survival. Mutations in the RAS and RAF genes, which are upstream regulators of the MAPK pathway, are associated with liver cancer.

4. **TGF-β Signaling Pathway**: The TGF-β (transforming growth factor-beta) signaling pathway has a complex role in liver cancer. In the early stages of liver cancer, TGF-β acts as a tumor sup-

pressor by inhibiting cell proliferation and inducing apoptosis. However, in advanced stages, it promotes tumor progression by inducing epithelial-mesenchymal transition (EMT), a process that enhances cancer cell invasion and metastasis. The dual role of TGF-β in liver cancer makes it a challenging but promising target for therapy.

5. **Angiogenesis Pathway**: Angiogenesis, the formation of new blood vessels, is a critical process in liver cancer development and progression. The vascular endothelial growth factor (VEGF) pathway is the primary regulator of angiogenesis in tumors. Overexpression of VEGF and its receptors (VEGFR) leads to increased blood vessel formation, providing nutrients and oxygen to the growing tumor. Anti-angiogenic therapies, such as bevacizumab (a VEGF inhibitor), have been explored as treatments for liver cancer.

Known Causes of Liver Cancer Related to Animal Products

Dietary factors, particularly the consumption of animal products, have been implicated in the development of liver cancer. Several components of animal products can contribute to liver cancer through different mechanisms.

1. **Aflatoxins**: Aflatoxins are potent carcinogens produced by certain molds, particularly Aspergillus species, which can contaminate food products such as peanuts, corn, and grains. These toxins are commonly found in animal products, especially in regions with poor food storage conditions. Aflatoxins cause DNA mutations, particularly in the TP53 gene, leading to liver cancer. While aflatoxins themselves are not found in animal tissues, livestock that consume contaminated feed can have higher levels of aflatoxins in their tissues, which can then be transferred to humans through the consumption of these animal products.

2. **Heme Iron**: Heme iron, found in red meat, has been associated with an increased risk of liver cancer. Heme iron can catalyze the formation of free radicals through the Fenton reaction, leading to oxidative stress and DNA damage in liver cells. This oxidative stress can initiate and promote the development of liver cancer. In contrast, non-heme iron, found in plant-based foods, is not associated with this increased risk, as it is absorbed differently and does not catalyze the same level of oxidative stress.

3. **Dioxins and PCBs**: Dioxins and polychlorinated biphenyls (PCBs) are environmental pollutants that can accumulate in animal fats. These chemicals are known to be carcinogenic and have been linked to liver cancer. Dioxins and PCBs can induce oxidative stress, disrupt endocrine signaling, and promote the activation of oncogenic pathways in liver cells. Consumption of animal products, particularly those high in fat, can increase the exposure to these toxic compounds.

4. **Saturated Fats**: High intake of saturated fats, primarily found in animal products, has been linked to non-alcoholic fatty liver disease (NAFLD), a condition characterized by excessive fat accumulation in the liver. NAFLD is a major risk factor for liver cancer, as it can progress to non-alcoholic steatohepatitis (NASH), cirrhosis, and eventually HCC. Saturated fats promote liver inflammation, insulin resistance, and oxidative stress, all of which contribute to liver cancer development.

5. **Processed Meats**: Processed meats, such as bacon, sausages, and hot dogs, contain nitrosamines and other carcinogenic compounds formed during processing and cooking. These compounds have been linked to an increased risk of liver cancer. Nitrosamines can cause DNA alkylation and mutations, leading to the initiation of cancer in liver cells.

How a Plant-Based Diet Can Help Reverse Liver Cancer

A plant-based diet, rich in fruits, vegetables, whole grains, legumes, nuts, and seeds, offers numerous benefits for liver health and may help in the reversal of liver cancer. The following are the key mechanisms by which a plant-based diet can exert protective and therapeutic effects against liver cancer.

1. **Antioxidant Properties**: Plant-based foods are rich in antioxidants such as vitamins C and E, polyphenols, flavonoids, and carotenoids. These antioxidants neutralize free radicals and reduce oxidative stress, which is a major driver of liver cancer development. By reducing oxidative damage to DNA, proteins, and lipids, a plant-based diet can help prevent the initiation and progression of liver cancer.

2. **Anti-Inflammatory Effects**: Chronic inflammation is a key factor in liver cancer development. Plant-based foods, particularly those rich in omega-3 fatty acids, phytochemicals, and fiber, have potent anti-inflammatory properties. Omega-3 fatty acids, found in flaxseeds, chia seeds, and walnuts, can reduce the production of pro-inflammatory cytokines and inhibit the NF-κB signaling pathway, which is involved in inflammation and cancer. Additionally, the fiber in plant-based foods promotes gut health and reduces systemic inflammation.

3. **Detoxification Support**: The liver is the primary organ responsible for detoxifying harmful substances, including carcinogens. A plant-based diet can enhance the liver's detoxification capacity by providing essential nutrients such as B vitamins, selenium, and sulfur compounds. Cruciferous vegetables, such as broccoli, cauliflower, and Brussels sprouts, contain glucosinolates, which are converted into bioactive compounds that induce phase II detoxification enzymes. These enzymes help to neutralize and eliminate carcinogens from the body.

4. **Regulation of Cell Proliferation**: Several plant-based compounds have been shown to regulate cell proliferation and induce apoptosis in cancer cells. For example, curcumin, found in turmeric, can inhibit the PI3K/AKT/mTOR pathway and promote the apoptosis of liver cancer cells. Similarly, resveratrol, found in grapes, can inhibit the Wnt/β-catenin pathway and reduce the proliferation of cancer cells. These compounds can help to slow down the growth of liver cancer and promote its regression.

5. **Reduction of Insulin Resistance**: Insulin resistance is a major factor in the development of NAFLD and liver cancer. A plant-based diet, particularly one low in refined carbohydrates and high in fiber, can improve insulin sensitivity and reduce the risk of liver cancer. Whole grains, legumes, and vegetables have a low glycemic index and help to stabilize blood sugar levels, reducing the demand for insulin and lowering the risk of liver cancer.

6. **Weight Management**: Obesity is a significant risk factor for liver cancer, particularly in the context of NAFLD and NASH. A plant-based diet, which is typically lower in calories and higher in fiber, can help with weight management and reduce the risk of liver cancer. By promoting satiety and reducing calorie intake, a plant-based diet can help to prevent obesity and its associated metabolic disorders.

7. **Gut Microbiome Modulation**: The gut microbiome plays a crucial role in liver health and the development of liver cancer. A plant-based diet, rich in fiber and prebiotics, can promote a healthy gut microbiome and reduce the production of harmful metabolites such as secondary bile acids and trimethylamine N-oxide (TMAO). These metabolites have been linked to liver inflammation and cancer. By supporting a diverse and healthy gut microbiome, a plant-based diet can protect against liver cancer.

8. **Epigenetic Modulation**: Certain plant-based compounds can influence epigenetic mechanisms, such as DNA methylation and

histone modification, which play a role in liver cancer. For example, green tea polyphenols, particularly epigallocatechin gallate (EGCG), have been shown to inhibit DNA methyltransferases and histone deacetylases, leading to the reactivation of tumor suppressor genes and the inhibition of cancer cell growth. These epigenetic effects can contribute to the reversal of liver cancer.

Liver cancer is a complex and multifactorial disease involving genetic mutations, epigenetic alterations, and dysregulated signaling pathways. The consumption of animal products, particularly those containing aflatoxins, heme iron, dioxins, saturated fats, and processed meats, has been associated with an increased risk of liver cancer. In contrast, a plant-based diet offers numerous protective and therapeutic benefits against liver cancer, including antioxidant, anti-inflammatory, detoxification, and epigenetic effects. By reducing oxidative stress, inflammation, and insulin resistance, a plant-based diet can help prevent the development of liver cancer and promote its reversal. The growing body of evidence supports the role of a plant-based diet in liver cancer prevention and management, making it a valuable approach for those at risk of or diagnosed with this disease.

Lung Cancer

Lung cancer is one of the most prevalent and deadly forms of cancer worldwide, with millions of new cases diagnosed each year.

Function of Lung Cancer

Lung cancer originates in the tissues of the lungs, typically in the cells lining the air passages. It occurs when abnormal cells grow uncontrollably, forming tumors that interfere with normal lung function. The primary function of the lungs is to exchange oxygen and carbon dioxide between the air and the bloodstream. Lung cancer disrupts this process by damaging the lung tissue and obstructing the airways.

Lung cancer can be categorized into two main types: non-small cell lung cancer (NSCLC) and small cell lung cancer (SCLC). NSCLC is the most common type, accounting for approximately 85% of all cases. It includes subtypes such as adenocarcinoma, squamous cell carcinoma, and large cell carcinoma. SCLC, on the other hand, is more aggressive and accounts for about 15% of lung cancer cases. Each type of lung cancer has distinct characteristics and behaviors, but all share the potential to metastasize (spread) to other parts of the body, further complicating treatment and prognosis.

Production of Lung Cancer

The production of lung cancer involves a complex interplay of genetic, environmental, and lifestyle factors. The development of lung cancer typically follows a multistep process, beginning with the initiation of genetic mutations and progressing through stages of promotion, progression, and metastasis.

Genetic Mutations

Lung cancer begins with genetic mutations that alter the normal functioning of cells. These mutations can be caused by various factors, including exposure to carcinogens, inherited genetic predispositions, and random errors in DNA replication. The most common genetic mutations associated with lung cancer occur in oncogenes and tumor suppressor genes.

Oncogenes are genes that promote cell growth and division. When mutated, they can become overactive and lead to uncontrolled cell proliferation. Common oncogenes implicated in lung cancer include the epidermal growth factor receptor (EGFR), KRAS, and ALK genes. Mutations in these genes drive the growth and survival of cancer cells.

Tumor suppressor genes, on the other hand, function to inhibit cell growth and promote cell death (apoptosis) when necessary. Mutations in tumor suppressor genes, such as TP53 and RB1, can disable these protective mechanisms, allowing cancer cells to evade apoptosis and continue growing.

Environmental and Lifestyle Factors

Environmental and lifestyle factors play a significant role in the production of lung cancer. The most well-known risk factor is smoking, which is responsible for approximately 85% of all lung cancer cases. Tobacco smoke contains over 7,000 chemicals, many of which are carcinogenic. These carcinogens can directly damage the DNA in lung cells, leading to the mutations that initiate cancer development.

Secondhand smoke, or passive smoking, also increases the risk of lung cancer. Non-smokers exposed to tobacco smoke are at a higher risk of developing lung cancer due to the inhalation of the same carcinogens present in tobacco smoke.

In addition to smoking, other environmental factors contribute to lung cancer production. These include exposure to radon gas, asbestos, air pollution, and certain occupational hazards. Radon, a naturally occurring radioactive gas, can seep into homes and buildings from the ground, and long-term exposure increases the risk of lung cancer. Asbestos, a group of naturally occurring fibrous minerals, was once widely used in construction and manufacturing. Inhalation of asbestos fibers can cause lung cancer, particularly mesothelioma, a rare and aggressive form of cancer that affects the lining of the lungs.

Air pollution, especially fine particulate matter (PM2.5), is another significant risk factor for lung cancer. Long-term exposure to polluted air, particularly in urban areas, can lead to chronic inflammation and DNA damage in lung cells, increasing the likelihood of cancer development.

Promotion and Progression

Once genetic mutations have occurred, the promotion stage of lung cancer involves the clonal expansion of mutated cells. This stage is char-

acterized by the increased proliferation of cells with oncogenic mutations, leading to the formation of a detectable tumor. Tumor cells can
acquire additional mutations that further enhance their growth and survival.

The progression stage involves the accumulation of more genetic alterations, enabling the tumor to invade surrounding tissues and metastasize to distant organs. Tumors can also develop resistance to the
body's immune system and to treatments, making lung cancer more
challenging to manage.

Regulation of Lung Cancer

The regulation of lung cancer involves multiple cellular pathways
that control cell growth, differentiation, and death. Dysregulation of
these pathways contributes to the development and progression of lung
cancer. Understanding these pathways is crucial for developing targeted
therapies and treatment strategies.

Epidermal Growth Factor Receptor (EGFR) Pathway

The EGFR pathway plays a central role in the regulation of lung cancer, particularly in NSCLC. EGFR is a receptor tyrosine kinase that,
when activated by binding to its ligands (such as epidermal growth factor), triggers a cascade of intracellular signaling pathways, including the
RAS-RAF-MEK-ERK and PI3K-AKT pathways. These pathways promote cell proliferation, survival, and angiogenesis (formation of new
blood vessels).

Mutations in the EGFR gene can lead to constitutive activation of
the receptor, driving uncontrolled cell growth and survival. Targeted
therapies known as EGFR tyrosine kinase inhibitors (TKIs), such as erlotinib and gefitinib, have been developed to block this pathway and are
used to treat patients with EGFR-mutant NSCLC.

KRAS Pathway

KRAS is a GTPase that acts as a molecular switch in cell signaling.
It is frequently mutated in lung cancer, particularly in adenocarcinomas. KRAS mutations lead to the continuous activation of downstream

signaling pathways, such as the RAF-MEK-ERK and PI3K-AKT pathways, promoting cell proliferation and survival.

KRAS mutations are associated with poor prognosis and resistance to certain therapies. While direct targeting of KRAS has been challenging, recent advances have led to the development of KRAS inhibitors, such as sotorasib, which show promise in treating KRAS-mutant lung cancer.

TP53 Pathway

TP53, commonly known as the "guardian of the genome," is a tumor suppressor gene that plays a critical role in regulating cell cycle arrest, DNA repair, and apoptosis. Mutations in TP53 are found in approximately 50% of lung cancers and are associated with more aggressive disease and resistance to therapy.

When TP53 is mutated or inactivated, cells lose the ability to undergo apoptosis in response to DNA damage, allowing cancer cells to survive and proliferate despite the accumulation of genetic alterations.

PI3K-AKT-mTOR Pathway

The PI3K-AKT-mTOR pathway is another key regulatory pathway in lung cancer. This pathway promotes cell growth, survival, and metabolism. Aberrant activation of the PI3K-AKT-mTOR pathway is common in lung cancer, particularly through mutations in the PI3KCA gene or loss of the tumor suppressor PTEN.

Inhibitors targeting this pathway, such as mTOR inhibitors (e.g., everolimus) and PI3K inhibitors (e.g., alpelisib), are being investigated as potential therapies for lung cancer.

Pathways Involved in Lung Cancer Development

The development of lung cancer is driven by multiple signaling pathways that control cell growth, differentiation, and survival. These pathways are often dysregulated in cancer, leading to uncontrolled cell proliferation and tumor growth.

RAS-RAF-MEK-ERK Pathway

The RAS-RAF-MEK-ERK pathway, also known as the MAPK pathway, is a critical signaling cascade involved in cell proliferation and differentiation. It is activated by various growth factors, including EGFR, and transmits signals from the cell surface to the nucleus.

In lung cancer, mutations in RAS (particularly KRAS) and RAF (particularly BRAF) can lead to constitutive activation of this pathway, driving uncontrolled cell growth. Targeting this pathway with inhibitors, such as MEK inhibitors (e.g., trametinib), has shown promise in treating certain subtypes of lung cancer.

PI3K-AKT-mTOR Pathway

The PI3K-AKT-mTOR pathway is involved in regulating cell growth, survival, and metabolism. Activation of this pathway occurs through receptor tyrosine kinases, such as EGFR, and is often dysregulated in lung cancer due to mutations in PI3KCA or loss of PTEN.

This pathway promotes cell survival by inhibiting apoptosis and promoting protein synthesis and glucose metabolism. Dysregulation of the PI3K-AKT-mTOR pathway contributes to the growth and survival of lung cancer cells, making it a target for therapeutic intervention.

Wnt/β-Catenin Pathway

The Wnt/β-catenin pathway is involved in regulating cell proliferation, differentiation, and stem cell maintenance. In lung cancer, aberrant activation of the Wnt/β-catenin pathway has been implicated in tumor growth, metastasis, and resistance to therapy.

This pathway is regulated by Wnt ligands binding to Frizzled receptors, leading to the stabilization and accumulation of β-catenin in the nucleus. β-catenin then activates transcription of target genes involved in cell proliferation and survival.

Hedgehog Pathway

The Hedgehog pathway is another signaling pathway involved in regulating cell growth and differentiation. In lung cancer, aberrant activation of the Hedgehog pathway has been associated with tumor growth, metastasis, and resistance to chemotherapy.

The pathway is activated by Hedgehog ligands binding to the Patched receptor, relieving inhibition of the Smoothened receptor and leading to the activation of GLI transcription factors. These transcription factors promote the expression of genes involved in cell proliferation and survival.

Known Causes Related to Animal Products

While smoking remains the leading cause of lung cancer, emerging evidence suggests that certain animal products may also contribute to lung cancer risk. Diets high in saturated fats, cholesterol, and red and processed meats have been associated with an increased risk of lung cancer.

Red and Processed Meats

Several studies have linked the consumption of red and processed meats to an increased risk of lung cancer. Processed meats, such as sausages, bacon, and ham, contain high levels of nitrates and nitrites, which can form carcinogenic compounds called nitrosamines during cooking or digestion.

A meta-analysis published in the journal *Cancer Epidemiology, Biomarkers & Prevention* found that higher intake of red and processed meats was associated with a significantly increased risk of lung cancer, particularly among smokers. The carcinogenic compounds in processed meats, combined with the inflammatory effects of saturated fats, may contribute to lung cancer development.

Saturated Fats and Cholesterol

Diets high in saturated fats and cholesterol, commonly found in animal products such as meat, dairy, and eggs, have been linked to an increased risk of lung cancer. Saturated fats can promote inflammation and oxidative stress, which are key drivers of cancer development.

A study published in *JAMA Oncology* found that higher intake of saturated fats and cholesterol was associated with a higher risk of lung cancer, particularly among smokers. The study suggested that these dietary components might contribute to lung cancer through their effects on inflammation and immune function.

Dairy Products

Dairy products, including milk, cheese, and butter, have also been implicated in lung cancer risk. Some studies suggest that high consumption of dairy products may be associated with an increased risk of lung cancer, particularly in women.

The potential link between dairy consumption and lung cancer may be due to the presence of hormones and growth factors in dairy products, such as insulin-like growth factor 1 (IGF-1). IGF-1 is known to promote cell growth and proliferation, and elevated levels of IGF-1 have been associated with an increased risk of various cancers, including lung cancer.

How a Plant-Based Diet Can Help with Reversal

A plant-based diet, rich in fruits, vegetables, whole grains, legumes, nuts, and seeds, has been shown to have numerous health benefits, including the potential to reduce the risk of lung cancer and aid in its reversal. Plant-based diets are naturally low in saturated fats and cholesterol and high in fiber, antioxidants, and phytonutrients, which can help protect against cancer.

Antioxidants and Phytonutrients

Plants are rich in antioxidants, such as vitamins C and E, and phytonutrients, such as flavonoids and carotenoids, which help neutralize free radicals and reduce oxidative stress. Oxidative stress is a key driver of cancer development, as it can lead to DNA damage and the activation of oncogenic pathways.

A study published in *Cancer Epidemiology, Biomarkers & Prevention* found that higher intake of fruits and vegetables was associated with a lower risk of lung cancer, particularly among smokers. The protective effects of plant-based foods may be due to their high antioxidant content, which helps protect cells from oxidative damage.

Fiber

Dietary fiber, found in plant-based foods such as fruits, vegetables, whole grains, and legumes, has been shown to reduce the risk of lung cancer. Fiber helps promote healthy digestion and gut microbiota, which play a role in immune function and inflammation regulation.

A meta-analysis published in *The Lancet* found that higher intake of dietary fiber was associated with a lower risk of lung cancer. The study suggested that fiber might help protect against lung cancer by reducing inflammation and promoting the elimination of carcinogens from the body.

Inflammation Reduction

Chronic inflammation is a key driver of cancer development, including lung cancer. A plant-based diet, rich in anti-inflammatory foods, can help reduce inflammation and lower the risk of cancer.

A study published in *The Journal of Nutrition* found that a plant-based diet was associated with lower levels of inflammatory markers, such as C-reactive protein (CRP), in the blood. The anti-inflammatory effects of a plant-based diet may help protect against lung cancer by reducing chronic inflammation and its associated damage to lung tissue.

Immune System Support

A plant-based diet can also support the immune system, which plays a crucial role in detecting and eliminating cancer cells. Certain plant foods, such as mushrooms, garlic, and turmeric, have been shown to enhance immune function and promote the activity of natural killer (NK) cells, which can target and destroy cancer cells.

A study published in *The American Journal of Clinical Nutrition* found that a diet rich in fruits and vegetables was associated with enhanced immune function, including increased activity of NK cells. The immune-boosting effects of a plant-based diet may help prevent the development and progression of lung cancer.

Specific Plant Foods and Their Effects

Several specific plant foods have been shown to have protective effects against lung cancer:

- **Cruciferous Vegetables:** Vegetables such as broccoli, cauliflower, and Brussels sprouts are rich in sulforaphane, a compound that has been shown to inhibit cancer cell growth and promote apoptosis in lung cancer cells.
- **Berries:** Berries, such as blueberries, strawberries, and raspberries, are rich in antioxidants and have been shown to reduce oxidative stress and inflammation, which can help protect against lung cancer.
- **Garlic:** Garlic contains organosulfur compounds, such as allicin, which have been shown to have anti-cancer effects. A study published in *Cancer Prevention Research* found that higher garlic intake was associated with a lower risk of lung cancer.
- **Turmeric:** Turmeric contains curcumin, a compound with potent anti-inflammatory and antioxidant properties. Curcumin has been shown to inhibit the growth of lung cancer cells and promote apoptosis.
- **Green Tea:** Green tea is rich in catechins, a type of antioxidant that has been shown to have anti-cancer effects. A study published in *Carcinogenesis* found that green tea consumption was associated with a lower risk of lung cancer.

Lung cancer is a complex and multifactorial disease with significant morbidity and mortality. Its development is driven by genetic mutations, environmental and lifestyle factors, and dysregulation of critical cellular pathways. While smoking remains the primary cause of lung cancer, emerging evidence suggests that certain animal products may also contribute to lung cancer risk.

A plant-based diet, rich in antioxidants, fiber, and anti-inflammatory compounds, offers a promising approach to reducing the risk of lung cancer and supporting its reversal. Specific plant foods, such as cruciferous vegetables, berries, garlic, turmeric, and green tea, have been shown to have protective effects against lung cancer.

Non-Hodgkin Lymphoma (NHL)

Non-Hodgkin Lymphoma (NHL) is a complex and diverse group of blood cancers that originate in the lymphatic system, which is a crucial part of the body's immune defense. Understanding NHL involves exploring its function, the biological mechanisms driving its production and regulation, and the pathways involved in its development. Moreover, exploring the link between diet—particularly the consumption of animal products—and the onset of NHL is vital for understanding potential preventive measures. Finally, the role of a plant-based diet in the potential reversal of NHL is increasingly recognized, warranting detailed discussion.

Function and Characteristics of Non-Hodgkin Lymphoma

Non-Hodgkin Lymphoma is a malignancy that originates from lymphocytes, a type of white blood cell crucial to the immune system. Unlike other lymphomas, NHL encompasses a wide variety of subtypes, each with distinct biological characteristics and clinical behaviors. The primary function of lymphocytes, the cells affected in NHL, is to protect the body against infections and foreign invaders. However, in NHL, these cells undergo malignant transformation, leading to uncontrolled growth and proliferation, which hampers their normal immune function.

Lymphocytes are broadly categorized into B cells and T cells, both of which can give rise to NHL. B-cell lymphomas are the most common, accounting for approximately 85% of NHL cases, while T-cell lymphomas are less common but often more aggressive. The abnormal proliferation of these lymphocytes can occur in any part of the lymphatic system, including the lymph nodes, spleen, thymus, and bone marrow, as well as extranodal sites such as the gastrointestinal tract, skin, and brain.

Production of Non-Hodgkin Lymphoma

The production or development of Non-Hodgkin Lymphoma is the result of a multistep process involving genetic mutations, chromosomal translocations, and epigenetic alterations that lead to the malignant transformation of lymphocytes. The pathogenesis of NHL is complex and multifactorial, involving both intrinsic genetic factors and extrinsic environmental influences.

1. **Genetic Mutations and Chromosomal Translocations**: Genetic mutations play a central role in the development of NHL. Mutations in oncogenes (genes that promote cell growth) and tumor suppressor genes (genes that inhibit cell growth) can lead to the unchecked proliferation of lymphocytes. For example, mutations in the BCL2 gene, which encodes a protein that prevents apoptosis (programmed cell death), are commonly seen in follicular lymphoma, a subtype of NHL. This mutation results in the overexpression of the BCL2 protein, allowing lymphocytes to evade apoptosis and accumulate abnormally.

   Chromosomal translocations are another key feature in the production of NHL. A well-known example is the t(14;18) translocation, which involves the BCL2 gene on chromosome 18 and the immunoglobulin heavy chain gene on chromosome 14. This translocation leads to the overexpression of the BCL2 protein, contributing to the pathogenesis of follicular lymphoma. Similarly, the t(8;14) translocation involving the MYC oncogene and the immunoglobulin gene is characteristic of Burkitt lymphoma, a highly aggressive form of NHL.

2. **Epigenetic Alterations**: Epigenetic changes, such as DNA methylation and histone modifications, also play a crucial role in the development of NHL. These alterations can silence tumor suppressor genes or activate oncogenes without changing the underlying DNA sequence. For instance, the hypermethylation of the CDKN2A gene, which encodes the tumor suppressor proteins p16INK4a and p14ARF, is frequently observed in NHL and contributes to uncontrolled cell cycle progression and tumor growth.

3. **Microenvironmental Factors**: The tumor microenvironment, which includes various non-malignant cells, signaling molecules, and extracellular matrix components, is integral to the production of NHL. Interactions between malignant lymphocytes and the microenvironment can promote tumor growth, survival, and resistance to therapy. For example, in the microenvironment of follicular lymphoma, the secretion of cytokines such as interleukin-4 (IL-4) and interleukin-10 (IL-10) by surrounding immune cells can support the survival and proliferation of lymphoma cells.

Regulation of Non-Hodgkin Lymphoma

The regulation of Non-Hodgkin Lymphoma involves multiple cellular and molecular mechanisms that control the growth, survival, and dissemination of malignant lymphocytes. These regulatory mechanisms include signaling pathways, immune evasion strategies, and the influence of external factors such as diet and environmental exposures.

1. **Signaling Pathways**: Several signaling pathways are dysregulated in NHL, contributing to the uncontrolled proliferation and survival of lymphoma cells. Among the most important are:
   - **B-cell receptor (BCR) signaling**: BCR signaling is crucial for normal B-cell development and function. In NHL, aberrant activation of the BCR signaling pathway can lead to increased cell survival and proliferation. This pathway involves various kinases, including Bruton's tyrosine kinase (BTK) and phosphatidylinositol 3-kinase (PI3K), which are frequently overactive in NHL subtypes such as diffuse large B-cell lymphoma (DLBCL).
   - **NF-κB pathway**: The nuclear factor kappa-light-chain-enhancer of activated B cells (NF-κB) pathway is involved in the regulation of immune responses and cell survival. In NHL, constitutive activation of NF-κB signaling, often due to mutations in upstream regulators such as CARD11 or MYD88, promotes the survival and proliferation of lymphoma cells.
   - **PI3K/AKT/mTOR pathway**: The PI3K/AKT/mTOR pathway is a key regulator of cell growth, survival, and metabolism. In NHL, dysregulation of this pathway, often through mutations in the PI3KCA gene or loss of function of the PTEN tumor suppressor, leads to enhanced cell survival and resistance to apoptosis.
   - **JAK/STAT pathway**: The Janus kinase/signal transducer and activator of transcription (JAK/STAT) pathway is involved in cytokine signaling and the regulation of immune responses. In NHL, mutations in the JAK2 or STAT3 genes can result in constitutive activation of this pathway, promoting tumor cell survival and proliferation.
2. **Immune Evasion**: NHL cells employ various strategies to evade the immune system, which allows them to persist and grow despite the presence of immune surveillance. One common mech-

anism is the expression of immune checkpoint proteins such as PD-L1 (programmed death-ligand 1) on the surface of lymphoma cells. PD-L1 binds to the PD-1 receptor on T cells, inhibiting their function and allowing the tumor cells to escape immune attack. This immune evasion mechanism has been targeted by immune checkpoint inhibitors, which have shown promise in the treatment of certain NHL subtypes.

3. **External Factors**: External factors, including diet and environmental exposures, can influence the regulation of NHL. Additionally, exposure to agricultural chemicals, such as pesticides, has been linked to an increased risk of NHL.

Pathways Involved in Non-Hodgkin Lymphoma

The development and progression of Non-Hodgkin Lymphoma involve several intricate biological pathways that contribute to the malignant behavior of lymphoma cells. These pathways are interconnected and often involve the dysregulation of normal cellular processes such as cell cycle control, apoptosis, and immune signaling.

1. **Apoptosis Pathways**: Apoptosis, or programmed cell death, is a critical mechanism that prevents the accumulation of damaged or abnormal cells. In NHL, dysregulation of apoptosis pathways is a common feature that allows lymphoma cells to survive and proliferate. The BCL2 family of proteins plays a central role in regulating apoptosis. Overexpression of the anti-apoptotic protein BCL2, as seen in follicular lymphoma, inhibits apoptosis and promotes tumor cell survival. Conversely, mutations or deletions in pro-apoptotic genes such as BAX or BAK can also contribute to the resistance of lymphoma cells to apoptosis.

2. **Cell Cycle Pathways**: The cell cycle is tightly regulated by a series of checkpoints that ensure proper cell division and prevent the proliferation of abnormal cells. In NHL, these checkpoints

are often disrupted, leading to uncontrolled cell division. The retinoblastoma (RB) pathway, which regulates the G1/S transition of the cell cycle, is frequently altered in NHL. Mutations in the RB1 gene or overexpression of cyclin D1, a key regulator of the cell cycle, can bypass these checkpoints, leading to unchecked cell proliferation.

3. **Immune Signaling Pathways**: Immune signaling pathways, particularly those involving cytokines and chemokines, are crucial for the regulation of immune responses. In NHL, dysregulation of these pathways can create a pro-tumorigenic microenvironment that supports the survival and proliferation of lymphoma cells. For example, the IL-6/STAT3 signaling pathway is often activated in NHL and promotes tumor growth by enhancing cell survival, proliferation, and angiogenesis.

4. **Angiogenesis Pathways**: Angiogenesis, the formation of new blood vessels, is essential for tumor growth and metastasis. In NHL, the vascular endothelial growth factor (VEGF) pathway is often upregulated, leading to increased angiogenesis and the provision of nutrients and oxygen to the tumor. VEGF expression is regulated by hypoxia-inducible factors (HIFs), which are activated under low oxygen conditions commonly found within tumors.

Known Causes Related to Animal Products

There is growing evidence that certain dietary factors, particularly the consumption of animal products, may contribute to the development of Non-Hodgkin Lymphoma. While the exact mechanisms are still under investigation, several hypotheses have been proposed to explain the potential link between animal products and NHL.

1. **High Saturated Fat Intake**: Diets high in saturated fats, which are predominantly found in animal products such as red meat

and dairy, have been associated with an increased risk of NHL. Saturated fats can promote chronic inflammation, oxidative stress, and the production of pro-inflammatory cytokines, all of which contribute to the development of cancer. Additionally, high-fat diets can lead to obesity, a known risk factor for NHL, by promoting insulin resistance and altering hormone levels.

2. **Heme Iron**: Heme iron, the form of iron found in animal products, has been implicated in the development of various cancers, including NHL. Unlike non-heme iron found in plant-based foods, heme iron can promote the formation of free radicals through the Fenton reaction, leading to DNA damage and increased cancer risk. Furthermore, excessive iron accumulation can contribute to a pro-oxidative and pro-inflammatory state, creating an environment conducive to tumor development.

3. **Carcinogens in Processed Meats**: Processed meats, such as sausages, bacon, and ham, contain carcinogenic compounds, including nitrosamines and polycyclic aromatic hydrocarbons (PAHs). These compounds can cause DNA damage and promote the development of NHL. The World Health Organization (WHO) has classified processed meats as Group 1 carcinogens, meaning there is sufficient evidence of their carcinogenicity in humans.

4. **Dairy Products and IGF-1**: Dairy products, particularly those with high-fat content, have been linked to an increased risk of NHL. One proposed mechanism involves the insulin-like growth factor 1 (IGF-1), a hormone found in dairy that promotes cell growth and proliferation. Elevated levels of IGF-1 have been associated with an increased risk of various cancers, including NHL, by promoting the survival and proliferation of malignant cells.

Plant-Based Diet Reversing Non-Hodgkin Lymphoma

A plant-based diet, rich in fruits, vegetables, whole grains, legumes, nuts, and seeds, has been shown to offer numerous health benefits, including a reduced risk of cancer. The potential for a plant-based diet to aid in the reversal of Non-Hodgkin Lymphoma is an area of growing interest, supported by emerging scientific evidence.

1. **Antioxidant and Anti-inflammatory Properties**: Plant-based foods are rich in antioxidants, such as vitamins C and E, polyphenols, and flavonoids, which can neutralize free radicals and reduce oxidative stress. This is particularly important in the context of NHL, where oxidative stress plays a significant role in the development and progression of the disease. Additionally, many plant-based foods have anti-inflammatory properties, which can help reduce chronic inflammation—a key driver of cancer.

   For example, cruciferous vegetables like broccoli, kale, and Brussels sprouts contain sulforaphane, a compound with potent anti-cancer properties. Sulforaphane has been shown to inhibit the growth of cancer cells, including those in NHL, by inducing apoptosis and blocking cell cycle progression. Similarly, berries are rich in polyphenols, which have been shown to reduce inflammation and oxidative stress, potentially lowering the risk of NHL.

2. **Fiber and Gut Microbiome**: A plant-based diet is high in dietary fiber, which plays a crucial role in maintaining a healthy gut microbiome. The gut microbiome, composed of trillions of microorganisms, is integral to immune function and the regulation of inflammation. A high-fiber diet promotes the growth of beneficial gut bacteria that produce short-chain fatty acids (SCFAs) like butyrate. SCFAs have anti-inflammatory and anti-cancer properties, which may help protect against the development and progression of NHL.

   Furthermore, a healthy gut microbiome can enhance the immune system's ability to detect and destroy malignant cells, providing another layer of defense against NHL. Conversely, diets low in fiber and high in animal products can disrupt the gut microbiome, leading to dysbiosis, chronic inflammation, and an increased risk of cancer.

3. **Phytonutrients and Chemoprevention**: Phytonutrients, naturally occurring compounds found in plants, have been extensively studied for their potential chemopreventive effects. These compounds, which include flavonoids, carotenoids, and lignans, have been shown to inhibit the growth of cancer cells, modulate signaling pathways, and induce apoptosis. In the context of NHL, phytonutrients may offer protective effects by targeting key pathways involved in the development and progression of the disease. For instance, curcumin, a compound found in turmeric, has been shown to inhibit the NF-κB signaling pathway, which is often dysregulated in NHL. By blocking this pathway, curcumin can reduce inflammation and inhibit the growth of lymphoma cells. Similarly, resveratrol, a phytonutrient found in grapes, has been shown to induce apoptosis and inhibit cell proliferation in various cancer cell lines, including those of NHL.

4. **Detoxification and Reduced Exposure to Carcinogens**: A plant-based diet can enhance the body's natural detoxification processes, helping to eliminate carcinogens and other harmful compounds. Many plant-based foods contain compounds that support the liver's detoxification pathways, such as glucosinolates in cruciferous vegetables and flavonoids in citrus fruits. These compounds can enhance the activity of detoxifying enzymes, such as glutathione S-transferase, which helps neutralize and eliminate carcinogens from the body.

Additionally, by reducing or eliminating the consumption of animal products, a plant-based diet can significantly lower exposure to dietary carcinogens such as nitrosamines, PAHs, and heme iron. This reduction in carcinogen exposure can decrease the risk of NHL and support the body's ability to repair DNA damage and prevent the progression of malignant cells.

5. **Weight Management and Hormonal Balance**: Obesity is a known risk factor for NHL, and maintaining a healthy weight is crucial for reducing the risk of cancer. A plant-based diet, which is typically lower in calories and higher in nutrients than an animal-based diet, can help promote weight loss and prevent obesity. Furthermore, plant-based diets have been shown to improve insulin sensitivity and reduce levels of circulating insulin and IGF-1, hormones that can promote the growth of cancer cells.

   By promoting hormonal balance and preventing obesity, a plant-based diet may reduce the risk of NHL and improve outcomes for individuals diagnosed with the disease. Moreover, weight management is essential for reducing the risk of relapse and improving overall survival in NHL patients.

Non-Hodgkin Lymphoma is a complex and multifaceted disease with various subtypes, each with unique characteristics and behaviors. The production and regulation of NHL involve intricate genetic, epigenetic, and microenvironmental factors, with multiple signaling pathways contributing to the development and progression of the disease. While traditional risk factors such as genetic mutations and chronic infections are well recognized, emerging evidence suggests that diet, particularly the consumption of animal products, may also play a significant role in the development of NHL.

High saturated fat intake, heme iron, carcinogens in processed meats, and dairy products have all been implicated in increasing the risk of NHL. Conversely, a plant-based diet offers numerous protective benefits, including antioxidant and anti-inflammatory effects, support for a healthy gut microbiome, and the presence of phytonutrients with chemopreventive properties. By reducing exposure to dietary carcinogens and promoting weight management and hormonal balance, a plant-based diet may not only lower the risk of NHL but also support the reversal of the disease in individuals who have been diagnosed.

As research continues to explore the connections between diet and cancer, the potential of a plant-based diet to prevent and reverse Non-Hodgkin Lymphoma offers a promising avenue for improving public health and patient outcomes. Further studies are needed to elucidate the specific mechanisms by which a plant-based diet exerts its protective effects and to develop targeted dietary interventions for individuals at risk of or diagnosed with NHL.

Ovarian Cancer

Ovarian cancer is one of the most challenging cancers to detect and treat, primarily because its symptoms are often vague and only present in advanced stages. Understanding the function, production, and regulation of ovarian cancer, including the pathways involved, is crucial for developing effective strategies for prevention, early detection, and treatment.

Function of Ovarian Cancer

Ovarian cancer arises from the uncontrolled growth of cells within the ovaries, the female reproductive organs responsible for producing eggs (ova), and secreting hormones such as estrogen and progesterone. The primary function of the ovaries is to regulate the menstrual cycle and support pregnancy. However, when ovarian cells undergo malignant transformation, they lose their ability to function normally and begin to proliferate uncontrollably. This leads to the formation of tumors, which can invade surrounding tissues and metastasize to distant organs.

The progression of ovarian cancer is categorized into four stages, with stage I being confined to the ovaries and stage IV indicating distant metastasis. The function of ovarian cancer cells is characterized by their ability to evade apoptosis (programmed cell death), sustain proliferative signaling, induce angiogenesis (formation of new blood vessels), and develop resistance to therapeutic agents.

Production of Ovarian Cancer

The production of ovarian cancer involves a complex interplay of genetic, environmental, and hormonal factors. While the exact cause of ovarian cancer remains unclear, several risk factors have been identified that contribute to its development:

1. **Genetic Mutations**: Mutations in certain genes, such as BRCA1 and BRCA2, significantly increase the risk of developing ovarian cancer. These genes are involved in DNA repair, and mutations can lead to the accumulation of genetic damage, promoting cancerous growth.

2. **Hormonal Imbalances**: Estrogen exposure, particularly unopposed estrogen (without progesterone), has been linked to an increased risk of ovarian cancer. This is because estrogen promotes cell division in the ovaries, and excessive cell division increases the likelihood of mutations.

3. **Chronic Inflammation**: Inflammation in the pelvic region, often due to conditions such as endometriosis or pelvic inflammatory disease, can create an environment conducive to cancer development. Inflammatory cytokines can induce oxidative stress and DNA damage, leading to malignant transformation.

4. **Age and Reproductive History**: The risk of ovarian cancer increases with age, particularly after menopause. Women who have never been pregnant, have had late pregnancies, or have not used oral contraceptives are also at higher risk, possibly due to the

continuous ovulation that occurs throughout their reproductive years.

5. **Environmental Factors**: Exposure to environmental toxins, such as asbestos and talc, has been implicated in the production of ovarian cancer. These substances can induce inflammation and oxidative stress, contributing to the development of malignancies.

Regulation of Ovarian Cancer

The regulation of ovarian cancer involves a network of signaling pathways that control cell proliferation, apoptosis, angiogenesis, and metastasis. Dysregulation of these pathways plays a critical role in the initiation and progression of ovarian cancer:

1. **PI3K/AKT/mTOR Pathway**: This pathway is crucial for cell survival and proliferation. In ovarian cancer, mutations or overexpression of components of this pathway can lead to uncontrolled cell growth and resistance to apoptosis. The PI3K/AKT/mTOR pathway is often hyperactivated in ovarian cancer, making it a potential target for therapeutic intervention.

2. **RAS/RAF/MEK/ERK Pathway**: This pathway is involved in regulating cell division and differentiation. Mutations in the RAS family of genes can lead to the activation of this pathway, promoting tumor growth. In ovarian cancer, the RAS/RAF/MEK/ERK pathway is frequently altered, contributing to the malignancy's aggressive nature.

3. **p53 Tumor Suppressor Pathway**: The p53 protein plays a crucial role in maintaining genomic stability by inducing cell cycle arrest or apoptosis in response to DNA damage. In ovarian cancer, mutations in the TP53 gene, which encodes p53, are common and lead to the loss of its tumor-suppressive function, allowing cancer cells to proliferate unchecked.

4. **Notch Signaling Pathway**: The Notch pathway regulates cell fate determination, proliferation, and apoptosis. Dysregulation of Notch signaling has been observed in ovarian cancer, where it promotes tumor growth, metastasis, and chemoresistance.

5. **Angiogenesis Pathway**: The formation of new blood vessels (angiogenesis) is essential for tumor growth and metastasis. Ovarian cancer cells often overexpress vascular endothelial growth factor (VEGF), which stimulates angiogenesis and provides the tumor with the necessary nutrients and oxygen for continued growth.

6. **Wnt/β-catenin Pathway**: This pathway is involved in cell proliferation and differentiation. Aberrant activation of the Wnt/β-catenin pathway has been linked to ovarian cancer development, as it promotes the expression of genes that drive tumorigenesis.

Detailed Pathways Involved in Ovarian Cancer

Understanding the molecular pathways involved in ovarian cancer provides insights into its pathogenesis and potential therapeutic targets. Here, we delve into some of the key pathways implicated in ovarian cancer:

1. PI3K/AKT/mTOR Pathway

The PI3K/AKT/mTOR pathway is one of the most frequently dysregulated pathways in ovarian cancer. This pathway is activated by various growth factors and cytokines, leading to the phosphorylation of phosphatidylinositol-3,4,5-trisphosphate (PIP3) by PI3K. PIP3, in turn, recruits and activates AKT, a serine/threonine kinase. Activated AKT phosphorylates downstream targets, including mTOR, which promotes cell growth, survival, and metabolism.

In ovarian cancer, mutations in PIK3CA (encoding the PI3K catalytic subunit) or loss of function of the tumor suppressor PTEN (which antagonizes PI3K activity) result in hyperactivation of this pathway. The consequence is enhanced cell proliferation, inhibition of apoptosis, and increased angiogenesis, all of which contribute to tumor growth and progression.

2. RAS/RAF/MEK/ERK Pathway

The RAS/RAF/MEK/ERK pathway, also known as the MAPK pathway, is another critical signaling cascade involved in ovarian cancer. This pathway is activated by receptor tyrosine kinases (RTKs) in response to growth factors, leading to the activation of RAS, a small GTPase. RAS then recruits and activates RAF, which phosphorylates and activates MEK, followed by the activation of ERK.

Activated ERK translocates to the nucleus, where it regulates the expression of genes involved in cell proliferation, differentiation, and survival. Mutations in RAS genes, particularly KRAS, are common in ovarian cancer and result in the constitutive activation of this pathway, driving tumorigenesis.

3. p53 Tumor Suppressor Pathway

The p53 protein, encoded by the TP53 gene, is often referred to as the "guardian of the genome" due to its role in preventing genomic instability. p53 responds to various cellular stresses, including DNA damage, by inducing cell cycle arrest, DNA repair, or apoptosis. In ovarian cancer, mutations in TP53 are among the most common genetic alterations, leading to the loss of p53's tumor-suppressive functions.

As a result, cells with damaged DNA are allowed to proliferate, accumulating further mutations that drive cancer progression. The loss of p53 function also contributes to chemoresistance, as cancer cells can evade apoptosis in response to DNA-damaging agents.

4. Notch Signaling Pathway

The Notch signaling pathway is a key regulator of cell fate decisions, including differentiation, proliferation, and apoptosis. Notch receptors are activated upon binding to their ligands, leading to the cleavage of the Notch intracellular domain (NICD), which translocates to the nucleus and regulates the expression of target genes.

In ovarian cancer, aberrant Notch signaling has been implicated in tumor growth, metastasis, and resistance to therapy. Overexpression of

Notch receptors or ligands, as well as mutations in pathway components, can lead to the constitutive activation of this pathway, promoting oncogenesis.

5. Angiogenesis Pathway

Angiogenesis, the formation of new blood vessels, is a critical process for tumor growth and metastasis. Ovarian cancer cells often overexpress VEGF, a potent angiogenic factor, which binds to its receptors on endothelial cells and stimulates the proliferation and migration of these cells, leading to the formation of new blood vessels.

The angiogenesis pathway is tightly regulated by a balance between pro-angiogenic and anti-angiogenic factors. In ovarian cancer, this balance is disrupted in favor of angiogenesis, providing the tumor with the necessary blood supply to support its growth and spread.

6. Wnt/β-catenin Pathway

The Wnt/β-catenin pathway is involved in regulating cell proliferation, differentiation, and migration. In this pathway, Wnt proteins bind to Frizzled receptors, leading to the stabilization and accumulation of β-catenin in the cytoplasm. β-catenin then translocates to the nucleus, where it regulates the expression of target genes.

Dysregulation of the Wnt/β-catenin pathway has been observed in ovarian cancer, where it promotes the expression of oncogenes and contributes to tumorigenesis. Mutations in pathway components, such as APC or CTNNB1 (encoding β-catenin), can lead to the constitutive activation of this pathway, driving cancer progression.

Known Causes Related to Animal Products

Dietary factors, particularly the consumption of animal products, have been implicated in the development of ovarian cancer. Several mechanisms have been proposed to explain the association between animal product consumption and increased cancer risk:

1. Hormone Exposure

Animal products, particularly red meat and dairy, are often associated with increased levels of hormones such as estrogen and insulin-like growth factor-1 (IGF-1). These hormones can promote cell proliferation and inhibit apoptosis, creating an environment conducive to cancer development. For example, high-fat diets rich in animal products can increase estrogen levels, which may stimulate the growth of estrogen-responsive ovarian cells.

2. Inflammatory Responses

The consumption of animal products, especially processed meats, has been linked to chronic inflammation, a known risk factor for cancer. Processed meats contain nitrosamines and other carcinogenic compounds that can induce oxidative stress and DNA damage. Additionally, the high levels of saturated fat in animal products can promote inflammation through the activation of pro-inflammatory pathways.

3. Oxidative Stress

Animal products are often high in heme iron, a type of iron found in red meat. Heme iron can catalyze the formation of free radicals, leading to oxidative stress and DNA damage. This oxidative stress can contribute to the initiation and progression of ovarian cancer by inducing mutations in critical genes involved in cell proliferation and survival.

4. Insulin Resistance and Obesity

Diets high in animal products, particularly those rich in saturated fats and cholesterol, are associated with an increased risk of obesity and insulin resistance. Both obesity and insulin resistance are risk factors for ovarian cancer, as they can lead to chronic inflammation, hormonal imbalances, and the activation of oncogenic pathways.

5. Endocrine Disrupting Chemicals (EDCs)

Animal products, particularly dairy, can contain endocrine-disrupting chemicals (EDCs) such as pesticides, dioxins, and polychlorinated biphenyls (PCBs). These chemicals can interfere with hormone signaling, leading to the dysregulation of pathways involved in cell proliferation and apoptosis. EDCs have been implicated in the development of hormone-related cancers, including ovarian cancer.

How a Plant-Based Diet Can Help with Reversal

A plant-based diet, rich in fruits, vegetables, whole grains, nuts, seeds, and legumes, offers a promising approach to the prevention and reversal of ovarian cancer. Several mechanisms explain how a plant-based diet can mitigate the risk and progression of this malignancy:

1. Antioxidant and Anti-Inflammatory Effects

Plant-based foods are rich in antioxidants, such as vitamins C and E, carotenoids, and polyphenols, which can neutralize free radicals and reduce oxidative stress. These antioxidants play a critical role in protecting cells from DNA damage, thereby reducing the risk of mutations that can lead to cancer. Additionally, many plant-based foods contain anti-inflammatory compounds, such as flavonoids and omega-3 fatty acids, which can inhibit pro-inflammatory pathways and reduce chronic inflammation, a known risk factor for cancer.

2. Hormone Regulation

A plant-based diet is associated with lower levels of circulating estrogen and IGF-1, both of which are linked to the development of ovarian cancer. Plant-based diets are typically lower in fat and higher in fiber, which can help reduce estrogen levels by promoting its excretion through the digestive system. Furthermore, certain plant compounds, such as lignans found in flaxseeds and isoflavones in soy, have weak estrogenic activity and can compete with endogenous estrogen for receptor binding, potentially reducing the risk of hormone-driven cancers.

3. Enhanced Detoxification

Cruciferous vegetables, such as broccoli, kale, and Brussels sprouts, contain compounds like sulforaphane and indole-3-carbinol, which can enhance the body's detoxification processes. These compounds activate phase II detoxification enzymes, which help neutralize and eliminate carcinogens from the body. By promoting the detoxification of harmful substances, a plant-based diet can reduce the overall carcinogenic burden and lower the risk of ovarian cancer.

4. Regulation of Cell Proliferation and Apoptosis

Plant-based foods contain a wide array of phytochemicals that can regulate cell proliferation and apoptosis. For example, curcumin, found in turmeric, has been shown to inhibit the PI3K/AKT/mTOR pathway, thereby suppressing cell growth and inducing apoptosis in ovarian cancer cells. Similarly, resveratrol, a polyphenol found in grapes, can inhibit the Wnt/β-catenin pathway, reducing the expression of oncogenes and promoting cell death in cancer cells.

5. Weight Management and Insulin Sensitivity

A plant-based diet is typically lower in calories and higher in fiber, which can aid in weight management and improve insulin sensitivity. Maintaining a healthy weight and preventing insulin resistance are crucial for reducing the risk of ovarian cancer, as obesity and insulin resistance are associated with chronic inflammation and hormonal imbalances that can promote cancer development.

6. Gut Microbiome Modulation

The gut microbiome plays a significant role in modulating inflammation, immune function, and hormone metabolism, all of which are relevant to cancer risk. A plant-based diet, rich in fiber and prebiotics, supports a diverse and healthy gut microbiome. Certain gut bacteria can metabolize dietary fibers into short-chain fatty acids (SCFAs), such as butyrate, which have anti-inflammatory and anti-cancer properties. By promoting a healthy gut microbiome, a plant-based diet can contribute to the prevention and reversal of ovarian cancer.

7. Avoidance of Harmful Animal Products

By adopting a plant-based diet, individuals can avoid the harmful effects associated with animal products, such as exposure to hormones, heme iron, and EDCs. This dietary shift can reduce the risk of ovarian cancer by minimizing the intake of substances that contribute to oxidative stress, inflammation, and hormonal imbalances.

Ovarian cancer is a complex disease influenced by genetic, hormonal, environmental, and dietary factors. Understanding the pathways involved in its development and progression provides valuable insights into potential therapeutic targets. The consumption of animal products has been linked to an increased risk of ovarian cancer through mechanisms such as hormone exposure, chronic inflammation, oxidative stress, and the presence of EDCs.

Conversely, a plant-based diet offers a multitude of benefits for the prevention and reversal of ovarian cancer. Its rich content of antioxidants, anti-inflammatory compounds, and phytochemicals supports the regulation of cell proliferation, apoptosis, and detoxification processes. Additionally, a plant-based diet promotes healthy weight management, insulin sensitivity, and gut microbiome modulation, all of which contribute to a reduced cancer risk.

By embracing a plant-based diet, individuals can take proactive steps toward reducing their risk of ovarian cancer and supporting overall health. This dietary approach not only addresses the root causes of cancer but also provides a sustainable and holistic way to nourish the body and promote long-term well-being.

Pancreatic Cancer

Pancreatic cancer is one of the most aggressive and deadly forms of cancer, characterized by its rapid progression and poor prognosis. Understanding its function, production, regulation, and the pathways involved is essential for developing effective prevention and treatment strategies. Furthermore, the impact of dietary choices, particularly the consumption of animal products versus a plant-based diet, plays a significant role in the etiology and potential reversal of this disease.

Function of Pancreatic Cancer

The pancreas is a vital organ located behind the stomach that plays crucial roles in digestion and blood sugar regulation. It produces digestive enzymes that help break down food in the small intestine and hormones like insulin that regulate blood sugar levels. Pancreatic cancer occurs when malignant cells develop in the tissues of the pancreas, leading to the formation of tumors that can interfere with the organ's function.

Pancreatic cancer typically arises from two main types of cells in the pancreas: exocrine cells and endocrine cells. The most common type, accounting for about 95% of cases, is pancreatic ductal adenocarcinoma (PDAC), which originates in the exocrine cells responsible for producing digestive enzymes. Less common are neuroendocrine tumors (NETs), which arise from the endocrine cells that produce hormones such as insulin and glucagon.

The function of pancreatic cancer, like all cancers, is marked by uncontrolled cellular proliferation. This unchecked growth leads to the formation of tumors that can invade nearby tissues and metastasize to other parts of the body. The aggressive nature of pancreatic cancer makes it particularly lethal, with a high potential for early metastasis and resistance to conventional treatments.

Production of Pancreatic Cancer

Pancreatic cancer production is a multistep process that involves genetic mutations, environmental factors, and lifestyle choices. The initiation and progression of pancreatic cancer are driven by a series of genetic alterations that transform normal pancreatic cells into malignant ones.

1. **Genetic Mutations:** The most common genetic mutations associated with pancreatic cancer occur in the KRAS gene, which is involved in cell signaling pathways that regulate cell growth and division. Mutations in the KRAS gene are present in over 90% of pancreatic ductal adenocarcinomas. Other frequently mutated genes in pancreatic cancer include TP53, CDKN2A, and

SMAD4. These genes play roles in tumor suppression, cell cycle regulation, and signal transduction, and their mutations contribute to the uncontrolled growth characteristic of cancer.

2. **Environmental and Lifestyle Factors:** Environmental and lifestyle factors also play significant roles in the production of pancreatic cancer. Tobacco smoking is the most established risk factor, accounting for approximately 20-30% of pancreatic cancer cases. Chronic pancreatitis, often resulting from heavy alcohol consumption or gallstones, is another known risk factor, as it leads to prolonged inflammation of the pancreas, creating an environment conducive to malignant transformation.

3. **Dietary Factors:** Diet plays a crucial role in the production of pancreatic cancer. High consumption of red and processed meats, which are rich in saturated fats and carcinogenic compounds like nitrosamines, has been linked to an increased risk of pancreatic cancer. Conversely, diets rich in fruits, vegetables, and whole grains, which provide antioxidants, fiber, and phytochemicals, have been associated with a reduced risk.

Regulation of Pancreatic Cancer

The regulation of pancreatic cancer involves complex interactions between genetic, epigenetic, and environmental factors. Several signaling pathways and cellular mechanisms are involved in the regulation of cell growth, apoptosis (programmed cell death), and metastasis.

1. **KRAS Pathway:** The KRAS gene encodes a protein that is part of the RAS/MAPK signaling pathway, which regulates cell proliferation, differentiation, and survival. In normal cells, this pathway is tightly regulated, but in pancreatic cancer, mutations in KRAS lead to constitutive activation of the pathway, driving un-

controlled cell growth. The KRAS pathway is a critical regulator of pancreatic cancer and a key target for therapeutic interventions.

2. **PI3K/AKT/mTOR Pathway:** The PI3K/AKT/mTOR pathway is another crucial regulator of cell growth and survival in pancreatic cancer. This pathway is often dysregulated in pancreatic cancer, leading to enhanced cell proliferation and resistance to apoptosis. Targeting this pathway with inhibitors has been explored as a potential therapeutic strategy in pancreatic cancer.

3. **TGF-β Pathway:** The transforming growth factor-beta (TGF-β) pathway plays a dual role in cancer. In normal cells, TGF-β acts as a tumor suppressor by inhibiting cell proliferation and promoting apoptosis. However, in pancreatic cancer, the TGF-β pathway can be hijacked to promote tumor progression and metastasis. This paradoxical role of TGF-β makes it a complex regulator of pancreatic cancer.

4. **Epigenetic Regulation:** Epigenetic modifications, such as DNA methylation and histone acetylation, also play significant roles in the regulation of gene expression in pancreatic cancer. These modifications can lead to the silencing of tumor suppressor genes or the activation of oncogenes, contributing to the development and progression of the disease.

Detailed Pathways in Pancreatic Cancer

Several key pathways are involved in the development and progression of pancreatic cancer, each contributing to the disease's aggressive nature and resistance to treatment.

1. **KRAS/MAPK Pathway:** The KRAS/MAPK pathway is one of the most critical pathways in pancreatic cancer. Mutations in the KRAS gene lead to the activation of downstream signaling molecules, including RAF, MEK, and ERK, which promote cell pro-

liferation and survival. This pathway is frequently dysregulated in pancreatic cancer, making it a central driver of tumor growth.

2. **PI3K/AKT/mTOR Pathway:** The PI3K/AKT/mTOR pathway is another crucial signaling pathway involved in pancreatic cancer. Activation of this pathway promotes cell growth, survival, and metabolism, contributing to the aggressive nature of the disease. Inhibitors targeting this pathway have shown promise in preclinical studies, but their efficacy in clinical trials has been limited.

3. **TGF-β/SMAD Pathway:** The TGF-β/SMAD pathway plays a complex role in pancreatic cancer. While TGF-β initially acts as a tumor suppressor, it can switch to a pro-tumorigenic role in advanced stages of the disease. This pathway is involved in epithelial-mesenchymal transition (EMT), a process that enhances the invasiveness and metastatic potential of cancer cells.

4. **Hedgehog Pathway:** The Hedgehog signaling pathway is another important pathway in pancreatic cancer, particularly in the tumor microenvironment. This pathway regulates the interactions between cancer cells and stromal cells, contributing to the dense stroma characteristic of pancreatic tumors. Inhibition of the Hedgehog pathway has been explored as a potential therapeutic strategy to disrupt the tumor-stroma interactions.

5. **Notch Pathway:** The Notch signaling pathway plays a role in cell differentiation, proliferation, and apoptosis. In pancreatic cancer, aberrant activation of the Notch pathway contributes to tumor growth and resistance to chemotherapy. Targeting the Notch pathway has shown potential in preclinical models, but clinical trials have faced challenges due to the pathway's complex role in normal tissue homeostasis.

Known Causes Related to Animal Products

Dietary choices, particularly the consumption of animal products, have been implicated in the etiology of pancreatic cancer. Several studies have shown that high intake of red and processed meats is associated with an increased risk of pancreatic cancer.

1. **Red and Processed Meats:** Red meat, such as beef, pork, and lamb, and processed meats, including bacon, sausages, and ham, are rich in saturated fats and contain carcinogenic compounds such as nitrosamines and polycyclic aromatic hydrocarbons (PAHs). These compounds are formed during the processing and cooking of meat, particularly at high temperatures. Nitrosamines, for example, are potent carcinogens that can induce DNA damage and promote the development of cancer.

2. **Saturated Fats:** High intake of saturated fats, which are abundant in animal products, has been linked to an increased risk of pancreatic cancer. Saturated fats can lead to the production of inflammatory molecules and oxidative stress, creating an environment conducive to cancer development. Additionally, diets high in saturated fats are associated with obesity, a known risk factor for pancreatic cancer.

3. **Heme Iron:** Heme iron, found in animal products, particularly red meat, has been shown to promote the formation of N-nitroso compounds, which are known carcinogens. Heme iron can also catalyze the production of reactive oxygen species (ROS), leading to oxidative damage to DNA and other cellular components, contributing to cancer development.

4. **Hormones and Growth Factors:** Animal products, particularly dairy, contain hormones and growth factors that can promote the growth of cancer cells. For example, insulin-like growth factor-1 (IGF-1), found in dairy products, has been shown to stimulate cell proliferation and inhibit apoptosis, contributing to cancer progression.

5. **Cooking Methods:** The method of cooking animal products can also influence the risk of pancreatic cancer. High-temperature cooking methods, such as grilling, barbecuing, and frying, can lead to the formation of carcinogenic compounds like heterocyclic amines (HCAs) and polycyclic aromatic hydrocarbons (PAHs). These compounds have been shown to induce DNA mutations and promote the development of cancer.

How a Plant-Based Diet Can Help with Reversal

A plant-based diet, rich in fruits, vegetables, whole grains, legumes, nuts, and seeds, offers numerous benefits that can help in the prevention and potential reversal of pancreatic cancer. This diet is naturally low in saturated fats and free from the carcinogenic compounds found in animal products, making it a powerful tool in cancer prevention and management.

1. **Antioxidants:** Fruits and vegetables are rich in antioxidants, such as vitamins C and E, carotenoids, and flavonoids, which help neutralize free radicals and reduce oxidative stress, a key contributor to cancer development. Antioxidants also play a role in repairing DNA damage and preventing the mutations that lead to cancer.

2. **Phytochemicals:** Plant-based foods are abundant in phytochemicals, such as polyphenols, glucosinolates, and isoflavones, which have been shown to have anti-cancer properties. These compounds can inhibit the growth of cancer cells, induce apoptosis, and modulate signaling pathways involved in cancer progression.

3. **Fiber:** A plant-based diet is high in dietary fiber, which has been associated with a reduced risk of pancreatic cancer. Fiber helps regulate blood sugar levels, reduces inflammation, and promotes a healthy gut microbiome, all of which contribute to cancer pre-

vention. Additionally, fiber aids in the elimination of carcinogens from the digestive tract.

4. **Low Glycemic Index:** Plant-based diets are typically low in glycemic index, which helps in maintaining stable blood sugar levels. High blood sugar levels and insulin resistance are risk factors for pancreatic cancer, and a diet that helps regulate blood sugar can reduce the risk of cancer development.

5. **Anti-inflammatory Effects:** Chronic inflammation is a key driver of cancer, including pancreatic cancer. A plant-based diet is rich in anti-inflammatory foods, such as leafy greens, berries, nuts, and seeds, which can help reduce inflammation and lower the risk of cancer.

6. **Reduced Exposure to Carcinogens:** By eliminating animal products, a plant-based diet reduces exposure to carcinogenic compounds such as nitrosamines, HCAs, and PAHs, which are formed during the processing and cooking of meat. This reduction in exposure to carcinogens is a crucial factor in cancer prevention.

7. **Improved Immune Function:** A plant-based diet can enhance immune function, making the body more capable of detecting and eliminating cancer cells. Nutrients such as vitamin C, beta-carotene, and zinc, which are abundant in plant-based foods, support the immune system's ability to fight cancer.

8. **Weight Management:** Obesity is a significant risk factor for pancreatic cancer, and a plant-based diet is effective in promoting weight loss and maintaining a healthy weight. This is due to the diet's low-calorie density, high fiber content, and ability to improve metabolic health.

9. **Detoxification:** Plant-based diets support the body's natural detoxification processes by providing essential nutrients that aid in the elimination of toxins and carcinogens. Cruciferous vegetables, such as broccoli and kale, contain compounds that activate

detoxification enzymes, helping the body rid itself of harmful substances.

Pancreatic cancer is a complex and aggressive disease with a high mortality rate. Understanding its function, production, and regulation, along with the pathways involved, is crucial for developing effective prevention and treatment strategies. The consumption of animal products, particularly red and processed meats, has been implicated in the etiology of pancreatic cancer due to the presence of carcinogenic compounds, high levels of saturated fats, and other harmful factors.

In contrast, a plant-based diet offers numerous benefits that can help in the prevention and potential reversal of pancreatic cancer. This diet is rich in antioxidants, phytochemicals, and fiber, all of which contribute to cancer prevention by reducing oxidative stress, modulating signaling pathways, and promoting overall health. Additionally, a plant-based diet reduces exposure to carcinogens and supports weight management, detoxification, and immune function, making it a powerful tool in the fight against pancreatic cancer.

Parathyroid Cancer

Parathyroid cancer is an exceptionally rare malignancy that affects the parathyroid glands, small endocrine glands located behind the thyroid gland in the neck. These glands are responsible for regulating calcium levels in the body through the secretion of parathyroid hormone (PTH). Parathyroid cancer can lead to hypercalcemia, a condition characterized by elevated calcium levels in the blood, which can cause various health issues.

Function of the Parathyroid Glands and Parathyroid Hormone (PTH)

The primary function of the parathyroid glands is to regulate the body's calcium and phosphorus levels. Calcium is essential for many physiological processes, including bone formation, muscle contraction, and nerve function. Phosphorus, on the other hand, is critical for energy production, cell membrane integrity, and DNA synthesis. The parathyroid glands maintain calcium homeostasis by secreting parathyroid hormone (PTH) in response to low blood calcium levels.

PTH exerts its effects through three primary mechanisms:

1. **Bone Resorption**: PTH stimulates osteoclasts, the cells responsible for bone resorption, to break down bone tissue, releasing calcium and phosphate into the bloodstream. This process increases blood calcium levels but decreases bone density over time.
2. **Renal Calcium Reabsorption**: PTH increases calcium reabsorption in the kidneys, reducing the amount of calcium excreted in the urine. Simultaneously, it decreases phosphate reabsorption, leading to increased phosphate excretion.
3. **Activation of Vitamin D**: PTH stimulates the conversion of 25-hydroxyvitamin D (the inactive form of vitamin D) to 1,25-dihydroxyvitamin D (the active form) in the kidneys. Active vitamin D enhances calcium absorption in the intestines, further contributing to the elevation of blood calcium levels.

These functions are tightly regulated to ensure that blood calcium levels remain within a narrow range. Disruption in the regulation of PTH, as seen in parathyroid cancer, can lead to severe hypercalcemia and its associated complications.

Production of Parathyroid Hormone (PTH) and Its Regulation

PTH production is regulated by a feedback loop involving blood calcium levels and the calcium-sensing receptors (CaSR) located on the surface of parathyroid cells. When blood calcium levels decrease, the CaSRs detect this change and stimulate the release of PTH. Conversely, when blood calcium levels are high, PTH secretion is suppressed. This negative feedback loop ensures that calcium homeostasis is maintained.

In parathyroid cancer, the normal regulatory mechanisms are often disrupted. Parathyroid cancer cells may produce excessive amounts of PTH, leading to hypercalcemia. Unlike benign parathyroid adenomas, which are the most common cause of primary hyperparathyroidism, parathyroid carcinoma is characterized by the invasive growth of cancerous cells, which can spread to adjacent tissues and distant organs.

Pathways Involved in Parathyroid Cancer

The molecular pathways involved in the development of parathyroid cancer are complex and not yet fully understood. However, several key pathways and genetic mutations have been identified as contributing factors:

1. **HRPT2/CDC73 Gene Mutation**: The most well-established genetic abnormality associated with parathyroid cancer is a mutation in the HRPT2 gene, also known as the CDC73 gene. This gene encodes the protein parafibromin, which plays a role in tumor suppression. Mutations in HRPT2/CDC73 result in the loss of parafibromin function, leading to uncontrolled cell growth and tumor development in the parathyroid glands. This mutation is present in a significant proportion of parathyroid carcinomas.

2. **Wnt/β-Catenin Pathway**: The Wnt/β-catenin signaling pathway is involved in cell proliferation, differentiation, and survival. Aberrant activation of this pathway has been implicated in var-

ious cancers, including parathyroid cancer. Mutations or alterations in components of the Wnt/β-catenin pathway can lead to the accumulation of β-catenin in the nucleus, promoting the expression of genes that drive cell proliferation and tumor growth.

3. **PI3K/Akt/mTOR Pathway**: The PI3K/Akt/mTOR pathway is another critical signaling pathway involved in cell growth and survival. Dysregulation of this pathway, through mutations or overactivation, can contribute to the development and progression of parathyroid cancer. The pathway promotes cell proliferation and inhibits apoptosis, leading to the unchecked growth of cancer cells.

4. **Cyclin D1 Overexpression**: Cyclin D1 is a cell cycle regulator that promotes the transition from the G1 phase to the S phase of the cell cycle, facilitating cell division. Overexpression of cyclin D1 has been observed in some cases of parathyroid cancer, contributing to uncontrolled cell proliferation.

5. **Angiogenesis**: Angiogenesis, the formation of new blood vessels, is a critical process in tumor growth and metastasis. Tumors, including parathyroid carcinomas, secrete various factors such as vascular endothelial growth factor (VEGF) that promote angiogenesis, ensuring an adequate blood supply to support tumor growth and dissemination.

Causes and Risk Factors

Parathyroid cancer is a rare condition, and its exact cause is often unknown. However, several risk factors and potential causes have been identified, including:

1. **Genetic Predisposition**: As mentioned earlier, mutations in the HRPT2/CDC73 gene are strongly associated with parathyroid cancer. Individuals with familial hyperparathyroidism-jaw tumor syndrome (HPT-JT), which is caused by germline mutations in

HRPT2/CDC73, have an increased risk of developing parathyroid cancer.

2. **Radiation Exposure**: Exposure to ionizing radiation, particularly during childhood, has been linked to an increased risk of developing various thyroid and parathyroid disorders, including cancer. This association is primarily due to radiation-induced DNA damage, which can lead to mutations and carcinogenesis.

3. **Chronic Kidney Disease**: Patients with chronic kidney disease (CKD) often develop secondary hyperparathyroidism due to impaired kidney function and the inability to excrete phosphate effectively. Over time, this condition can progress to tertiary hyperparathyroidism, characterized by autonomous PTH secretion. While tertiary hyperparathyroidism is more commonly associated with benign parathyroid hyperplasia or adenomas, there is a potential risk for malignant transformation, particularly in patients with long-standing disease.

4. **Dietary Factors**: While the role of diet in the development of parathyroid cancer is not as well-established as in other cancers, some studies suggest that dietary factors, particularly the consumption of animal products, may influence the risk of developing parathyroid disorders, including cancer. High intake of dietary calcium, particularly from dairy products, has been associated with an increased risk of hyperparathyroidism, a condition that can predispose individuals to parathyroid cancer.

Animal Products and Parathyroid Cancer: Potential Links

The consumption of animal products has been linked to various types of cancer, primarily due to the presence of carcinogens, hormones, and other bioactive compounds that may promote tumorigenesis. Several mechanisms through which animal products may contribute to the development of parathyroid cancer include:

1. **High Dietary Calcium**: Dairy products are a significant source of dietary calcium. While calcium is essential for bone health, excessive intake, particularly from animal sources, may increase the risk of hyperparathyroidism. Elevated calcium levels can lead to the overproduction of PTH and potentially contribute to the development of parathyroid cancer in susceptible individuals.

2. **Hormonal Contaminants**: Animal products, particularly meat and dairy, often contain exogenous hormones, such as estrogens and growth hormones, which can disrupt endocrine function and promote the growth of hormone-sensitive tissues, including the parathyroid glands. Chronic exposure to these hormones may increase the risk of tumorigenesis.

3. **Inflammation and Oxidative Stress**: The consumption of red and processed meats has been associated with increased inflammation and oxidative stress, both of which are known to contribute to cancer development. Chronic inflammation can lead to DNA damage, promote cell proliferation, and inhibit apoptosis, creating an environment conducive to cancer formation.

4. **Phosphate Additives**: Many processed animal products contain phosphate additives, which are used as preservatives and flavor enhancers. High phosphate intake has been linked to disruptions in phosphate and calcium metabolism, potentially leading to secondary hyperparathyroidism and increasing the risk of parathyroid gland abnormalities, including cancer.

5. **IGF-1 Pathway Activation**: Insulin-like growth factor 1 (IGF-1) is a hormone that plays a crucial role in cell growth and proliferation. High levels of IGF-1, which can be stimulated by the consumption of animal protein, have been linked to an increased risk of several cancers, including those of the endocrine system. IGF-1 promotes cell division and inhibits apoptosis, potentially contributing to the growth of parathyroid tumors.

Plant-Based Diet and Reversal of Parathyroid Cancer

A plant-based diet, rich in fruits, vegetables, whole grains, legumes, nuts, and seeds, offers several potential benefits in reducing the risk and aiding the reversal of parathyroid cancer. The following mechanisms highlight how a plant-based diet can be protective and therapeutic:

1. **Lower Dietary Calcium**: Plant-based diets tend to be lower in dietary calcium compared to diets rich in dairy products. This may reduce the risk of hypercalcemia and hyperparathyroidism, which are predisposing factors for parathyroid cancer. Calcium from plant sources, such as leafy greens and fortified plant milks, is absorbed differently from that in dairy products, potentially offering a more balanced approach to calcium intake without over-stimulating PTH production.

2. **Anti-inflammatory Effects**: A diet rich in plant foods is naturally anti-inflammatory due to the presence of phytochemicals, antioxidants, and dietary fiber. Chronic inflammation is a known risk factor for cancer development, and reducing inflammation through diet may help prevent the initiation and progression of parathyroid cancer. For example, compounds like curcumin (found in turmeric), resveratrol (found in grapes), and quercetin (found in onions and apples) have been shown to exhibit anti-inflammatory and anti-cancer properties.

3. **Antioxidant Defense**: Oxidative stress, caused by an imbalance between free radicals and antioxidants, can lead to DNA damage and cancer development. Plant-based diets are rich in antioxidants, such as vitamins C and E, carotenoids, and polyphenols, which neutralize free radicals and protect cells from oxidative damage. By enhancing the body's antioxidant defense, a plant-based diet may help reduce the risk of parathyroid cancer.

4. **Hormone Regulation**: A plant-based diet can help regulate hormone levels, particularly by reducing exposure to exogenous hormones found in animal products. Phytoestrogens, which are

plant-derived compounds found in foods like soy, flaxseeds, and legumes, can have a modulating effect on estrogen receptors, potentially reducing the risk of hormone-sensitive cancers, including those of the parathyroid glands.

5. **Alkaline Diet**: Many plant-based foods contribute to an alkaline diet, which may help in maintaining optimal blood pH levels. An acidic environment, often associated with high consumption of animal products, can lead to calcium leaching from bones and increased PTH production to maintain calcium balance. By promoting an alkaline environment, a plant-based diet may reduce the need for excessive PTH secretion and lower the risk of parathyroid gland hyperplasia or cancer.

6. **Lower Phosphate Levels**: Plant-based diets are generally lower in phosphate compared to diets high in animal products. This can help prevent disruptions in phosphate and calcium metabolism, reducing the risk of secondary hyperparathyroidism and parathyroid cancer. Additionally, plant-based foods are less likely to contain phosphate additives, further contributing to balanced mineral metabolism.

7. **Modulation of IGF-1 Levels**: A plant-based diet, particularly one low in animal protein, has been shown to reduce circulating levels of IGF-1. Lower IGF-1 levels are associated with a reduced risk of cancer, including endocrine-related cancers like parathyroid cancer. The reduction in IGF-1 may decrease cell proliferation and promote apoptosis, helping to prevent the growth and spread of parathyroid tumors.

8. **Enhanced Detoxification Pathways**: A diet rich in cruciferous vegetables, such as broccoli, cauliflower, and Brussels sprouts, can enhance the body's detoxification pathways. These vegetables contain compounds like sulforaphane, which support the liver's ability to detoxify carcinogens and other harmful substances. By enhancing detoxification, a plant-based diet may reduce the bur-

den of toxins that could potentially contribute to parathyroid cancer development.

Clinical Evidence Supporting Plant-Based Diets

While direct studies on the impact of plant-based diets on parathyroid cancer are limited due to the rarity of the disease, evidence from related research on diet and endocrine health supports the potential benefits of a plant-based approach:

1. **Dietary Patterns and Hyperparathyroidism**: Studies have shown that diets high in fruits and vegetables are associated with a lower risk of hyperparathyroidism, a condition that can lead to parathyroid cancer. The Nurses' Health Study, for example, found that a higher intake of dietary fiber and antioxidant-rich foods was inversely associated with the risk of developing hyperparathyroidism.

2. **Plant-Based Diets and Hormone Regulation**: Research has demonstrated that plant-based diets can help regulate hormone levels, particularly by reducing circulating levels of IGF-1 and improving insulin sensitivity. These hormonal changes may reduce the risk of developing hormone-related cancers, including those of the parathyroid glands.

3. **Cancer Prevention**: Numerous studies have highlighted the role of plant-based diets in cancer prevention. For instance, the Adventist Health Study-2 found that vegetarians had a significantly lower risk of developing various cancers compared to non-vegetarians. The anti-inflammatory, antioxidant, and hormone-modulating effects of plant-based diets likely contribute to this protective effect.

4. **Reversal of Hypercalcemia**: There is some evidence to suggest that dietary interventions can help manage hypercalcemia, a key feature of parathyroid cancer. A case report published in the Jour-

nal of Clinical Endocrinology and Metabolism described a patient with hypercalcemia who achieved significant improvement in calcium levels after adopting a plant-based diet, highlighting the potential of dietary modification in managing parathyroid disorders.

Parathyroid cancer is a rare but serious condition characterized by the uncontrolled growth of parathyroid cells and the overproduction of parathyroid hormone. The development of parathyroid cancer is influenced by genetic mutations, particularly in the HRPT2/CDC73 gene, as well as by disruptions in key signaling pathways such as the Wnt/β-catenin and PI3K/Akt/mTOR pathways. While the role of diet in the etiology of parathyroid cancer is still being explored, evidence suggests that the consumption of animal products, particularly those high in calcium, hormones, and phosphate, may increase the risk of developing this malignancy.

In contrast, a plant-based diet offers numerous protective benefits against parathyroid cancer and other related conditions. By reducing inflammation, oxidative stress, and hormone disruption, and by promoting balanced calcium and phosphate metabolism, a plant-based diet may help prevent the onset of parathyroid cancer and support the reversal of hypercalcemia and other related disorders. Although further research is needed to establish direct links between plant-based diets and parathyroid cancer prevention or reversal, the existing evidence strongly supports the adoption of a plant-based diet as part of a comprehensive approach to endocrine health and cancer prevention.

Prostate Cancer

Prostate cancer is one of the most common types of cancer among men worldwide, particularly in Western countries. It arises in the prostate gland, which is a small, walnut-shaped gland in men that produces seminal fluid. This fluid is crucial for nourishing and transporting sperm during ejaculation. Prostate cancer often grows slowly and initially remains confined to the prostate gland, where it may not cause serious harm. However, some types of prostate cancer are more aggressive and can spread quickly.

Function and Production of Prostate Cancer

The primary function of the prostate gland is to produce fluid that, together with sperm cells from the testes and fluids from other glands, makes up semen. The prostate gland surrounds the urethra, the tube through which urine and semen exit the body. The prostate's growth and function are largely controlled by androgens, primarily testosterone, which is produced in the testes.

Prostate cancer develops when the cells in the prostate begin to grow uncontrollably. Like all cancers, prostate cancer is a result of genetic mutations that cause normal cells to become cancerous. These mutations often occur in the DNA of a single prostate cell, causing it to divide more rapidly than normal cells and to survive longer than it should. As these abnormal cells accumulate, they form a tumor, which can grow and invade surrounding tissues or spread to other parts of the body, a process known as metastasis.

Pathways Involved in Prostate Cancer Development

Prostate cancer is influenced by several molecular pathways, many of which involve hormones, growth factors, and signaling proteins. Here are some of the key pathways involved in prostate cancer:

1. Androgen Receptor Signaling Pathway

Androgens, such as testosterone and dihydrotestosterone (DHT), play a crucial role in prostate cancer development and progression.

These hormones bind to the androgen receptor (AR), a type of nuclear receptor that, once activated, translocates to the cell nucleus and regulates the expression of genes involved in cell growth, differentiation, and survival. In prostate cancer, the AR signaling pathway is often dysregulated, leading to uncontrolled cell proliferation.

Androgen deprivation therapy (ADT), which reduces androgen levels or blocks their interaction with the AR, is a common treatment for prostate cancer. However, many tumors eventually become resistant to ADT, often due to mutations in the AR gene that allow the receptor to remain active even in low-androgen environments.

2. PI3K/AKT/mTOR Pathway

The PI3K/AKT/mTOR signaling pathway is another critical pathway in prostate cancer. This pathway is involved in cell growth, survival, and metabolism. In prostate cancer, it is often activated due to mutations or loss of the PTEN tumor suppressor gene. Activation of the PI3K/AKT/mTOR pathway leads to increased cell proliferation and survival, contributing to tumor growth and progression.

Targeting the PI3K/AKT/mTOR pathway is a potential therapeutic strategy for prostate cancer, especially in cases where the AR pathway is no longer effective.

3. Wnt/β-catenin Pathway

The Wnt/β-catenin pathway is involved in regulating cell fate, migration, and proliferation. In prostate cancer, this pathway can be aberrantly activated, leading to increased β-catenin levels in the cell nucleus, where it promotes the expression of genes that drive tumor growth. Mutations in components of the Wnt/β-catenin pathway are found in some prostate cancers, particularly in more aggressive forms of the disease.

4. Inflammatory Pathways

Chronic inflammation is thought to play a role in prostate cancer development. Inflammatory cytokines and chemokines can create a tumor-promoting environment by inducing oxidative stress, DNA damage, and promoting cell survival and proliferation. Pathways such as

NF-κB and STAT3, which are involved in the inflammatory response, have been implicated in prostate cancer progression.

5. Cell Cycle and Apoptosis Regulation

Cell cycle dysregulation and evasion of apoptosis (programmed cell death) are hallmarks of cancer. In prostate cancer, alterations in genes that regulate the cell cycle, such as p53 and RB1, can lead to uncontrolled cell division. Similarly, mutations in genes involved in apoptosis, such as BCL-2, can allow cancer cells to survive when they should normally undergo programmed death.

Known Causes Related to Animal Products

Diet plays a significant role in the risk of developing prostate cancer, and a substantial body of evidence links the consumption of certain animal products to an increased risk of the disease. The following are some of the animal-derived foods that have been implicated in prostate cancer:

1. Red and Processed Meats

Red meat, particularly when cooked at high temperatures, produces carcinogenic compounds such as heterocyclic amines (HCAs) and polycyclic aromatic hydrocarbons (PAHs). These compounds have been shown to cause DNA damage in prostate cells, leading to mutations that can initiate cancer development. Processed meats, which are preserved through smoking, curing, or adding chemical preservatives, contain nitrates and nitrites that can also form carcinogenic compounds in the body.

Studies have consistently shown that a high intake of red and processed meats is associated with an increased risk of prostate cancer, particularly aggressive forms of the disease. The World Health Organization (WHO) has classified processed meat as a Group 1 carcinogen, meaning there is sufficient evidence to link it to cancer in humans, and

red meat as a Group 2A carcinogen, indicating that it is probably carcinogenic to humans.

2. Dairy Products

Dairy products, including milk, cheese, and yogurt, are another cate-
gory of animal-derived foods that have been associated with an increased
risk of prostate cancer. The high calcium content in dairy products is
thought to be a contributing factor, as excessive calcium intake can suppress the production of 1,25-dihydroxyvitamin D3 (the active form of
vitamin D), a hormone that has protective effects against prostate cancer.

Moreover, dairy products are rich in hormones, such as insulin-like
growth factor 1 (IGF-1), which promotes cell growth and inhibits apoptosis. Elevated levels of IGF-1 have been linked to an increased risk of
several cancers, including prostate cancer. Some studies have also suggested that dairy products may increase oxidative stress and inflammation, further contributing to cancer risk.

3. Saturated Fats

Diets high in saturated fats, commonly found in animal products
like fatty cuts of meat, butter, and full-fat dairy products, have been
linked to a higher risk of prostate cancer. Saturated fats can increase the
production of cholesterol, which is a precursor to androgens like testosterone. Elevated androgen levels can stimulate the growth of prostate
cancer cells.

In addition, saturated fats can promote inflammation and oxidative
stress, which are known to contribute to cancer development. Studies
have shown that men who consume diets high in saturated fats have a
higher risk of developing prostate cancer and dying from the disease.

4. Animal Protein

Animal protein, particularly from red meat, can increase the production of certain hormones and growth factors, such as IGF-1, that
promote the growth of cancer cells. Furthermore, the consumption of
animal protein leads to the production of higher levels of acid in the

body, which the kidneys neutralize by excreting calcium. This calcium loss can contribute to an environment that favors cancer development.

The Role of a Plant-Based Diet in Prostate Cancer Reversal

A plant-based diet, which emphasizes whole, unprocessed plant foods like fruits, vegetables, whole grains, legumes, nuts, and seeds, has been shown to have protective effects against prostate cancer. Such a diet is low in saturated fats and free of the carcinogens found in animal products, making it an effective strategy for both preventing and managing prostate cancer.

1. Antioxidant and Anti-Inflammatory Effects

Plant-based foods are rich in antioxidants, such as vitamins C and E, carotenoids, and polyphenols, which protect cells from oxidative stress by neutralizing free radicals. Oxidative stress can lead to DNA damage, a key step in cancer development. By reducing oxidative stress, a plant-based diet can help prevent the initiation and progression of prostate cancer.

In addition, many plant foods have anti-inflammatory properties. Chronic inflammation is a known risk factor for cancer, including prostate cancer. Phytochemicals found in fruits, vegetables, and other plant foods can reduce inflammation by inhibiting inflammatory pathways like NF-κB and reducing the production of pro-inflammatory cytokines.

2. Hormonal Regulation

A plant-based diet can also help regulate hormone levels, which is crucial in prostate cancer prevention and management. For example, consuming a diet rich in phytoestrogens, such as those found in soy products, can have a modulating effect on estrogen levels. Phytoestrogens can bind to estrogen receptors and exert weak estrogenic or anti-estrogenic effects, depending on the context. This can help reduce the risk of hormone-dependent cancers like prostate cancer.

Furthermore, a plant-based diet is typically lower in fats, particularly saturated fats, which can reduce the production of androgens like testosterone. Lowering androgen levels can slow the growth of prostate cancer cells and reduce the risk of cancer progression.

3. Impact on IGF-1 Levels

Insulin-like growth factor 1 (IGF-1) is a hormone that plays a significant role in cell growth and development. Elevated levels of IGF-1 have been linked to an increased risk of several cancers, including prostate cancer. A plant-based diet, particularly one that is low in animal protein, has been shown to reduce IGF-1 levels in the body. This reduction in IGF-1 can decrease the proliferation of cancer cells and inhibit tumor growth.

4. Epigenetic Modulation

Epigenetics refers to changes in gene expression that do not involve alterations in the DNA sequence. Diet and lifestyle factors can influence epigenetic mechanisms, such as DNA methylation and histone modification, which can either promote or suppress cancer development. A plant-based diet has been shown to positively affect epigenetic markers associated with cancer.

For example, certain phytochemicals, such as sulforaphane (found in cruciferous vegetables like broccoli) and curcumin (found in turmeric), can modulate epigenetic pathways and inhibit the expression of oncogenes (genes that promote cancer). By altering the epigenetic landscape, a plant-based diet can potentially reverse cancerous changes in prostate cells.

5. Microbiome Modulation

The gut microbiome, the community of microorganisms residing in the gastrointestinal tract, plays a crucial role in health and disease, including cancer. Diet is one of the most significant factors influencing the composition of the gut microbiome. A plant-based diet promotes a healthy gut microbiome rich in beneficial bacteria that produce short-chain fatty acids (SCFAs), such as butyrate.

SCFAs have anti-inflammatory and anti-cancer properties. They can inhibit the growth of cancer cells, induce apoptosis, and reduce inflammation in the prostate. Additionally, a healthy gut microbiome can enhance the immune system's ability to recognize and eliminate cancer cells.

Evidence Supporting a Plant-Based Diet for Prostate Cancer

Several clinical studies have explored the impact of a plant-based diet on prostate cancer, providing evidence of its protective and therapeutic effects.

1. Ornish Study

One of the most well-known studies in this area was conducted by Dr. Dean Ornish and colleagues. The Ornish study involved men with early-stage prostate cancer who chose active surveillance (monitoring the cancer rather than immediate treatment). Participants were placed on a comprehensive lifestyle intervention that included a low-fat, whole-food, plant-based diet, regular physical activity, stress management techniques, and social support.

The study found that after one year, the men who followed the plant-based diet had lower PSA levels (a marker of prostate cancer progression), reduced prostate cancer cell growth, and increased cancer cell apoptosis compared to the control group. Moreover, the intervention group showed favorable changes in gene expression related to cancer progression, highlighting the potential of a plant-based diet to slow or even reverse the course of prostate cancer.

2. Adventist Health Study

The Adventist Health Study, which includes a large cohort of Seventh-day Adventists (many of whom follow vegetarian or vegan diets), has provided valuable insights into the relationship between diet and prostate cancer risk. The study found that men who followed a vegan diet had a significantly lower risk of prostate cancer compared to those who consumed meat and dairy products.

The reduced risk was particularly notable for aggressive forms of prostate cancer, suggesting that a plant-based diet may be especially beneficial in preventing the most dangerous types of the disease.

3. Pritikin Program

The Pritikin Program, which promotes a low-fat, high-fiber, plant-based diet combined with exercise, has also been shown to benefit men with prostate cancer. Research has demonstrated that this program can reduce PSA levels and slow the progression of prostate cancer. The Pritikin Program's emphasis on whole, unprocessed plant foods and lifestyle modifications aligns with the broader evidence supporting the role of a plant-based diet in cancer prevention and management.

Adopting a Plant-Based Diet for Prostate Cancer

For men with prostate cancer or those at risk of developing the disease, adopting a plant-based diet can be a powerful strategy for improving health outcomes. Here are some practical considerations for making the transition:

1. Focus on Whole Foods

Emphasize whole, unprocessed plant foods in your diet, such as fruits, vegetables, whole grains, legumes, nuts, and seeds. These foods are rich in nutrients, fiber, and phytochemicals that support overall health and protect against cancer.

2. Eliminate Animal Products

To maximize the benefits of a plant-based diet, eliminate the consumption of animal products, including red meat, processed meats, dairy, and eggs. Replace these foods with plant-based alternatives, such as legumes, tofu, tempeh, and plant-based milks.

3. Include a Variety of Plant Foods

Eating a diverse range of plant foods ensures that you obtain a broad spectrum of nutrients and phytochemicals. Aim to include a variety of colors in your meals, as different colored fruits and vegetables contain different beneficial compounds.

4. Be Mindful of Protein Intake

While it is possible to meet your protein needs on a plant-based diet, it is essential to include protein-rich plant foods, such as legumes, tofu, tempeh, seitan, quinoa, and nuts. These foods provide all the essential amino acids necessary for health.

5. Consider Supplementing with Vitamin B12

Vitamin B12 is primarily found in animal products, so those following a strict plant-based diet should consider supplementing with vitamin B12 to prevent deficiency. Fortified foods, such as plant-based milks and cereals, can also provide B12.

6. Stay Hydrated

Adequate hydration is important for overall health and can support the body's natural detoxification processes. Drink plenty of water throughout the day, and consider incorporating herbal teas and water-rich fruits and vegetables into your diet.

7. Engage in Regular Physical Activity

In addition to following a plant-based diet, regular physical activity is crucial for maintaining a healthy weight, reducing inflammation, and improving overall health. Aim for at least 150 minutes of moderate-intensity exercise, such as brisk walking, each week.

8. Manage Stress

Chronic stress can have detrimental effects on health, including increasing the risk of cancer. Incorporate stress management techniques, such as mindfulness meditation, deep breathing exercises, and yoga, into your daily routine.

Prostate cancer is a complex disease influenced by a combination of genetic, hormonal, and environmental factors. The pathways involved in its development, such as the androgen receptor signaling pathway and the PI3K/AKT/mTOR pathway, highlight the intricate mechanisms that drive cancer progression. While certain animal products, including red and processed meats, dairy, and saturated fats, have been linked to an increased risk of prostate cancer, a plant-based diet offers a promising approach for both prevention and management.

By reducing exposure to carcinogens, modulating hormone levels, lowering IGF-1 levels, and promoting a healthy gut microbiome, a plant-based diet can help slow the progression of prostate cancer and potentially reverse the disease. Clinical studies, such as the Ornish study and the Adventist Health Study, provide compelling evidence supporting the protective effects of plant-based eating.

For men at risk of or diagnosed with prostate cancer, transitioning to a plant-based diet, coupled with lifestyle modifications like regular exercise and stress management, offers a holistic and evidence-based approach to improving outcomes. The growing body of research underscores the potential of plant-based nutrition to not only reduce the risk of prostate cancer but also to enhance overall health and longevity.

Retinoblastoma

Retinoblastoma is a rare form of eye cancer that primarily affects young children, usually under the age of five. It arises in the retina, the light-sensitive layer of tissue at the back of the eye. While the cancer can be life-threatening if not treated promptly, the majority of cases are curable, especially when detected early.

Function of Retinoblastoma

Retinoblastoma develops from the immature cells of the retina, known as retinoblasts. The retina is responsible for converting light into neural signals, which are then processed by the brain to create visual images. In Retinoblastoma, mutations in the genes that control cell division and differentiation lead to uncontrolled growth of these retinal cells, resulting in the formation of tumors.

The primary function of Retinoblastoma, from a pathological perspective, is the abnormal proliferation of retinal cells due to the loss of regulatory mechanisms that normally inhibit excessive cell growth. The cancerous cells fail to differentiate into mature retinal cells and instead continue to divide uncontrollably, forming a mass that can affect vision and, if untreated, metastasize to other parts of the body.

Production of Retinoblastoma

The production of Retinoblastoma is primarily driven by mutations in the RB1 gene, which is located on chromosome 13q14. The RB1 gene is a tumor suppressor gene that encodes the retinoblastoma protein (pRB). This protein plays a critical role in regulating the cell cycle, particularly the transition from the G1 phase to the S phase, where DNA replication occurs.

In a healthy cell, pRB functions to prevent excessive cell division by inhibiting the activity of transcription factors like E2F, which are necessary for the progression of the cell cycle. When pRB is phosphorylated, it releases E2F, allowing the cell to proceed with DNA replication and division. However, when the RB1 gene is mutated, the production of functional pRB is impaired, leading to a loss of cell cycle control and the unchecked proliferation of retinal cells.

Retinoblastoma can occur in two forms: hereditary and sporadic. In hereditary Retinoblastoma, a germline mutation in one copy of the RB1 gene is inherited from a parent, while the second copy undergoes somatic mutation later in life, leading to tumor development. This form of Retinoblastoma typically presents in both eyes (bilateral). In sporadic Retinoblastoma, both copies of the RB1 gene are mutated in a single retinal cell, leading to tumor formation in one eye (unilateral).

Regulation of Retinoblastoma

The regulation of Retinoblastoma is closely tied to the molecular mechanisms that govern cell cycle progression and apoptosis (programmed cell death). The RB1 gene and its protein product, pRB, are central to this regulation.

1. **Cell Cycle Regulation**: The pRB protein exerts its regulatory effect by binding to and inhibiting the E2F family of transcription factors, which are essential for the transcription of genes required for DNA synthesis. In its hypophosphorylated state, pRB is active and binds E2F, preventing the cell from entering the S phase. When pRB is phosphorylated by cyclin-dependent kinases (CDKs), it releases E2F, allowing the cell cycle to progress. In Retinoblastoma, mutations in the RB1 gene result in the production of a dysfunctional pRB protein that cannot effectively regulate the cell cycle, leading to uncontrolled cell division.

2. **Apoptosis Regulation**: pRB also plays a role in apoptosis by interacting with various proteins that promote cell death in response to DNA damage or other cellular stresses. When pRB is inactivated due to RB1 mutations, the cell loses its ability to undergo apoptosis in response to signals that would normally trigger cell death, contributing to tumor formation.

3. **Epigenetic Regulation**: Epigenetic modifications, such as DNA methylation and histone acetylation, also play a role in the regulation of the RB1 gene and the development of Retinoblastoma. Hypermethylation of the RB1 promoter region can lead to the silencing of the gene, further contributing to the loss of pRB function and the development of the disease.

Molecular Pathways in Retinoblastoma

Several key molecular pathways are involved in the development and progression of Retinoblastoma:

1. **RB1 Pathway**: The RB1 pathway is the primary pathway implicated in Retinoblastoma. The loss of function of the RB1 gene leads to the deregulation of the cell cycle and the unchecked proliferation of retinal cells. This pathway is also involved in maintaining genomic stability, and its disruption can lead to additional genetic alterations that contribute to tumorigenesis.

2. **p53 Pathway**: The p53 protein is another critical tumor suppressor that plays a role in the cellular response to DNA damage. In Retinoblastoma, the p53 pathway may be indirectly affected by the loss of pRB function, as pRB and p53 interact in the regulation of cell cycle arrest and apoptosis. Mutations in the TP53 gene, although less common in Retinoblastoma compared to other cancers, can further compromise the cell's ability to respond to DNA damage and contribute to tumor progression.

3. **MYCN Pathway**: Amplification of the MYCN oncogene is observed in a subset of Retinoblastoma cases. MYCN is a transcription factor that drives cell proliferation and is often associated with aggressive forms of cancer. In Retinoblastoma, MYCN amplification is linked to a more aggressive disease phenotype and poor prognosis.

4. **Wnt Signaling Pathway**: The Wnt signaling pathway is involved in cell proliferation, differentiation, and apoptosis. Aberrant activation of the Wnt pathway has been implicated in Retinoblastoma, where it may contribute to the unchecked proliferation of retinal cells and resistance to apoptosis.

5. **Hedgehog Signaling Pathway**: The Hedgehog signaling pathway plays a role in embryonic development and the maintenance of stem cells. Dysregulation of this pathway has been associated with various cancers, including Retinoblastoma. Abnormal activation of Hedgehog signaling can promote the proliferation of cancer stem cells and contribute to tumor growth.

Known Causes and Animal Products

While Retinoblastoma can be caused by genetic mutations, environmental factors, including diet, may also influence the development and progression of the disease. Research has suggested that certain components of animal products may contribute to cancer risk by promoting inflammation, oxidative stress, and the activation of oncogenic pathways.

1. **Saturated Fats**: Diets high in saturated fats, commonly found in animal products such as red meat, butter, and cheese, have been associated with increased cancer risk. Saturated fats can promote inflammation and oxidative stress, leading to DNA damage and the activation of oncogenic pathways, including those involved in Retinoblastoma.

2. **Heme Iron**: Heme iron, found in red meat, has been implicated in cancer development due to its ability to generate free radicals through the Fenton reaction. These free radicals can cause oxidative damage to DNA, leading to mutations in critical genes such as RB1. Additionally, heme iron may promote the proliferation of cancer cells by increasing the availability of iron, which is essential for DNA synthesis and cell division.

3. **Dairy Products**: Some studies have suggested a potential link between the consumption of dairy products and an increased risk of certain cancers, including Retinoblastoma. The presence of growth factors, such as insulin-like growth factor-1 (IGF-1), in dairy products may promote cell proliferation and inhibit apoptosis, contributing to tumor development.

4. **Processed Meats**: Processed meats, such as bacon, sausages, and hot dogs, contain nitrates and nitrites, which can be converted into carcinogenic compounds known as nitrosamines. These compounds can cause DNA damage and have been associated with an increased risk of various cancers, including those affecting the retina.

Plant-Based Diet and Retinoblastoma Reversal

A plant-based diet, rich in fruits, vegetables, whole grains, legumes, nuts, and seeds, has been shown to have numerous health benefits, including a reduced risk of cancer. Several mechanisms by which a plant-based diet may help in the prevention and reversal of Retinoblastoma include:

1. **Antioxidant Properties**: Fruits and vegetables are rich in antioxidants, such as vitamins C and E, carotenoids, and flavonoids, which can neutralize free radicals and reduce oxidative stress. By protecting against DNA damage, antioxidants may help prevent the mutations that lead to Retinoblastoma.

2. **Anti-Inflammatory Effects**: A plant-based diet is typically lower in pro-inflammatory compounds found in animal products, such as saturated fats and arachidonic acid. Plant foods are also rich in anti-inflammatory compounds, such as omega-3 fatty acids, polyphenols, and fiber. By reducing inflammation, a plant-based diet may lower the risk of cancer development and progression.

3. **Regulation of Cell Cycle and Apoptosis**: Certain plant compounds, such as sulforaphane (found in cruciferous vegetables), resveratrol (found in grapes), and curcumin (found in turmeric), have been shown to modulate cell cycle regulation and promote apoptosis in cancer cells. These compounds may help restore the normal regulation of cell division and prevent the unchecked proliferation of retinal cells.

4. **Modulation of Epigenetic Changes**: Epigenetic modifications, such as DNA methylation and histone acetylation, play a role in the regulation of gene expression. Plant-based diets, which are high in folate, fiber, and phytochemicals, may influence these epigenetic changes and contribute to the reactivation of tumor suppressor genes like RB1.

5. **Reduction of IGF-1 Levels**: A plant-based diet has been associated with lower levels of insulin-like growth factor-1 (IGF-1), a
hormone that promotes cell growth and inhibits apoptosis. High
levels of IGF-1, often seen with the consumption of animal products, have been linked to an increased risk of various cancers, including Retinoblastoma. By reducing IGF-1 levels, a plant-based
diet may help prevent the development and progression of the
disease.

6. **Gut Microbiome and Cancer Prevention**: The gut microbiome, which is influenced by diet, plays a crucial role in overall
health, including cancer prevention. A plant-based diet promotes
a healthy gut microbiome by providing fiber and other prebiotics
that support the growth of beneficial bacteria. These bacteria can
produce short-chain fatty acids (SCFAs), such as butyrate, which
have anti-inflammatory and anti-cancer properties. A healthy gut
microbiome may contribute to the prevention of Retinoblastoma by modulating immune function and reducing inflammation.

7. **Detoxification Pathways**: Many plant foods contain compounds that enhance the body's natural detoxification processes,
helping to eliminate carcinogens and other harmful substances.
For example, cruciferous vegetables like broccoli and kale are rich
in glucosinolates, which are converted into isothiocyanates—compounds that activate detoxification enzymes and
protect against cancer.

Retinoblastoma is a complex cancer with a well-established genetic
basis, primarily involving mutations in the RB1 gene. However, environmental factors, including diet, may also influence the risk and
progression of the disease. Animal products, particularly those high in
saturated fats, heme iron, and growth factors, may contribute to can-

cer risk through mechanisms such as inflammation, oxidative stress, and disruption of cell cycle regulation.

In contrast, a plant-based diet offers numerous protective benefits, including antioxidant and anti-inflammatory properties, regulation of cell cycle and apoptosis, modulation of epigenetic changes, reduction of IGF-1 levels, and support of a healthy gut microbiome. By incorporating a variety of plant foods rich in nutrients and phytochemicals, individuals may reduce their risk of Retinoblastoma and support the body's natural defenses against cancer.

Skin Cancer

Skin cancer is the most common type of cancer, affecting millions of people worldwide each year. It develops when skin cells undergo abnormal growth, often due to exposure to ultraviolet (UV) radiation from the sun or tanning beds. There are several types of skin cancer, including basal cell carcinoma, squamous cell carcinoma, and melanoma, each with unique characteristics, causes, and treatment options. While the causes of skin cancer are multifactorial, emerging research suggests that diet, particularly a plant-based diet, may play a significant role in the prevention and reversal of this condition.

Function of Skin Cancer

Skin cancer primarily functions by disrupting the normal processes of cell growth and differentiation in the skin. The skin, being the largest organ of the body, consists of three main layers: the epidermis (outermost layer), the dermis (middle layer), and the hypodermis (deepest layer). Skin cancer typically originates in the epidermis, where the most common cells are keratinocytes, melanocytes, and basal cells.

1. **Basal Cell Carcinoma (BCC):** BCC is the most common type of skin cancer, originating in the basal cells at the bottom of the epidermis. These cells are responsible for producing new skin cells as old ones die. BCC usually grows slowly and rarely spreads to other parts of the body. However, it can cause significant local damage if left untreated.
2. **Squamous Cell Carcinoma (SCC):** SCC originates in the squamous cells, which are flat cells located near the surface of the epidermis. This type of skin cancer is more aggressive than BCC and can spread to other parts of the body if not treated early.
3. **Melanoma:** Melanoma is the deadliest form of skin cancer and originates in the melanocytes, the cells responsible for producing melanin, the pigment that gives skin its color. Melanoma can spread rapidly to other organs if not detected and treated early.

Production of Skin Cancer

The production of skin cancer involves a series of genetic mutations that lead to uncontrolled cell growth. These mutations can be triggered by various factors, including environmental, genetic, and lifestyle factors. The process of skin cancer development can be divided into several stages:

1. **Initiation:** The initiation phase occurs when DNA damage occurs in the skin cells. This damage is often caused by UV radiation from the sun or tanning beds, leading to mutations in critical genes that control cell growth and repair. The most commonly affected genes in skin cancer are the tumor suppressor gene p53 and the proto-oncogene BRAF.
2. **Promotion:** During the promotion phase, the mutated cells begin to multiply abnormally. This phase is often influenced by factors such as chronic UV exposure, inflammation, and immune

system suppression. The mutated cells evade normal cellular control mechanisms and continue to proliferate.

3. **Progression:** In the progression phase, the abnormal cells accumulate further mutations, leading to the formation of a tumor. This tumor can invade surrounding tissues and, in some cases, metastasize to other parts of the body.

Regulation of Skin Cancer

The body has several mechanisms in place to regulate cell growth and prevent the development of cancer. However, these mechanisms can be compromised in individuals with skin cancer. The regulation of skin cancer involves both intrinsic and extrinsic factors:

Intrinsic Factors:

- **DNA Repair Mechanisms:** The skin has inherent DNA repair mechanisms that can correct damage caused by UV radiation. Enzymes such as nucleotide excision repair enzymes play a crucial role in identifying and repairing DNA damage. However, if these repair mechanisms are overwhelmed or faulty, mutations can accumulate, leading to skin cancer.

- **Tumor Suppressor Genes:** Tumor suppressor genes, such as p53, play a critical role in regulating cell growth and preventing cancer. The p53 gene, often referred to as the "guardian of the genome," can induce cell cycle arrest, DNA repair, or apoptosis (cell death) in response to DNA damage. Mutations in the p53 gene are common in skin cancer and can lead to uncontrolled cell growth.

- **Cell Cycle Control:** The cell cycle is tightly regulated by a series of checkpoints that ensure cells do not divide uncontrollably. Cyclins, cyclin-dependent kinases (CDKs), and CDK inhibitors are key regulators of the cell cycle. In skin cancer, mutations in these regulatory proteins can lead to unchecked cell division.

Extrinsic Factors:

- **Immune System:** The immune system plays a vital role in identifying and eliminating cancerous cells. However, skin cancer cells can evade immune surveillance through various mechanisms, such as downregulating major histocompatibility complex (MHC) molecules or secreting immunosuppressive cytokines. Immunotherapy, which enhances the immune system's ability to recognize and destroy cancer cells, has shown promise in treating advanced skin cancer.

- **Hormones and Growth Factors:** Hormones and growth factors, such as epidermal growth factor (EGF) and vascular endothelial growth factor (VEGF), can promote the growth and survival of skin cancer cells. Targeting these growth factors with specific inhibitors is a therapeutic strategy in skin cancer treatment.

Pathways Involved in Skin Cancer

The development and progression of skin cancer involve several key signaling pathways. Understanding these pathways provides insight into the molecular mechanisms of skin cancer and potential therapeutic targets.

1. **MAPK/ERK Pathway:** The mitogen-activated protein kinase (MAPK) pathway, also known as the extracellular signal-regulated kinase (ERK) pathway, is a key signaling cascade involved in cell proliferation, differentiation, and survival. Mutations in the BRAF gene, which encodes a protein kinase in the MAPK path-

way, are commonly found in melanoma. The V600E mutation in BRAF leads to constitutive activation of the MAPK pathway, driving uncontrolled cell growth. Targeted therapies, such as BRAF inhibitors, have been developed to treat melanoma with BRAF mutations.

2. **PI3K/AKT/mTOR Pathway:** The phosphoinositide 3-kinase (PI3K) pathway is another critical signaling pathway involved in cell growth, survival, and metabolism. Activation of PI3K leads to the phosphorylation and activation of AKT, which in turn activates the mammalian target of rapamycin (mTOR). This pathway is often dysregulated in skin cancer, leading to increased cell proliferation and survival. Inhibitors of the PI3K/AKT/mTOR pathway are being explored as potential treatments for skin cancer.

3. **Wnt/β-Catenin Pathway:** The Wnt/β-catenin pathway plays a crucial role in cell proliferation, differentiation, and migration. Aberrant activation of this pathway has been implicated in the development of various cancers, including skin cancer. In particular, mutations in the CTNNB1 gene, which encodes β-catenin, can lead to the accumulation of β-catenin in the nucleus, promoting the expression of genes involved in cell proliferation. Targeting the Wnt/β-catenin pathway is an area of active research in cancer therapy.

4. **Hedgehog Pathway:** The Hedgehog signaling pathway is essential for embryonic development and tissue regeneration. Dysregulation of this pathway, often due to mutations in the PTCH1 or SMO genes, can lead to the development of basal cell carcinoma.

Known Causes Related to Animal Products

While UV radiation is the primary cause of skin cancer, dietary factors, particularly those related to animal products, have been increasingly recognized as contributing factors. Several mechanisms through which animal products may promote skin cancer include:

1. **High-Fat Diets:** Diets high in saturated fats, commonly found in animal products, have been linked to an increased risk of various cancers, including skin cancer. Saturated fats can promote inflammation, oxidative stress, and insulin resistance, all of which are factors that contribute to cancer development. Moreover, a high-fat diet can lead to obesity, a known risk factor for skin cancer.

2. **Heme Iron:** Heme iron, predominantly found in red meat, has been associated with an increased risk of cancer, including skin cancer. Heme iron can promote the formation of reactive oxygen species (ROS), leading to oxidative damage to DNA, proteins, and lipids. This oxidative stress can result in mutations and contribute to the initiation and progression of skin cancer.

3. **Heterocyclic Amines (HCAs) and Polycyclic Aromatic Hydrocarbons (PAHs):** HCAs and PAHs are carcinogenic compounds formed when meat is cooked at high temperatures, such as grilling or frying. These compounds can cause DNA mutations and promote cancer development. Regular consumption of well-done or charred meat has been associated with an increased risk of skin cancer.

4. **Dairy Products:** Dairy consumption has been linked to an increased risk of various cancers, including skin cancer. Dairy products contain insulin-like growth factor 1 (IGF-1), a hormone that promotes cell growth and has been implicated in cancer development. High levels of IGF-1 can stimulate the proliferation of skin cells and contribute to the progression of skin cancer.

5. **Processed Meats:** Processed meats, such as bacon, sausages, and hot dogs, contain nitrates and nitrites, which can form carcinogenic N-nitroso compounds. These compounds have been associated with an increased risk of skin cancer and other malignancies.

Additionally, processed meats are often high in sodium and saturated fats, further contributing to cancer risk.

The Role of a Plant-Based Diet in Reversal

A plant-based diet, rich in fruits, vegetables, whole grains, legumes, nuts, and seeds, has been shown to have protective effects against various cancers, including skin cancer. Several mechanisms through which a plant-based diet may help reverse or prevent skin cancer include:

1. **Antioxidant-Rich Foods:** Plant-based foods are rich in antioxidants, such as vitamins C and E, beta-carotene, and polyphenols, which help neutralize free radicals and reduce oxidative stress. Antioxidants can protect skin cells from DNA damage caused by UV radiation and other environmental factors, thereby reducing the risk of skin cancer.

2. **Anti-Inflammatory Properties:** Many plant-based foods have anti-inflammatory properties that can help reduce chronic inflammation, a key driver of cancer development. For example, omega-3 fatty acids found in flaxseeds, walnuts, and chia seeds have been shown to reduce inflammation and inhibit the growth of cancer cells. Similarly, phytochemicals such as curcumin in turmeric and resveratrol in grapes have potent anti-inflammatory effects.

3. **Fiber-Rich Diet:** A plant-based diet is typically high in dietary fiber, which has been associated with a reduced risk of various cancers, including skin cancer. Fiber helps regulate blood sugar levels, reduce insulin resistance, and promote a healthy gut microbiome, all of which are factors that can influence cancer risk. Additionally, fiber binds to toxins and carcinogens in the digestive tract, facilitating their elimination from the body.

4. **Phytochemicals and Flavonoids:** Phytochemicals and flavonoids, found in a wide variety of plant foods, have been

shown to have anticancer properties. These compounds can inhibit the growth and proliferation of cancer cells, induce apoptosis, and modulate signaling pathways involved in cancer development. For example, quercetin, found in apples and onions, has been shown to inhibit the growth of melanoma cells, while sulforaphane, found in cruciferous vegetables like broccoli and kale, has been shown to induce phase II detoxification enzymes that protect against cancer.

5. **Low Glycemic Index:** Plant-based diets tend to have a lower glycemic index, meaning they cause a slower and more gradual rise in blood sugar levels. High glycemic index foods, often found in processed and refined animal products, can lead to spikes in insulin and IGF-1 levels, promoting cancer cell growth. By contrast, a low glycemic index diet helps maintain stable blood sugar levels and reduces the risk of insulin resistance, a factor associated with an increased risk of skin cancer.

6. **Weight Management:** A plant-based diet is typically lower in calories and higher in nutrient density, making it an effective strategy for weight management. Obesity is a known risk factor for various cancers, including skin cancer, as excess body fat can lead to chronic inflammation, hormonal imbalances, and insulin resistance. By promoting healthy weight loss and maintaining a healthy weight, a plant-based diet can reduce the risk of skin cancer.

7. **Detoxification:** Many plant-based foods, particularly cruciferous vegetables like broccoli, cabbage, and Brussels sprouts, contain compounds that support the body's natural detoxification processes. These foods can enhance the activity of detoxification enzymes in the liver, helping to eliminate carcinogens and reduce the risk of skin cancer. Additionally, the high water content of many plant-based foods helps to flush out toxins and keep the skin hydrated and healthy.

8. **Sun Protection:** Certain plant-based foods have been shown to offer natural sun protection by boosting the skin's resilience to UV radiation. For example, lycopene, found in tomatoes and watermelon, has been shown to protect the skin from sunburn and reduce the risk of skin cancer. Similarly, polyphenols in green tea have been shown to protect the skin from UV-induced damage and inhibit the growth of cancer cells.

Skin cancer is a complex disease influenced by a combination of genetic, environmental, and lifestyle factors. While UV radiation is the primary cause of skin cancer, dietary factors, particularly those related to animal products, can also play a significant role in its development. A diet high in saturated fats, heme iron, HCAs, PAHs, dairy products, and processed meats can increase the risk of skin cancer by promoting inflammation, oxidative stress, and insulin resistance.

Conversely, a plant-based diet rich in antioxidants, anti-inflammatory compounds, fiber, phytochemicals, and flavonoids can help prevent and even reverse skin cancer by protecting the skin from DNA damage, reducing inflammation, regulating blood sugar levels, and promoting healthy weight management. Additionally, plant-based foods that support detoxification and offer natural sun protection can further reduce the risk of skin cancer.

As research continues to uncover the complex interactions between diet and cancer, it is becoming increasingly clear that a plant-based diet offers significant protective benefits against skin cancer and other malignancies. By adopting a diet rich in whole, plant-based foods, individuals can take proactive steps to reduce their risk of skin cancer and support overall health and well-being.

Stomach Cancer

Stomach cancer, also known as gastric cancer, is a malignancy that originates in the cells lining the stomach. This type of cancer typically develops over many years and is influenced by a variety of factors, including diet, genetics, environmental factors, and infections. Understanding the function, production, and regulation of stomach cancer is crucial for developing effective prevention and treatment strategies.

Function of Stomach Cancer

Stomach cancer, like other forms of cancer, results from the uncontrolled growth and division of abnormal cells. These cells can invade and destroy normal tissue, leading to the formation of a tumor. The stomach plays a critical role in digestion, and when cancer develops in this organ, it can interfere with its ability to function properly. As the tumor grows, it can obstruct the passage of food, leading to symptoms such as difficulty swallowing, weight loss, nausea, vomiting, and a feeling of fullness after eating small amounts of food.

In the early stages, stomach cancer may not cause any symptoms, which is why it is often diagnosed at a more advanced stage. As the disease progresses, it can spread to other parts of the body through the lymphatic system or bloodstream, a process known as metastasis. This can further complicate treatment and reduce the chances of survival.

Production of Stomach Cancer

The production of stomach cancer involves a series of cellular and molecular changes that lead to the transformation of normal gastric cells into cancerous ones. The development of stomach cancer is a multistep process that can be divided into several stages:

1. **Initiation**: This stage involves the initial genetic mutations that occur in the cells lining the stomach. These mutations can be caused by various factors, including exposure to carcinogens, such as certain chemicals in processed meats or infections like *He-*

licobacter pylori (H. pylori). The genetic alterations can lead to the activation of oncogenes (genes that promote cell growth) or the inactivation of tumor suppressor genes (genes that inhibit cell growth), setting the stage for cancer development.

2. **Promotion**: In this stage, the mutated cells begin to proliferate abnormally. This abnormal growth is often triggered by chronic inflammation, which can be caused by persistent H. pylori infection or other factors such as chronic gastritis. The inflammatory environment promotes further genetic and epigenetic changes, leading to the clonal expansion of precancerous cells.

3. **Progression**: As the abnormal cells continue to grow and divide, they accumulate additional mutations that allow them to invade surrounding tissues and, eventually, metastasize to other parts of the body. This stage is characterized by the formation of a malignant tumor, which can be detected through various imaging techniques or biopsies.

4. **Metastasis**: In the final stage, cancer cells break away from the primary tumor and spread to other organs, such as the liver, lungs, or lymph nodes. Metastatic stomach cancer is more challenging to treat and is often associated with a poor prognosis.

Regulation of Stomach Cancer

The regulation of stomach cancer involves a complex interplay of genetic, epigenetic, and environmental factors. Several key pathways and regulatory mechanisms are involved in the development and progression of stomach cancer:

1. **Genetic Mutations**: Genetic mutations play a central role in the initiation and progression of stomach cancer. Mutations in genes such as TP53, CDH1, and KRAS are commonly associated with gastric cancer. TP53 is a tumor suppressor gene that regulates cell cycle arrest, DNA repair, and apoptosis (programmed cell death).

Mutations in TP53 can lead to the loss of these protective mechanisms, allowing cancer cells to survive and proliferate. CDH1 encodes E-cadherin, a protein involved in cell adhesion. Mutations in CDH1 can disrupt cell-cell adhesion, promoting invasion and metastasis. KRAS is an oncogene that regulates cell growth and division. Mutations in KRAS can lead to uncontrolled cell proliferation.

2. **Epigenetic Changes**: Epigenetic changes, such as DNA methylation and histone modification, also play a critical role in stomach cancer. These changes can alter gene expression without changing the underlying DNA sequence. For example, hypermethylation of the promoter region of tumor suppressor genes can silence their expression, contributing to cancer development. Conversely, hypomethylation of oncogenes can lead to their overexpression, further driving tumor growth.

3. **Inflammatory Pathways**: Chronic inflammation is a key driver of stomach cancer. Inflammation can be caused by persistent H. pylori infection, which is the most significant risk factor for gastric cancer. H. pylori infection triggers an immune response that leads to the production of pro-inflammatory cytokines, such as interleukin-1β (IL-1β), tumor necrosis factor-α (TNF-α), and interleukin-8 (IL-8). These cytokines promote a pro-inflammatory environment that supports the survival and proliferation of precancerous cells. Additionally, inflammation can induce oxidative stress, leading to DNA damage and further genetic mutations.

4. **Signaling Pathways**: Several signaling pathways are involved in the regulation of stomach cancer, including the Wnt/β-catenin, Hedgehog, and Notch pathways. The Wnt/β-catenin pathway is critical for cell proliferation and differentiation. Dysregulation of this pathway can lead to the accumulation of β-catenin in the nucleus, where it activates the transcription of genes that promote cell growth and survival. The Hedgehog pathway is involved in tissue patterning during embryogenesis, but its reactivation in

adult tissues can contribute to cancer development. The Notch pathway regulates cell fate determination, and its dysregulation has been implicated in various cancers, including stomach cancer.

Detailed Pathways Involved in Stomach Cancer

Understanding the pathways involved in stomach cancer is essential for developing targeted therapies and improving patient outcomes. Some of the key pathways implicated in stomach cancer include:

1. **Wnt/β-catenin Pathway**: The Wnt/β-catenin pathway is one of the most well-studied pathways in gastric cancer. Under normal conditions, β-catenin is bound to the cytoplasmic protein complex and is degraded by the ubiquitin-proteasome system. However, in the presence of Wnt ligands, this degradation is inhibited, leading to the accumulation of β-catenin in the cytoplasm. β-catenin then translocates to the nucleus, where it binds to T-cell factor/lymphoid enhancer-binding factor (TCF/LEF) transcription factors and activates the expression of target genes involved in cell proliferation and survival. Dysregulation of this pathway can result in uncontrolled cell growth and contribute to the development of gastric cancer.

2. **PI3K/AKT/mTOR Pathway**: The PI3K/AKT/mTOR pathway is another critical pathway involved in stomach cancer. Activation of this pathway promotes cell growth, proliferation, and survival by inhibiting apoptosis and promoting protein synthesis. Mutations or amplifications of genes encoding components of this pathway, such as PI3K, AKT, and mTOR, are frequently observed in gastric cancer. Additionally, the pathway can be activated by growth factor receptors, such as EGFR and HER2, which are overexpressed in some gastric cancers. Inhibitors targeting this pathway are being explored as potential therapeutic options for gastric cancer.

3. **NF-κB Pathway**: The NF-κB pathway is a key regulator of inflammation and immune responses. In gastric cancer, this pathway is often activated by chronic inflammation, particularly in the context of H. pylori infection. Activation of NF-κB leads to the transcription of genes involved in inflammation, cell survival, and proliferation. The persistent activation of NF-κB in the gastric mucosa can contribute to the development and progression of gastric cancer. Targeting the NF-κB pathway has been proposed as a potential strategy for treating inflammation-associated gastric cancer.

4. **Hedgehog Pathway**: The Hedgehog signaling pathway is involved in embryonic development and tissue patterning. In adult tissues, this pathway is typically inactive, but its aberrant activation has been implicated in various cancers, including gastric cancer. The Hedgehog pathway regulates the expression of genes involved in cell proliferation, differentiation, and survival. In gastric cancer, mutations in components of the Hedgehog pathway, such as PTCH1 or SMO, can lead to its constitutive activation, promoting tumor growth. Inhibitors of the Hedgehog pathway are being investigated as potential therapies for gastric cancer.

5. **Notch Pathway**: The Notch signaling pathway plays a crucial role in cell fate determination, differentiation, and proliferation. Dysregulation of this pathway has been associated with gastric cancer. In the Notch pathway, interaction between a Notch receptor and its ligand on neighboring cells leads to the cleavage of the Notch receptor's intracellular domain, which translocates to the nucleus and activates the transcription of target genes. Abnormal activation of the Notch pathway can promote the proliferation and survival of gastric cancer cells. Inhibitors targeting the Notch pathway are being explored as potential therapeutic agents for gastric cancer.

Known Causes Related to Animal Products

Dietary factors play a significant role in the development of stomach cancer, and the consumption of certain animal products has been associated with an increased risk of this disease. Several mechanisms have been proposed to explain the link between animal products and stomach cancer:

1. **Processed Meats**: The consumption of processed meats, such as sausages, bacon, and hot dogs, has been strongly linked to an increased risk of stomach cancer. Processed meats often contain nitrites and nitrates, which are used as preservatives and color fixatives. In the acidic environment of the stomach, these compounds can be converted into N-nitroso compounds, which are potent carcinogens. N-nitroso compounds can cause DNA damage, leading to mutations that contribute to the development of stomach cancer.

2. **Red Meat**: High consumption of red meat, such as beef, pork, and lamb, has also been associated with an increased risk of stomach cancer. Red meat contains heme iron, which can promote the formation of N-nitroso compounds in the stomach. Additionally, cooking red meat at high temperatures, such as grilling or barbecuing, can lead to the formation of heterocyclic amines (HCAs) and polycyclic aromatic hydrocarbons (PAHs), both of which are carcinogenic. These compounds can cause DNA damage and contribute to the development of stomach cancer.

3. **Salted and Smoked Foods**: The consumption of salted and smoked foods, which are common in some traditional diets, has been linked to an increased risk of stomach cancer. Salted foods can cause damage to the stomach lining, leading to chronic inflammation and an increased risk of cancer. Smoked foods contain PAHs, which are formed during the smoking process and are known carcinogens. The combination of salt and PAHs can create a pro-carcinogenic environment in the stomach.

4. **High-Fat Dairy Products**: Some studies have suggested that high-fat dairy products, such as butter and cheese, may be associated with an increased risk of stomach cancer. These products contain saturated fats, which can promote inflammation and oxidative stress, contributing to the development of cancer. Additionally, dairy products can contain hormones, such as insulin-like growth factor-1 (IGF-1), which can promote the proliferation of cancer cells.

5. **H. pylori Infection and Animal Products**: H. pylori infection is a major risk factor for stomach cancer. Some studies have suggested that the consumption of animal products, particularly red meat and processed meats, may increase the risk of H. pylori infection. The exact mechanism is not well understood, but it may be related to the impact of these foods on the gut microbiome or the production of N-nitroso compounds that promote the survival of H. pylori.

How a Plant-Based Diet Can Help with Reversal

A plant-based diet, which emphasizes the consumption of whole plant foods such as fruits, vegetables, legumes, whole grains, nuts, and seeds, has been shown to offer significant protective effects against stomach cancer. Several mechanisms have been proposed to explain how a plant-based diet can help with the reversal of stomach cancer:

1. **Antioxidant and Anti-Inflammatory Properties**: Plant-based foods are rich in antioxidants, such as vitamins C and E, carotenoids, and polyphenols, which can neutralize free radicals and reduce oxidative stress. Oxidative stress is a key factor in the development of cancer, as it can cause DNA damage and promote genetic mutations. Additionally, many plant foods have anti-inflammatory properties, which can reduce chronic inflammation and lower the risk of cancer.

2. **Fiber-Rich Diet**: A plant-based diet is naturally high in dietary fiber, which has been shown to have protective effects against stomach cancer. Fiber can bind to potential carcinogens in the digestive tract, reducing their absorption and promoting their excretion. Additionally, fiber supports a healthy gut microbiome, which can enhance the immune response and protect against infections like H. pylori.

3. **Phytochemicals**: Plant-based foods contain a wide range of phytochemicals, such as flavonoids, glucosinolates, and lignans, which have been shown to have anti-cancer properties. These compounds can inhibit the growth and proliferation of cancer cells, induce apoptosis (programmed cell death), and prevent angiogenesis (the formation of new blood vessels that supply tumors). For example, sulforaphane, a compound found in cruciferous vegetables like broccoli and Brussels sprouts, has been shown to inhibit the growth of gastric cancer cells.

4. **Low in Saturated Fats**: A plant-based diet is typically low in saturated fats, which can promote inflammation and oxidative stress. By reducing the intake of saturated fats, a plant-based diet can help lower the risk of stomach cancer and support the body's natural defenses against cancer.

5. **Reduction of Carcinogen Exposure**: By avoiding or minimizing the consumption of animal products, particularly red and processed meats, a plant-based diet can reduce exposure to carcinogens such as N-nitroso compounds, HCAs, and PAHs. This reduction in carcinogen exposure can lower the risk of stomach cancer and support the body's ability to repair damaged DNA and prevent the progression of cancer.

6. **Immune System Support**: A plant-based diet can enhance the immune system's ability to recognize and destroy cancer cells. Many plant foods contain nutrients, such as vitamin C, zinc, and selenium, that are essential for immune function. Additionally,

the fiber in plant foods can support a healthy gut microbiome, which plays a crucial role in regulating the immune response.

7. **Weight Management**: Obesity is a known risk factor for stomach cancer, and a plant-based diet can help with weight management. Plant-based diets are typically lower in calories and higher in fiber, which can promote satiety and prevent overeating. By maintaining a healthy weight, individuals can reduce their risk of developing stomach cancer and improve their overall health.

8. **Inhibition of Tumor Growth**: Some plant-based compounds have been shown to directly inhibit the growth of gastric cancer cells. For example, curcumin, a compound found in turmeric, has been shown to inhibit the proliferation of gastric cancer cells by blocking the NF-κB pathway. Similarly, resveratrol, a compound found in grapes and berries, has been shown to induce apoptosis in gastric cancer cells by activating the p53 pathway.

9. **Detoxification Support**: A plant-based diet can support the body's natural detoxification processes, helping to eliminate harmful toxins and carcinogens. For example, cruciferous vegetables like broccoli and cauliflower contain compounds that activate phase II detoxification enzymes, which can help the body metabolize and excrete carcinogens.

Stomach cancer is a complex disease with multiple contributing factors, including genetic mutations, chronic inflammation, and dietary influences. The consumption of certain animal products, such as processed meats, red meat, and high-fat dairy products, has been associated with an increased risk of stomach cancer due to the formation of carcinogens like N-nitroso compounds, HCAs, and PAHs. However, adopting a plant-based diet can offer significant protective effects against stomach cancer and may even help with the reversal of the disease. A plant-based diet is rich in antioxidants, anti-inflammatory compounds, fiber, and phytochemicals, all of which can support the body's natural

defenses against cancer. By reducing exposure to carcinogens, supporting the immune system, and promoting healthy weight management,
a plant-based diet can play a crucial role in preventing and managing
stomach cancer.

Testicular Cancer

Testicular cancer is a relatively rare form of cancer that originates
in the testicles, the male reproductive glands responsible for producing
sperm and testosterone. Despite its rarity, testicular cancer is the most
common cancer in young men aged 15 to 35 years. This type of cancer
is highly treatable, especially when detected early, but understanding its
function, production, regulation, and the impact of diet—particularly
a plant-based diet—on its development and potential reversal is crucial
for better outcomes.

Function of the Testicles

The testicles, or testes, are two oval-shaped organs located within the
scrotum, a loose pouch of skin below the penis. They have two main
functions: producing sperm (spermatogenesis) and producing testosterone, the primary male sex hormone.

Spermatogenesis is a highly regulated process that occurs within the
seminiferous tubules of the testicles. It involves the division and maturation of germ cells into spermatozoa, which are then stored in the epi-
didymis until ejaculation. This process is crucial for male fertility and is
influenced by a complex interplay of hormones, including follicle-stimulating hormone (FSH) and luteinizing hormone (LH), both of which
are regulated by the pituitary gland.

Testosterone production in the Leydig cells of the testicles is another
vital function. Testosterone is responsible for the development of male
secondary sexual characteristics, such as facial hair, deepening of the

voice, and muscle mass. It also plays a role in maintaining libido, mood, and overall energy levels. The production of testosterone is regulated by the hypothalamic-pituitary-gonadal axis, a feedback loop involving the hypothalamus, pituitary gland, and testicles.

Production and Regulation of Testicular Cancer

Testicular cancer arises when cells in the testicles grow uncontrollably, forming a malignant tumor. The majority of testicular cancers originate in the germ cells, which are responsible for producing sperm. These cancers are classified into two main types: seminomas and non-seminomas. Seminomas tend to grow slowly and are more sensitive to radiation therapy, while non-seminomas are more aggressive and often require chemotherapy.

The exact cause of testicular cancer is not fully understood, but several risk factors have been identified. These include:

1. **Cryptorchidism (Undescended Testicle):** Men with a history of cryptorchidism, where one or both testicles fail to descend into the scrotum, have a significantly higher risk of developing testicular cancer. The risk is present even if surgery is performed to correct the condition.
2. **Family History:** A family history of testicular cancer increases the risk, suggesting a genetic predisposition. Specific genetic mutations, such as those affecting the KIT gene or the BAK1 gene, have been linked to an increased risk.
3. **Age and Ethnicity:** Testicular cancer is most common in young men between the ages of 15 and 35 and is more prevalent in Caucasians than in African Americans or Asians.
4. **History of Testicular Cancer:** Men who have had testicular cancer in one testicle are at an increased risk of developing it in the other testicle.

The development of testicular cancer involves several key molecular pathways and genetic alterations. One of the most significant pathways implicated in testicular cancer is the KIT signaling pathway. The KIT gene encodes a receptor tyrosine kinase that plays a critical role in the survival, proliferation, and differentiation of germ cells. Mutations in the KIT gene or its downstream signaling components can lead to uncontrolled cell growth and tumor formation.

Another important pathway is the WNT signaling pathway, which is involved in regulating cell fate, proliferation, and migration. Dysregulation of WNT signaling has been observed in various cancers, including testicular cancer, and is associated with the development of germ cell tumors.

Additionally, alterations in the p53 tumor suppressor pathway, which plays a crucial role in preventing cancer by inducing cell cycle arrest, apoptosis, or senescence in response to cellular stress, have been identified in testicular cancer. Mutations in the p53 gene can lead to the loss of its tumor-suppressive functions, allowing cancer cells to proliferate unchecked.

Known Causes Related to Animal Products

Emerging research suggests that diet, particularly the consumption of animal products, may play a role in the development of testicular cancer. While the exact mechanisms are still being explored, several hypotheses have been proposed based on epidemiological studies and experimental data.

1. **Dairy Products:** The consumption of dairy products has been associated with an increased risk of testicular cancer in some studies. Dairy products contain high levels of insulin-like growth factor 1 (IGF-1), a hormone that promotes cell growth and has been implicated in the development of several cancers, including testicular cancer. Additionally, dairy products may contain estrogens

and other hormones that could potentially disrupt the hormonal balance in the body and contribute to cancer development.

2. **Red and Processed Meat:** Red and processed meats have been linked to an increased risk of various cancers, including testicular cancer. These meats contain high levels of saturated fats and cholesterol, which can promote inflammation and oxidative stress, leading to DNA damage and cancer development. Furthermore, the cooking of red meat at high temperatures can produce carcinogenic compounds such as heterocyclic amines and polycyclic aromatic hydrocarbons, which have been shown to induce mutations in the DNA of germ cells.

3. **Animal Fat:** A diet high in animal fat has been associated with an increased risk of testicular cancer. Animal fats are rich in saturated fatty acids, which can promote inflammation and increase the levels of free radicals in the body. These free radicals can damage the DNA in germ cells, leading to mutations and cancer development. Additionally, animal fats can disrupt the balance of sex hormones in the body, potentially promoting the growth of hormone-sensitive tumors.

4. **Cholesterol:** Cholesterol is a key component of cell membranes and is essential for the production of steroid hormones, including testosterone. However, high levels of cholesterol, particularly low-density lipoprotein (LDL) cholesterol, have been associated with an increased risk of testicular cancer. Cholesterol can be metabolized into oxysterols, which are known to promote cancer cell proliferation and metastasis. Furthermore, cholesterol can activate signaling pathways such as the Hedgehog pathway, which is involved in the development of germ cell tumors.

5. **Hormones in Meat:** The use of synthetic hormones in meat production has raised concerns about their potential role in cancer development. These hormones, including estrogen, progesterone, and testosterone, are used to promote growth in livestock and can remain in the meat products consumed by humans. The

presence of these hormones in the diet could disrupt the endocrine system and promote the development of hormone-sensitive cancers, including testicular cancer.

Pathways Implicated in Testicular Cancer

Several key molecular pathways are implicated in the development and progression of testicular cancer. Understanding these pathways provides insights into potential targets for therapy and the role of diet in modulating cancer risk.

1. **KIT Signaling Pathway:** The KIT signaling pathway is crucial for the survival and proliferation of germ cells. The KIT receptor is activated by its ligand, stem cell factor (SCF), leading to the activation of downstream signaling pathways such as the PI3K/AKT and MAPK/ERK pathways. These pathways promote cell survival, proliferation, and migration. Mutations in the KIT gene or overexpression of KIT can lead to uncontrolled cell growth and tumor formation in the testicles.

2. **WNT Signaling Pathway:** The WNT signaling pathway plays a critical role in regulating cell fate, proliferation, and migration. In the context of testicular cancer, dysregulation of WNT signaling can lead to the development of germ cell tumors. Activation of WNT signaling promotes the stabilization and nuclear translocation of β-catenin, which acts as a transcriptional coactivator for genes involved in cell proliferation and survival. Aberrant activation of WNT signaling has been observed in testicular cancer, suggesting its role in tumorigenesis.

3. **p53 Tumor Suppressor Pathway:** The p53 tumor suppressor pathway is a key regulator of the cellular response to stress, including DNA damage, hypoxia, and oncogene activation. The p53 protein induces cell cycle arrest, apoptosis, or senescence in response to cellular stress, thereby preventing the propagation of

damaged cells. Mutations in the p53 gene, which are common in many cancers, can lead to the loss of its tumor-suppressive functions, allowing cancer cells to proliferate unchecked. In testicular cancer, alterations in the p53 pathway have been implicated in tumor development and resistance to therapy.

4. **Hedgehog Signaling Pathway:** The Hedgehog signaling pathway is involved in embryonic development and tissue regeneration. Dysregulation of this pathway has been implicated in the development of several cancers, including testicular cancer. Activation of Hedgehog signaling promotes the expression of genes involved in cell proliferation and survival, contributing to tumor growth and metastasis. Cholesterol, which is a key modulator of Hedgehog signaling, may play a role in the activation of this pathway in testicular cancer.

5. **PI3K/AKT/mTOR Pathway:** The PI3K/AKT/mTOR pathway is a central regulator of cell growth, proliferation, and survival. Activation of this pathway leads to the phosphorylation and activation of downstream targets involved in protein synthesis, cell cycle progression, and metabolism. Dysregulation of the PI3K/AKT/mTOR pathway has been observed in testicular cancer, contributing to tumor growth and resistance to apoptosis. This pathway is also influenced by dietary factors, including the intake of animal products rich in saturated fats and cholesterol.

The Role of a Plant-Based Diet in Reversing Testicular Cancer

A plant-based diet, which emphasizes the consumption of fruits, vegetables, whole grains, legumes, nuts, and seeds while minimizing or eliminating animal products, has been associated with a reduced risk of various cancers, including testicular cancer. Several mechanisms may explain the protective effects of a plant-based diet against cancer development and its potential role in reversing testicular cancer.

1. **Anti-Inflammatory Effects:** Chronic inflammation is a key driver of cancer development and progression. A plant-based diet is rich in anti-inflammatory compounds, including phytochemicals, antioxidants, and fiber, which can help reduce inflammation in the body. Fruits and vegetables, in particular, are high in antioxidants such as vitamins C and E, carotenoids, and flavonoids, which can neutralize free radicals and reduce oxidative stress, thereby preventing DNA damage and cancer development.

2. **Hormonal Balance:** A plant-based diet can help maintain hormonal balance by reducing the intake of exogenous hormones found in animal products and promoting the excretion of excess hormones through increased fiber intake. High-fiber foods, such as whole grains, legumes, and vegetables, can bind to estrogens and other hormones in the digestive tract, promoting their elimination from the body. This can reduce the levels of circulating hormones that may promote the growth of hormone-sensitive tumors, including testicular cancer.

3. **Regulation of IGF-1:** Insulin-like growth factor 1 (IGF-1) is a hormone that promotes cell growth and has been implicated in the development of several cancers, including testicular cancer. High levels of IGF-1 are associated with increased cancer risk and progression. A plant-based diet, particularly one low in animal protein, has been shown to reduce circulating levels of IGF-1, thereby reducing cancer risk. Plant proteins, such as those found in legumes, nuts, and seeds, do not stimulate IGF-1 production to the same extent as animal proteins, making them a healthier choice for cancer prevention and management.

4. **Antioxidant Defense:** Oxidative stress, caused by an imbalance between free radicals and antioxidants in the body, is a key factor in cancer development. A plant-based diet is rich in antioxidants that can protect cells from oxidative damage and reduce the risk of cancer. Berries, leafy greens, cruciferous vegetables, and nuts

are particularly high in antioxidants and have been shown to have protective effects against cancer.

5. **Epigenetic Modulation:** Epigenetics refers to changes in gene expression that do not involve alterations in the DNA sequence. Diet can influence epigenetic modifications, such as DNA methylation and histone acetylation, which can regulate the expression of genes involved in cancer development. A plant-based diet, rich in bioactive compounds such as polyphenols, can modulate epigenetic marks and promote the expression of tumor suppressor genes while inhibiting oncogenes. This epigenetic regulation may contribute to the reversal of testicular cancer by reprogramming cancer cells toward a less aggressive phenotype.

6. **Gut Microbiome:** The gut microbiome plays a crucial role in maintaining overall health and has been implicated in cancer development. A plant-based diet promotes a healthy and diverse gut microbiome, which can produce short-chain fatty acids (SCFAs) with anti-inflammatory and anticancer properties. SCFAs, such as butyrate, can inhibit the growth of cancer cells and promote apoptosis, thereby reducing the risk of cancer progression. Additionally, a healthy gut microbiome can enhance the immune system's ability to recognize and eliminate cancer cells.

7. **Weight Management:** Obesity is a known risk factor for several cancers, including testicular cancer. A plant-based diet is typically lower in calories and higher in fiber, which can promote weight loss and help maintain a healthy weight. By reducing body fat, a plant-based diet can lower the levels of circulating estrogens and other hormones that may promote cancer growth. Additionally, weight loss can improve insulin sensitivity and reduce the risk of insulin resistance, which is associated with increased cancer risk.

8. **Detoxification:** A plant-based diet supports the body's natural detoxification processes by providing essential nutrients and antioxidants that enhance liver function and promote the elimination of toxins. Cruciferous vegetables, such as broccoli,

cauliflower, and Brussels sprouts, contain compounds that support phase II detoxification enzymes in the liver, helping to neutralize and eliminate carcinogens from the body. This detoxification process can reduce the burden of environmental toxins that may contribute to cancer development.

9. **Apoptosis Induction:** Apoptosis, or programmed cell death, is a natural process that helps eliminate damaged or abnormal cells from the body. Cancer cells often evade apoptosis, allowing them to survive and proliferate. A plant-based diet can promote apoptosis in cancer cells through the action of bioactive compounds found in plant foods. For example, sulforaphane, a compound found in cruciferous vegetables, has been shown to induce apoptosis in cancer cells by activating the p53 pathway and inhibiting the NF-κB pathway. Other plant compounds, such as curcumin from turmeric and resveratrol from grapes, also have pro-apoptotic effects that can help reverse cancer.

10. **Immune System Enhancement:** A strong immune system is essential for recognizing and eliminating cancer cells. A plant-based diet can enhance immune function by providing essential nutrients, such as vitamins A, C, E, and zinc, as well as bioactive compounds with immunomodulatory effects. Mushrooms, for example, contain beta-glucans that can stimulate the activity of immune cells, such as natural killer cells and macrophages, which play a critical role in cancer surveillance and elimination. Additionally, the anti-inflammatory effects of a plant-based diet can help reduce chronic inflammation, which can suppress immune function and promote cancer growth.

Testicular cancer is a complex disease with multifactorial origins, including genetic, environmental, and dietary factors. While the exact causes of testicular cancer are not fully understood, emerging evidence suggests that diet, particularly the consumption of animal products, may play a role in its development. Animal products such as dairy, red and processed meats, and high-fat foods have been associated with increased cancer risk through mechanisms involving inflammation, hormonal disruption, oxidative stress, and epigenetic modifications.

In contrast, a plant-based diet offers numerous protective benefits that may reduce the risk of testicular cancer and potentially aid in its reversal. A diet rich in fruits, vegetables, whole grains, legumes, nuts, and seeds provides essential nutrients, antioxidants, and bioactive compounds that support overall health and modulate key pathways involved in cancer development. By reducing inflammation, promoting hormonal balance, enhancing antioxidant defense, modulating epigenetic marks, and supporting a healthy gut microbiome, a plant-based diet can create an internal environment that is less conducive to cancer growth.

Furthermore, the weight management benefits of a plant-based diet, along with its ability to enhance detoxification, induce apoptosis, and boost immune function, make it a powerful tool in cancer prevention and management.

Thyroid Cancer

Thyroid cancer is a malignant tumor that arises from the thyroid gland, a butterfly-shaped organ located at the base of the neck. It plays a crucial role in regulating metabolism, growth, and development through the production of thyroid hormones. Thyroid cancer represents a small percentage of all cancers but has seen a rising incidence in recent years, partly due to improved diagnostic techniques and increased exposure to risk factors, including dietary influences.

Function of the Thyroid Gland

The thyroid gland is essential for maintaining the body's metabolic rate, heart and digestive function, muscle control, brain development, and bone maintenance. It produces three hormones: thyroxine (T4), triiodothyronine (T3), and calcitonin. T4 and T3 are crucial for regulating the body's metabolism, while calcitonin plays a role in calcium homeostasis.

The production of T4 and T3 is regulated by the thyroid-stimulating hormone (TSH) produced by the pituitary gland. When the thyroid gland produces adequate levels of T4 and T3, a feedback loop reduces TSH production. Conversely, low levels of T4 and T3 stimulate the release of TSH to increase thyroid hormone production.

Types of Thyroid Cancer

Thyroid cancer can be classified into several types based on the origin of the cells involved. The main types include:

- **Papillary thyroid cancer (PTC)**: The most common type, accounting for about 80% of all cases. It usually grows slowly and often spreads to lymph nodes in the neck.
- **Follicular thyroid cancer (FTC)**: Represents about 10-15% of thyroid cancers. It can spread to other parts of the body, such as the lungs and bones.
- **Medullary thyroid cancer (MTC)**: Accounts for about 4% of thyroid cancers and originates from the parafollicular cells (C cells) of the thyroid, which produce calcitonin.
- **Anaplastic thyroid cancer (ATC)**: A rare, aggressive form of thyroid cancer that accounts for about 1-2% of cases. It grows rapidly and is often difficult to treat.
- **Hurthle cell carcinoma**: A subtype of follicular thyroid cancer characterized by distinct cellular features and a higher risk of metastasis.

Production and Regulation of Thyroid Cancer

Thyroid cancer develops when the DNA of thyroid cells undergoes mutations that lead to uncontrolled cell growth. These genetic mutations can be inherited or acquired due to environmental factors, such as exposure to ionizing radiation or dietary influences.

The regulation of thyroid cancer involves complex interactions between genetic, epigenetic, and environmental factors. Key regulatory pathways implicated in thyroid cancer include:

- **MAPK/ERK Pathway**: This pathway is frequently activated in thyroid cancer, particularly in papillary thyroid carcinoma. Mutations in the BRAF gene, which encodes a protein kinase in the MAPK/ERK pathway, are common in thyroid cancer and lead to uncontrolled cell proliferation.
- **PI3K/AKT Pathway**: The PI3K/AKT signaling pathway is also involved in thyroid cancer, particularly in follicular and anaplastic thyroid carcinomas. Mutations in genes such as RAS, PTEN, and PIK3CA can activate this pathway, promoting tumor growth and survival.
- **RET/PTC Rearrangement**: RET/PTC rearrangements are specific genetic alterations found in a significant percentage of papillary thyroid cancers. These rearrangements lead to the activation of the RET tyrosine kinase, which drives tumorigenesis through the MAPK/ERK pathway.
- **Wnt/β-Catenin Pathway**: Aberrations in the Wnt/β-catenin signaling pathway have been implicated in the development and progression of various thyroid cancers, particularly in anaplastic thyroid carcinoma.

Pathways Involved in Thyroid Cancer Progression

The progression of thyroid cancer involves multiple cellular pathways that regulate cell growth, apoptosis, angiogenesis, and metastasis. The major pathways include:

- **Apoptosis Pathway**: In cancer, the normal process of programmed cell death (apoptosis) is often disrupted, allowing cancer cells to survive and proliferate. In thyroid cancer, mutations in genes such as BCL2 and TP53 can inhibit apoptosis, leading to tumor growth.
- **Angiogenesis Pathway**: Tumors require a blood supply to grow beyond a certain size. Thyroid cancers can stimulate the formation of new blood vessels (angiogenesis) by secreting growth factors like VEGF (vascular endothelial growth factor). The VEGF/VEGFR pathway is a critical regulator of angiogenesis in thyroid cancer.
- **Epithelial-Mesenchymal Transition (EMT) Pathway**: EMT is a process by which epithelial cells acquire mesenchymal characteristics, including increased motility and invasiveness. This process is crucial for cancer metastasis. In thyroid cancer, EMT is driven by factors such as TGF-β, which can promote tumor invasion and spread.
- **Immune Evasion Pathway**: Thyroid cancers, like other malignancies, can evade the immune system through various mechanisms, including the expression of immune checkpoint proteins such as PD-L1. This allows cancer cells to escape immune surveillance and continue growing.

Known Causes of Thyroid Cancer Linked to Animal Products

Several dietary factors, particularly those associated with animal products, have been implicated in the development and progression of thyroid cancer. These include:

- **High Iodine Intake from Animal Sources**: While iodine is essential for thyroid function, excessive intake, particularly from animal sources like dairy products, can increase the risk of thyroid cancer. High iodine levels can lead to thyroid dysfunction and may promote the development of cancerous cells in the thyroid gland.
- **Dairy Products**: Dairy consumption has been linked to an increased risk of thyroid cancer, particularly due to its high content of saturated fats, hormones, and iodine. Dairy products can also contribute to the formation of goitrogens, which interfere with thyroid hormone production and increase the risk of cancerous growths.
- **Red and Processed Meats**: Diets high in red and processed meats are associated with an increased risk of various cancers, including thyroid cancer. These meats contain carcinogenic compounds such as heterocyclic amines (HCAs) and polycyclic aromatic hydrocarbons (PAHs) formed during cooking at high temperatures. Additionally, the high levels of saturated fats and cholesterol in these meats can contribute to cancer progression.
- **Fish and Seafood**: Although fish is often considered a healthy food, it can contain high levels of mercury and other environmental contaminants. Mercury exposure has been linked to thyroid dysfunction and an increased risk of thyroid cancer. Additionally, certain types of fish and seafood are high in iodine, which can contribute to thyroid cancer risk when consumed in excess.
- **Eggs**: Eggs are another animal product that has been associated with thyroid cancer risk. They are a source of dietary cholesterol and can contribute to oxidative stress, inflammation, and hormonal imbalances that may promote cancer development.

Plant-Based Diet for Reversal of Thyroid Cancer

A plant-based diet, rich in fruits, vegetables, whole grains, legumes, nuts, and seeds, offers numerous benefits in the prevention and reversal of thyroid cancer. Several mechanisms by which a plant-based diet can help include:

- **Antioxidant-Rich Foods**: Fruits and vegetables are rich in antioxidants, such as vitamins C and E, carotenoids, and flavonoids, which can neutralize free radicals and reduce oxidative stress—a key factor in cancer development. Antioxidants also help repair DNA damage and modulate signaling pathways involved in cell proliferation and apoptosis.

- **Anti-Inflammatory Effects**: Chronic inflammation is a significant contributor to cancer progression, including thyroid cancer. A plant-based diet is naturally anti-inflammatory, as it is low in pro-inflammatory compounds found in animal products, such as saturated fats and arachidonic acid. Foods like berries, leafy greens, and turmeric contain potent anti-inflammatory compounds that can reduce cancer risk.

- **Fiber and Gut Health**: A plant-based diet is high in dietary fiber, which promotes healthy digestion and supports a balanced gut microbiome. A healthy gut microbiome is crucial for modulating the immune system, reducing inflammation, and eliminating carcinogens. Fiber also binds to excess hormones and toxins in the gut, preventing their reabsorption and reducing the risk of hormone-driven cancers like thyroid cancer.

- **Phytoestrogens**: Certain plant-based foods, such as flaxseeds, soy, and whole grains, contain phytoestrogens—natural compounds that can modulate estrogen activity in the body. Phytoestrogens have been shown to have protective effects against hormone-related cancers, including thyroid cancer, by regulating estrogen metabolism and reducing the growth of cancer cells.

- **Low Glycemic Load**: Plant-based diets typically have a low glycemic load, which helps maintain stable blood sugar levels and reduces the risk of insulin resistance. Insulin resistance is associated with an increased risk of cancer, including thyroid cancer, due to its role in promoting cell proliferation and inhibiting apoptosis.

- **Detoxification Pathways**: A plant-based diet supports the body's natural detoxification processes, particularly in the liver. Cruciferous vegetables like broccoli, kale, and Brussels sprouts are rich in glucosinolates, which enhance the detoxification of carcinogens and reduce the risk of cancer development. These vegetables also contain compounds that inhibit the growth of cancer cells and induce apoptosis.

- **Hormonal Balance**: A plant-based diet helps maintain hormonal balance, which is crucial in preventing and reversing thyroid cancer. High consumption of animal products can lead to hormonal imbalances, such as elevated estrogen and insulin levels, which can promote cancer growth. Plant-based foods, on the other hand, support hormonal regulation by providing essential nutrients, reducing exposure to exogenous hormones, and modulating the body's natural hormone production.

- **Weight Management**: Obesity is a significant risk factor for thyroid cancer, as excess body fat can lead to hormonal imbalances, chronic inflammation, and insulin resistance—all of which promote cancer development. A plant-based diet is typically lower in calories and higher in nutrients, making it an effective strategy for weight management and reducing cancer risk.

Case Studies on a Plant-Based Diet and Thyroid Cancer

Several studies have demonstrated the benefits of a plant-based diet in reducing the risk of thyroid cancer and supporting overall thyroid health. For example:

- A study published in the **Journal of Clinical Endocrinology & Metabolism** found that higher consumption of fruits and vegetables was associated with a reduced risk of thyroid cancer, particularly among women. The protective effects were attributed to the high levels of antioxidants and fiber in plant-based foods, which help reduce oxidative stress and inflammation.
- Research published in **Cancer Epidemiology, Biomarkers & Prevention** highlighted the role of cruciferous vegetables in thyroid cancer prevention. The study found that individuals who consumed more cruciferous vegetables had a lower risk of developing thyroid cancer. The protective effect was linked to the presence of glucosinolates, which enhance detoxification and inhibit cancer cell growth.
- A case-control study in **Thyroid** Journal showed that a diet rich in plant-based foods, particularly those high in phytoestrogens, was associated with a lower risk of thyroid cancer. The study suggested that phytoestrogens may modulate estrogen metabolism and reduce the growth of estrogen-dependent tumors in the thyroid gland.
- Another study in **Nutrition and Cancer** found that a plant-based diet was associated with a reduced risk of thyroid cancer among individuals with a family history of the disease. The researchers concluded that the anti-inflammatory and antioxidant properties of plant-based foods could help mitigate genetic predispositions to thyroid cancer.

Thyroid cancer is a complex disease influenced by genetic, environmental, and dietary factors. While the exact causes of thyroid cancer are multifaceted, there is growing evidence that dietary patterns, particularly those involving high consumption of animal products, play a significant role in its development. On the other hand, a plant-based diet offers numerous protective benefits that can help prevent and even reverse thyroid cancer.

By adopting a diet rich in fruits, vegetables, whole grains, legumes, nuts, and seeds, individuals can harness the power of natural antioxidants, anti-inflammatory compounds, and essential nutrients to support thyroid health and reduce the risk of cancer. Moreover, the elimination of animal products, which are associated with increased cancer risk due to their content of carcinogens, hormones, and unhealthy fats, further enhances the protective effects of a plant-based diet.

As research continues to uncover the links between diet and thyroid cancer, it becomes increasingly clear that dietary interventions, particularly those centered around plant-based foods, should be a cornerstone of cancer prevention and treatment strategies. By making informed dietary choices, individuals can take proactive steps to protect their thyroid health and overall well-being.

Vaginal Cancer

Vaginal cancer is a relatively rare form of cancer that originates in the vaginal tissue. The vagina, a muscular tube connecting the external genitals to the uterus, plays an essential role in the female reproductive system. Understanding vaginal cancer involves exploring its function within the body, the pathways that lead to its production, the mechanisms regulating its growth and spread, and the influence of diet—particularly the potential of a plant-based diet—in mitigating and even reversing the disease.

Function of the Vagina and Vaginal Cancer

The vagina serves multiple functions within the female body. It is part of the reproductive system, allowing for the passage of menstrual blood, serving as the canal through which childbirth occurs, and facilitating sexual intercourse. The vaginal lining consists of squamous epithelial cells, which are crucial for its protective function. These cells help to form a barrier against infections and other harmful agents. Vaginal cancer occurs when cells within the vaginal lining undergo malignant transformation, leading to the formation of a tumor.

Vaginal cancer can disrupt these normal functions, causing symptoms such as abnormal bleeding, pain during intercourse, and changes in vaginal discharge. If left untreated, vaginal cancer can metastasize, spreading to other parts of the body, including the lymph nodes, liver, lungs, and bones. The severity and progression of vaginal cancer depend on various factors, including the type of cancer, the stage at diagnosis, and the individual's overall health.

Production and Regulation of Vaginal Cancer

The production of vaginal cancer involves several complex processes that result in the uncontrolled growth of malignant cells. The development of cancer, including vaginal cancer, is generally understood through the multi-step carcinogenesis model, which includes initiation, promotion, and progression stages.

1. **Initiation**: This stage involves the mutation of DNA in the cells of the vaginal lining. These mutations can occur due to various factors, including exposure to carcinogens, such as those found in tobacco smoke, and potentially harmful substances found in animal products. During initiation, normal cells undergo genetic changes that may not immediately result in cancer but make the cells more susceptible to further damage.

2. **Promotion**: In this stage, the initiated cells begin to proliferate. This process can be influenced by factors such as hormonal imbalances, chronic inflammation, and dietary factors. The repeated exposure to estrogen without the balance of progesterone is one such promoter, as it can lead to excessive growth of the vaginal lining, increasing the risk of malignant transformation. Similarly, certain compounds in animal products, such as saturated fats and hormones, may contribute to the promotion of these initiated cells.

3. **Progression**: During progression, the proliferating cells acquire more mutations that allow them to invade surrounding tissues and spread to distant sites in the body. The regulation of vaginal cancer at this stage is particularly challenging, as the cancer cells often become resistant to normal regulatory mechanisms, such as apoptosis (programmed cell death). The immune system's ability to recognize and destroy these cells may also be compromised, allowing the cancer to grow unchecked.

Pathways Leading to Vaginal Cancer

The pathways that lead to vaginal cancer involve a complex interplay of genetic, environmental, and lifestyle factors.

Another critical pathway involves the role of estrogen. Estrogen plays a vital role in regulating the growth and function of the vaginal lining. However, prolonged exposure to high levels of estrogen without the counteracting effects of progesterone can lead to the overgrowth of vaginal epithelial cells, increasing the risk of mutations and cancer. This pathway is particularly relevant in postmenopausal women, who may experience a decline in progesterone levels while maintaining or increasing estrogen levels due to hormone replacement therapy or other factors.

Inflammation is another pathway that can contribute to the development of vaginal cancer. Chronic inflammation, whether due to infections, irritants, or other factors, can lead to continuous cell turnover and DNA damage, increasing the risk of cancer. Inflammatory cytokines released during chronic inflammation can promote cell proliferation and survival, further contributing to the cancerous transformation of vaginal cells.

Known Causes Related to Animal Products

The consumption of animal products has been linked to several types of cancer, including vaginal cancer, through various mechanisms. One of the primary concerns is the presence of hormones and growth factors in animal products, particularly those derived from animals treated with synthetic hormones. These substances can mimic or interfere with the body's natural hormones, disrupting the delicate balance needed to regulate cell growth and division.

1. **Hormones in Animal Products**: Estrogens, both naturally occurring and synthetic, are commonly found in dairy products, meat, and other animal-derived foods. These hormones can contribute to the estrogenic load in the body, particularly in postmenopausal women, who are already at an increased risk of hormone-related cancers. The excess estrogen can promote the proliferation of vaginal epithelial cells, increasing the likelihood of mutations and cancer development.

2. **Saturated Fats and Inflammation**: Saturated fats, prevalent in animal products such as red meat and dairy, have been linked to increased levels of inflammation in the body. Chronic inflammation is a known risk factor for many cancers, including vaginal cancer. Saturated fats can also contribute to obesity, which is another risk factor for hormone-related cancers, as adipose tissue can produce estrogen.

3. **Carcinogenic Compounds**: Certain cooking methods commonly used for animal products, such as grilling and frying, can produce carcinogenic compounds like heterocyclic amines (HCAs) and polycyclic aromatic hydrocarbons (PAHs). These compounds can cause DNA mutations in vaginal epithelial cells, contributing to the initiation of cancer. Additionally, the consumption of processed meats, which often contain nitrates and nitrites, has been associated with an increased risk of several cancers, including those of the reproductive system.

4. **Animal Protein and IGF-1**: The consumption of animal protein has been linked to increased levels of insulin-like growth factor 1 (IGF-1) in the body. IGF-1 is a hormone that promotes cell growth and proliferation. Elevated levels of IGF-1 have been associated with an increased risk of several cancers, including those of the reproductive system. In the context of vaginal cancer, high IGF-1 levels can promote the growth of initiated cells, contributing to the progression of the disease.

The Role of a Plant-Based Diet in Reversal

A plant-based diet has been shown to offer numerous health benefits, including a reduced risk of various cancers. In the context of vaginal cancer, a plant-based diet can play a significant role in both prevention and reversal through several mechanisms.

1. **Antioxidant and Anti-Inflammatory Properties**: Plant-based foods are rich in antioxidants, such as vitamins C and E, and phytochemicals, such as flavonoids and carotenoids. These compounds help to neutralize free radicals, reducing oxidative stress and preventing DNA damage that can lead to cancer. Additionally, many plant-based foods have anti-inflammatory properties, which can help to reduce chronic inflammation, a known risk factor for cancer.

2. **Hormone Regulation**: A plant-based diet can help to regulate hormone levels, particularly estrogen. Certain plant foods, such as flaxseeds and soy, contain phytoestrogens, which are plant-derived compounds that can mimic or modulate the effects of estrogen in the body. Phytoestrogens can bind to estrogen receptors, potentially blocking the more potent effects of endogenous estrogen and reducing the risk of hormone-related cancers, including vaginal cancer.

3. **Fiber and Detoxification**: Plant-based foods are high in dietary fiber, which is essential for the proper functioning of the digestive system. Fiber helps to bind and eliminate excess hormones, toxins, and carcinogens from the body, reducing the overall estrogen load and the risk of cancer. Additionally, fiber supports a healthy gut microbiome, which plays a crucial role in the detoxification of harmful substances and the regulation of the immune system.

4. **Lowering IGF-1 Levels**: A plant-based diet, particularly one low in processed foods and animal products, has been shown to reduce levels of IGF-1 in the body. By lowering IGF-1 levels, a plant-based diet can help to slow the growth of cancer cells and reduce the risk of cancer progression. This effect is particularly important in the context of vaginal cancer, where elevated IGF-1 levels can contribute to the proliferation of malignant cells.

5. **Enhancing Immune Function**: A diet rich in fruits, vegetables, whole grains, and legumes provides essential nutrients that support the immune system. Vitamins A, C, and E, along with zinc and selenium, are particularly important for immune function. A strong immune system is better equipped to recognize and destroy cancer cells, preventing the growth and spread of vaginal cancer. Additionally, certain plant foods, such as garlic, turmeric, and green tea, contain compounds that have been shown to enhance immune function and exhibit anti-cancer properties.

6. **Weight Management**: Maintaining a healthy weight is crucial for reducing the risk of hormone-related cancers, including vagi-

nal cancer. A plant-based diet, which is typically lower in calories and saturated fats, can help individuals achieve and maintain a healthy weight. This is particularly important because excess body fat can increase estrogen production, contributing to the development and progression of vaginal cancer.

7. **Phytochemicals and Cancer-Fighting Compounds**: Numerous studies have highlighted the cancer-fighting properties of phytochemicals found in plant-based foods. For example, cruciferous vegetables such as broccoli, cauliflower, and kale contain glucosinolates, which are compounds that can inhibit cancer cell growth and promote apoptosis (programmed cell death) in cancer cells. Similarly, berries are rich in anthocyanins, which have been shown to have anti-cancer effects. By incorporating a variety of plant-based foods into the diet, individuals can benefit from a wide range of these cancer-fighting compounds.

Evidence Supporting a Plant-Based Diet for Cancer Reversal

Numerous studies have supported the role of a plant-based diet in reducing the risk of cancer and aiding in cancer reversal. A landmark study published in *The Journal of the American College of Nutrition* found that a plant-based diet significantly reduced the risk of developing cancer, including cancers of the reproductive system. The study highlighted that individuals who followed a plant-based diet had lower levels of circulating estrogen and other hormones associated with cancer risk.

Another study published in *Cancer Epidemiology, Biomarkers & Prevention* found that women who consumed a diet rich in fruits, vegetables, and whole grains had a lower risk of developing vaginal and cervical cancers. The study suggested that the protective effects of a plant-based diet were likely due to the high levels of antioxidants and anti-inflammatory compounds found in these foods.

Research published in *Nutrition and Cancer* also demonstrated the potential of a plant-based diet in reducing IGF-1 levels and inhibiting cancer cell growth. The study showed that individuals who adopted a plant-based diet experienced significant reductions in IGF-1 levels, which were associated with a decreased risk of cancer progression.

Implementing a Plant-Based Diet for Vaginal Cancer Reversal

For individuals diagnosed with vaginal cancer, adopting a plant-based diet can be a powerful tool in their treatment and recovery plan. While it is important to work with healthcare providers to develop a comprehensive treatment strategy, incorporating a plant-based diet can provide additional support in reversing the disease.

A plant-based diet should focus on whole, unprocessed foods that are rich in nutrients, fiber, and phytochemicals. Emphasizing a variety of fruits, vegetables, whole grains, legumes, nuts, and seeds will ensure that the body receives the essential nutrients needed to support immune function, regulate hormones, and reduce inflammation.

1. **Fruits and Vegetables**: Aim to include a wide range of colorful fruits and vegetables in the diet, as they are rich in antioxidants, vitamins, and minerals. Cruciferous vegetables, such as broccoli, Brussels sprouts, and cabbage, are particularly beneficial due to their cancer-fighting properties.
2. **Whole Grains**: Incorporate whole grains such as brown rice, quinoa, oats, and barley into meals. Whole grains are high in fiber, which supports detoxification and hormone regulation.
3. **Legumes**: Beans, lentils, chickpeas, and other legumes are excellent sources of plant-based protein and fiber. They also contain phytoestrogens, which can help regulate estrogen levels and reduce the risk of hormone-related cancers.
4. **Nuts and Seeds**: Flaxseeds, chia seeds, walnuts, and almonds are rich in omega-3 fatty acids, which have anti-inflammatory properties. Including these foods in the diet can help reduce inflammation and support overall health.

5. **Herbs and Spices**: Incorporate herbs and spices such as turmeric, garlic, ginger, and oregano into meals. These ingredients have been shown to have anti-inflammatory and anti-cancer properties.

6. **Green Tea**: Green tea is rich in catechins, which are compounds that have been shown to inhibit cancer cell growth. Drinking green tea regularly can provide additional support in cancer prevention and reversal.

Vaginal cancer, while rare, poses significant health challenges due to its potential to disrupt the normal functions of the female reproductive system and spread to other parts of the body. Understanding the pathways and mechanisms that lead to vaginal cancer is crucial for developing effective prevention and treatment strategies. The consumption of animal products, particularly those containing hormones, saturated fats, and carcinogenic compounds, has been linked to an increased risk of vaginal cancer. Conversely, a plant-based diet offers numerous protective benefits, including antioxidant and anti-inflammatory properties, hormone regulation, and support for the immune system.

By adopting a plant-based diet rich in fruits, vegetables, whole grains, legumes, nuts, and seeds, individuals can reduce their risk of developing vaginal cancer and support their body in reversing the disease if diagnosed. The scientific evidence supporting the role of a plant-based diet in cancer prevention and reversal continues to grow, offering hope and guidance for those seeking to improve their health through dietary choices.

5

Chemo/Radiation/Antibiotics

Chemotherapy, a cornerstone in the treatment of various cancers, has long been regarded as a double-edged sword. While it claims to target and destroy rapidly dividing cancer cells, it also inadvertently affects normal cells, leading to a host of side effects. Among the most concerning potential side effects is the possibility that chemotherapy, referred to here as "bad chemistry," can cause gene mutations that may lead to secondary cancers.

The Mechanism of Chemotherapy-Induced Gene Mutations

Chemotherapy works by targeting cells that are rapidly dividing, a hallmark characteristic of cancer cells. However, because many normal cells in the body also divide rapidly, such as those in the bone marrow, digestive tract, and hair follicles, they too can be affected by chemotherapy. The drugs used in chemotherapy are typically classified into several categories based on their mechanisms of action: alkylating agents, antimetabolites, topoisomerase inhibitors, mitotic inhibitors, and antitumor antibiotics. Each of these drugs can cause DNA damage, which may lead to mutations if not properly repaired.

Alkylating Agents and DNA Damage

Alkylating agents, such as cyclophosphamide and chlorambucil, work by adding alkyl groups to DNA, leading to the formation of cross-links between DNA strands. These cross-links prevent the DNA from being properly replicated during cell division, which triggers cell death. However, if the damage is not extensive enough to kill the cell, it can lead to mutations when the cell attempts to repair the damage. These mutations can accumulate over time and may result in the transformation of normal cells into cancerous ones.

Antimetabolites and Misincorporation into DNA

Antimetabolites, such as 5-fluorouracil and methotrexate, mimic the building blocks of DNA or RNA. When these drugs are incorporated into DNA or RNA, they cause errors in the genetic code, leading to mutations. For example, 5-fluorouracil is incorporated into RNA in place of uracil, leading to faulty RNA processing and translation. Methotrexate inhibits dihydrofolate reductase, an enzyme necessary for the synthesis of thymidine, a critical component of DNA. The resulting thymidine deficiency can lead to DNA breaks and mutations.

Topoisomerase Inhibitors and Chromosomal Breaks

Topoisomerase inhibitors, such as doxorubicin and etoposide, interfere with the enzyme topoisomerase, which helps to unwind DNA during replication. By inhibiting this enzyme, these drugs cause breaks in the DNA strands. While these breaks can kill cancer cells, they can also lead to chromosomal rearrangements and mutations in normal cells. These mutations can disrupt the normal regulation of cell growth and division, potentially leading to the development of secondary cancers.

Mitotic Inhibitors and Spindle Assembly Checkpoint Disruption

Mitotic inhibitors, such as paclitaxel and vincristine, disrupt the mitotic spindle, a structure necessary for the proper segregation of chromosomes during cell division. When the spindle is disrupted, cells may end up with an abnormal number of chromosomes, a condition known as aneuploidy. Aneuploidy is a common feature of cancer cells and can drive tumorigenesis by disrupting the balance of oncogenes and tumor suppressor genes.

Antitumor Antibiotics and Free Radical Formation

Antitumor antibiotics, such as bleomycin and mitomycin C, generate free radicals that cause extensive DNA damage. These free radicals can lead to double-strand breaks in DNA, which are particularly difficult for the cell to repair. If these breaks are not repaired correctly, they can result in mutations, chromosomal translocations, and other genetic abnormalities that contribute to cancer development.

Pathways Involved in Chemotherapy-Induced Mutations

The pathways through which chemotherapy-induced mutations occur are complex and involve multiple cellular processes. These include DNA repair pathways, cell cycle checkpoints, apoptosis, and the regulation of oxidative stress.

DNA Repair Pathways

The DNA repair pathways are crucial in maintaining genomic integrity. When chemotherapy drugs cause DNA damage, the cell activates these pathways to repair the damage. The most important DNA repair mechanisms include base excision repair (BER), nucleotide excision repair (NER), homologous recombination (HR), and non-homologous end joining (NHEJ).

- **Base Excision Repair (BER):** BER is responsible for repairing small, non-helix-distorting base lesions. If chemotherapy-induced damage results in small lesions, BER will attempt to correct these errors. However, if BER fails or is overwhelmed by the extent of the damage, mutations may occur.
- **Nucleotide Excision Repair (NER):** NER is involved in repairing bulky, helix-distorting DNA adducts, such as those caused by alkylating agents. If NER is defective or overwhelmed, the cell may incorporate incorrect nucleotides during repair, leading to mutations.
- **Homologous Recombination (HR):** HR repairs double-strand breaks using a homologous sequence as a template. When chemotherapy causes double-strand breaks, HR can repair them accurately. However, if HR is compromised, cells may rely on error-prone repair mechanisms, leading to mutations.

- **Non-Homologous End Joining (NHEJ):** NHEJ is another pathway that repairs double-strand breaks, but it does so without using a homologous template, making it more error-prone than HR. NHEJ can lead to chromosomal translocations and mutations, which are hallmarks of cancer cells.

Cell Cycle Checkpoints

Cell cycle checkpoints are mechanisms that ensure the proper progression of the cell cycle and prevent the propagation of damaged DNA. Chemotherapy-induced DNA damage activates these checkpoints, particularly the G1/S and G2/M checkpoints.

- **G1/S Checkpoint:** The G1/S checkpoint ensures that the cell does not enter the DNA synthesis phase (S phase) with damaged DNA. If chemotherapy induces DNA damage, this checkpoint can halt the cell cycle to allow for repair. However, if the damage is irreparable, the cell may bypass this checkpoint, leading to the replication of damaged DNA and the accumulation of mutations.
- **G2/M Checkpoint:** The G2/M checkpoint prevents the cell from entering mitosis (M phase) with damaged DNA. If chemotherapy causes extensive damage, this checkpoint can arrest the cell cycle to facilitate repair. However, like the G1/S checkpoint, if the damage is too severe, the cell may proceed through mitosis with damaged DNA, leading to chromosomal abnormalities and mutations.

Apoptosis and Chemotherapy

Apoptosis, or programmed cell death, is a mechanism by which cells with irreparable damage are eliminated to prevent the propagation of mutations. Chemotherapy can activate apoptosis in cancer cells, but it can also trigger apoptosis in normal cells. If the apoptotic pathways are defective, cells with chemotherapy-induced mutations may survive and proliferate, leading to cancer development.

The key regulators of apoptosis include the p53 tumor suppressor gene, Bcl-2 family proteins, and caspases.

- **p53 Tumor Suppressor Gene:** p53 is known as the "guardian of the genome" because of its role in maintaining genomic stability. It is activated in response to DNA damage and can induce cell cycle arrest, DNA repair, or apoptosis. Mutations in p53 are common in cancer cells and can impair the cell's ability to undergo apoptosis in response to chemotherapy, leading to the survival of mutated cells.
- **Bcl-2 Family Proteins:** The Bcl-2 family includes both pro-apoptotic and anti-apoptotic proteins that regulate the mitochondrial pathway of apoptosis. Chemotherapy can shift the balance towards pro-apoptotic signals, leading to cell death. However, if anti-apoptotic signals dominate, cells with DNA damage may survive and contribute to tumorigenesis.
- **Caspases:** Caspases are a family of proteases that execute apoptosis. Chemotherapy-induced activation of caspases leads to cell death. However, if caspase activation is impaired, cells with chemotherapy-induced mutations may evade apoptosis and continue to proliferate.

Oxidative Stress and Free Radical Formation

Chemotherapy drugs, particularly antitumor antibiotics, can generate reactive oxygen species (ROS) and free radicals, which cause oxidative damage to DNA, proteins, and lipids. This oxidative stress can overwhelm the cell's antioxidant defenses, leading to mutations and cell death.

- **ROS and DNA Damage:** ROS can cause a variety of DNA lesions, including base modifications, single-strand breaks, and double-strand breaks. If these lesions are not repaired correctly, they can lead to mutations and chromosomal instability.
- **Antioxidant Defense Mechanisms:** Cells have several antioxidant defense mechanisms, including superoxide dismutase (SOD), catalase, and glutathione peroxidase, which neutralize ROS. However, chemotherapy-induced oxidative stress can exceed the capacity of these defenses, leading to oxidative DNA damage and mutations.
- **Oxidative Stress-Induced Apoptosis:** High levels of oxidative stress can trigger apoptosis through the mitochondrial pathway. However, if apoptosis is evaded, cells with oxidative DNA damage may survive and contribute to cancer development.

Chemotherapy-Induced Secondary Cancers

One of the most concerning long-term effects of chemotherapy is the potential development of secondary cancers. These secondary cancers are distinct from the primary cancer that was initially treated and are thought to arise due to the mutagenic effects of chemotherapy.

Types of Secondary Cancers

The types of secondary cancers that are most commonly associated with chemotherapy include acute myeloid leukemia (AML), myelodysplastic syndromes (MDS), and solid tumors such as bladder, lung, and breast cancer.

- **Acute Myeloid Leukemia (AML) and Myelodysplastic Syndromes (MDS):** Alkylating agents and topoisomerase inhibitors are particularly associated with an increased risk of AML and MDS. These cancers arise from mutations in hematopoietic stem cells, leading to uncontrolled proliferation of abnormal blood cells.

- **Solid Tumors:** Chemotherapy can also increase the risk of developing solid tumors. For example, patients treated with cyclophosphamide for breast cancer have an increased risk of developing bladder cancer. Similarly, radiation therapy combined with chemotherapy can increase the risk of lung and breast cancers.

Molecular Mechanisms of Secondary Cancer Development

The molecular mechanisms underlying secondary cancer development involve the accumulation of mutations in key oncogenes and tumor suppressor genes. These mutations can arise directly from chemotherapy-induced DNA damage or indirectly through the disruption of DNA repair and apoptotic pathways.

- **Oncogene Activation:** Oncogenes are genes that promote cell growth and division. Mutations in these genes can lead to their overactivation, driving the uncontrolled proliferation of cancer cells. Chemotherapy-induced mutations can activate oncogenes, leading to the development of secondary cancers.
- **Tumor Suppressor Gene Inactivation:** Tumor suppressor genes, such as p53 and BRCA1/2, regulate cell cycle checkpoints, DNA repair, and apoptosis. Mutations in these genes can impair their function, allowing cells with DNA damage to survive and proliferate. Chemotherapy-induced mutations in tumor suppressor genes can contribute to the development of secondary cancers.
- **Chromosomal Instability:** Chromosomal instability, characterized by an increased rate of chromosomal rearrangements, is a hallmark of cancer. Chemotherapy-induced DNA damage can lead to chromosomal translocations, deletions, and amplifications, contributing to the development of secondary cancers.
- **Epigenetic Changes:** In addition to genetic mutations, chemotherapy can also induce epigenetic changes, such as DNA

methylation and histone modification, which can alter gene expression and contribute to cancer development. These epigenetic changes can be heritable and may play a role in the initiation and progression of secondary cancers.

Chemotherapy, which is a tool in the fight against cancer, is not without its risks. The very mechanisms that make it effective against cancer cells—DNA damage, disruption of cell division, and induction of apoptosis—also pose a threat to normal cells. The DNA damage caused by chemotherapy can lead to mutations, chromosomal instability, and the development of secondary cancers. Understanding the pathways involved in chemotherapy-induced gene mutations, such as DNA repair, cell cycle checkpoints, and oxidative stress, is crucial for developing strategies to minimize these risks.

Radiation

The Harmful Effects of Radiation Treatments in Cancer

Radiation therapy is one of the most common treatments for cancer, used in about half of all cancer cases. While it claims to be effective in killing cancer cells and shrinking tumors, radiation therapy also carries significant risks, particularly the potential to cause harm to healthy cells and tissues. This can lead to long-term complications, including the induction of secondary cancers.

Introduction to Radiation Therapy

Radiation therapy uses high doses of radiation to kill cancer cells or slow their growth by damaging their DNA. The goal is to target cancer cells while minimizing exposure to healthy cells. However, even with advanced techniques, some healthy cells are invariably affected. The damage to healthy cells can result in a range of side effects, from mild skin irritation to severe organ damage and the induction of secondary malignancies.

Mechanisms of Radiation-Induced Damage
DNA Damage

Radiation primarily exerts its effects by inducing DNA damage. Ionizing radiation, such as X-rays, gamma rays, and particle radiation, can break DNA strands directly or produce free radicals that indirectly cause DNA breaks. These breaks can result in mutations if not properly repaired.

1. **Direct DNA Damage**: Ionizing radiation can directly break the DNA strands. Double-strand breaks (DSBs) are particularly dangerous as they can lead to chromosomal aberrations if not correctly repaired.
2. **Indirect DNA Damage**: Radiation can ionize water molecules within cells, creating reactive oxygen species (ROS) such as hydroxyl radicals. These ROS can damage DNA, proteins, and lipids, leading to cellular dysfunction.

Cellular Pathways Affected by Radiation
DNA Repair Mechanisms

Cells have evolved complex mechanisms to repair DNA damage. The key pathways include:

1. **Non-Homologous End Joining (NHEJ)**: This is the predominant pathway for repairing DSBs in non-dividing cells. NHEJ is quick but error-prone, often leading to mutations.
2. **Homologous Recombination (HR)**: This pathway is used during cell division and is more accurate than NHEJ. HR uses a sister

chromatid as a template for repair, reducing the likelihood of mutations.

If these repair mechanisms fail or are overwhelmed by the extent of the damage, mutations can accumulate, potentially leading to cancer.

Apoptosis and Senescence

Severely damaged cells may undergo programmed cell death (apoptosis) or enter a state of permanent growth arrest (senescence) to prevent the propagation of damaged DNA. However, if these pathways are disrupted, it can lead to the survival of mutated cells, which may become cancerous.

1. **Apoptosis**: This process involves a series of biochemical events leading to cell death, which helps eliminate damaged cells.
2. **Senescence**: This is a state where cells stop dividing but do not die. Senescent cells can secrete inflammatory cytokines, growth factors, and proteases, contributing to a pro-tumorigenic environment.

Radiation-Induced Mutagenesis

Radiation can induce a variety of genetic mutations, including point mutations, deletions, insertions, and chromosomal rearrangements. These mutations can activate oncogenes or inactivate tumor suppressor genes, leading to uncontrolled cell growth and cancer.

Radiation-Induced Carcinogenesis

Radiation is a well-known carcinogen. Secondary cancers can arise years or even decades after the initial radiation treatment. The risk is particularly high for pediatric cancer patients and for those who receive high doses of radiation.

1. **Secondary Solid Tumors**: These can occur in any organ or tissue that received radiation. Common sites include the breast, lung, thyroid, and gastrointestinal tract.
2. **Leukemia**: Radiation can cause leukemia by inducing mutations in hematopoietic stem cells. The latency period for radiation-induced leukemia is typically shorter than for solid tumors.

Case Studies and Epidemiological Evidence
Atomic Bomb Survivors

Studies of atomic bomb survivors have provided critical insights into the long-term effects of radiation exposure. Increased incidences of leukemia and solid tumors have been observed in survivors, highlighting the carcinogenic potential of ionizing radiation.

Medical Radiation Workers

Epidemiological studies of medical radiation workers have shown an elevated risk of cancer, particularly for those with long-term exposure to low doses of radiation. These findings underscore the importance of minimizing occupational exposure.

Pediatric Cancer Patients

Children are more sensitive to radiation than adults due to their rapidly dividing cells and longer life expectancy. Studies have shown that pediatric cancer patients who undergo radiation therapy have a significantly higher risk of developing secondary cancers later in life.

Biological Pathways Involved in Radiation-Induced Cancer
The p53 Pathway

The tumor suppressor protein p53 plays a crucial role in maintaining genomic stability. It is activated in response to DNA damage and can induce cell cycle arrest, DNA repair, or apoptosis. Mutations in the p53 gene are common in radiation-induced cancers, leading to the loss of its tumor suppressor functions.

The RAS Pathway

Mutations in the RAS family of oncogenes are also implicated in radiation-induced carcinogenesis. Activated RAS proteins can promote cell proliferation and survival, contributing to the development of cancer.

The NF-κB Pathway

The NF-κB pathway is involved in the cellular response to stress, including radiation-induced DNA damage. It regulates the expression of genes involved in inflammation, cell survival, and proliferation. Dysregulation of this pathway can contribute to tumorigenesis.

The PI3K/AKT/mTOR Pathway

This pathway is critical for cell growth and survival. Radiation can activate the PI3K/AKT/mTOR pathway, leading to increased cell survival and proliferation, which can contribute to cancer development.

Clinical Implications and Recommendations

Minimizing Exposure

Efforts should be made to minimize radiation exposure to healthy tissues during cancer treatment. Techniques such as intensity-modulated radiation therapy (IMRT) and proton therapy can help achieve this goal.

Alternative Therapies

Exploring alternative cancer treatments that do not rely on ionizing radiation, such as a plant-based diet, may reduce the risk of radiation-induced secondary cancers.

Long-Term Monitoring

Patients who undergo radiation therapy should be closely monitored for the development of secondary cancers. This is particularly important for pediatric patients and those who receive high doses of radiation.

Radiation therapy remains a cornerstone of cancer treatment, but its potential to cause harm by mutating healthy cells and inducing secondary cancers cannot be overlooked. Understanding the biological pathways involved and implementing strategies to minimize these risks are essential for improving the safety and efficacy of cancer treatment.

Antibiotics

Antibiotics are used in the fight against bacterial infections. However, emerging evidence suggests that their use is not without long-term consequences, particularly concerning cancer development. Research shows the complex relationship between antibiotic use and cancer.

Antibiotics are used in combating bacterial infections. However, their widespread use has also led to unintended consequences, including antibiotic resistance, disruptions in gut microbiota, and potential links to various cancers.

The role of antibiotics in cancer development is an area of growing concern. Research indicates that antibiotics may influence cancer risk through several mechanisms, including alterations in the gut microbiome, immune system suppression, and direct effects on cellular processes. This report aims to provide a comprehensive review of the evidence linking antibiotics to cancer, focusing on the underlying biological pathways and the implications for public health.

The Gut Microbiome: A Key Player in Cancer Risk

One of the primary ways antibiotics may contribute to cancer is through their impact on the gut microbiome. The human gut is home to trillions of microorganisms, including bacteria, viruses, and fungi, collectively known as the microbiome. This complex ecosystem plays a crucial role in maintaining health by aiding digestion, regulating the immune system, and protecting against harmful pathogens.

Disruption of the Gut Microbiome

Antibiotics are designed to kill or inhibit the growth of bacteria, but their effects are not limited to the targeted pathogens. They also disrupt the balance of beneficial bacteria in the gut, leading to a condition known as dysbiosis. Dysbiosis is characterized by an imbalance in the microbial population, with a decrease in beneficial bacteria and an increase in harmful bacteria.

Research has shown that dysbiosis can contribute to cancer development by promoting chronic inflammation, altering metabolic processes, and affecting the immune response. For example, a study published in *Nature* found that long-term antibiotic use was associated with an increased risk of colorectal cancer, a finding that has been supported by other studies.

Chronic Inflammation and Cancer

Chronic inflammation is a well-established risk factor for cancer. Inflammation can lead to DNA damage, promote cell proliferation, and inhibit apoptosis, all of which are key steps in carcinogenesis. Dysbiosis induced by antibiotics can promote chronic inflammation by disrupting the balance of pro-inflammatory and anti-inflammatory bacteria in the gut.

A study published in *Gastroenterology* found that individuals with a history of prolonged antibiotic use had a higher risk of developing colorectal adenomas, which are precursors to colorectal cancer. The authors suggested that the pro-inflammatory environment created by dysbiosis could contribute to the development of these adenomas.

Metabolic Changes and Carcinogenesis

The gut microbiome plays a critical role in metabolism, including the processing of dietary components, the synthesis of vitamins, and the regulation of bile acids. Disruption of these metabolic processes by antibiotics can lead to the production of carcinogenic compounds.

For example, bile acids are synthesized in the liver and modified by gut bacteria. These modified bile acids can promote cancer by inducing DNA damage, altering gene expression, and promoting cell proliferation. A study published in *The Lancet* found that individuals with high levels of certain bile acids had an increased risk of developing hepatocellular carcinoma, a type of liver cancer.

Immune System Suppression

The gut microbiome is intricately linked to the immune system. Beneficial bacteria in the gut help regulate immune responses, promoting tolerance to harmless antigens while defending against pathogens. Antibiotics can disrupt this balance, leading to immune system dysfunction and increased susceptibility to cancer.

A study published in *Immunity* found that antibiotic-induced dysbiosis impaired the ability of the immune system to recognize and eliminate cancer cells. The authors suggested that the loss of beneficial bacteria could lead to a weakened immune response, allowing cancer cells to evade detection and grow unchecked.

Direct Effects of Antibiotics on Cellular Processes

In addition to their impact on the gut microbiome, antibiotics may also directly contribute to carcinogenesis through their effects on cellular processes. Several studies have investigated the potential genotoxic effects of antibiotics, exploring how these drugs may induce DNA damage, promote mutations, and alter cellular signaling pathways.

1. DNA Damage and Mutagenesis

One of the most concerning potential effects of antibiotics is their ability to cause DNA damage, which can lead to mutations and cancer. Some antibiotics, particularly those in the quinolone class, have been shown to induce DNA strand breaks and interfere with DNA repair mechanisms.

A study published in *Carcinogenesis* found that the antibiotic ciprofloxacin, a commonly used quinolone, induced DNA damage in human cells and increased the frequency of mutations. The authors concluded that the genotoxic effects of ciprofloxacin could contribute to cancer development, particularly with long-term or high-dose use.

2. Oxidative Stress and Carcinogenesis

Antibiotics can also promote cancer through the generation of oxidative stress. Oxidative stress occurs when there is an imbalance between the production of reactive oxygen species (ROS) and the body's ability to detoxify them. ROS are highly reactive molecules that can damage cellular components, including DNA, proteins, and lipids.

A study published in *Free Radical Biology and Medicine* found that certain antibiotics, including doxycycline and minocycline, increased ROS production in human cells. The authors suggested that the resulting oxidative stress could contribute to cancer by promoting DNA damage and activating pro-carcinogenic signaling pathways.

3. Alteration of Cellular Signaling Pathways

Antibiotics may also influence cancer risk by altering cellular signaling pathways that regulate cell growth, division, and apoptosis. For example, some antibiotics have been shown to activate the NF-κB pathway, a key regulator of inflammation and cell survival.

A study published in *Oncogene* found that the antibiotic tetracycline activated the NF-κB pathway in human cells, leading to increased cell proliferation and resistance to apoptosis. The authors suggested that the activation of this pathway by antibiotics could contribute to cancer development, particularly in tissues with pre-existing inflammation.

Evidence from Epidemiological Studies

Epidemiological studies provide additional evidence linking antibiotic use to cancer risk. Several large-scale studies have investigated the association between antibiotic use and the incidence of various cancers, with many finding a positive correlation.

1. Colorectal Cancer

Colorectal cancer is one of the most extensively studied cancers in relation to antibiotic use. Multiple studies have found that individuals with a history of frequent or long-term antibiotic use have an increased risk of developing colorectal cancer.

A study published in *Gut* analyzed data from over 20,000 patients and found that those who had used antibiotics for more than 10 days had a significantly higher risk of developing colorectal cancer compared to those who had not used antibiotics. The authors suggested that the disruption of the gut microbiome and the resulting chronic inflammation could be key factors in this increased risk.

2. Breast Cancer

Breast cancer is another cancer type that has been linked to antibiotic use. A study published in *JAMA* analyzed data from over 10,000 women and found that those who had used antibiotics for more than 500 days had a significantly higher risk of developing breast cancer compared to those who had used antibiotics for less than 15 days.

The study's authors hypothesized that the increased risk could be due to the immunosuppressive effects of antibiotics, as well as their impact on the gut microbiome. Dysbiosis may lead to increased estrogen production, which is a known risk factor for breast cancer.

3. Lung Cancer

The association between antibiotic use and lung cancer is less well-established but has been suggested by some studies. A study published in *Cancer Epidemiology, Biomarkers & Prevention* found that individuals with a history of frequent antibiotic use had a slightly increased risk of developing lung cancer.

The authors noted that while the association was modest, it was consistent with the hypothesis that antibiotic-induced immune suppression and chronic inflammation could contribute to cancer development.

4. Prostate Cancer

Prostate cancer has also been linked to antibiotic use, particularly in men with a history of recurrent urinary tract infections (UTIs). A study published in *The Lancet Oncology* found that men who had taken antibiotics for recurrent UTIs had a higher risk of developing prostate cancer compared to those who had not taken antibiotics.

The study's authors suggested that chronic inflammation of the prostate, combined with the immunosuppressive effects of antibiotics, could increase the risk of cancer in this population.

Mechanistic Pathways Linking Antibiotics to Cancer

The link between antibiotics and cancer is supported by several mechanistic pathways, including those related to the gut microbiome, immune system suppression, and direct effects on cellular processes. Understanding these pathways is critical for developing strategies to mitigate the potential risks associated with antibiotic use.

1. Microbial Dysbiosis and Inflammation

As previously discussed, the disruption of the gut microbiome by antibiotics can lead to dysbiosis, chronic inflammation, and an increased risk of cancer. This pathway is supported by both experimental and epidemiological evidence, particularly in the context of colorectal cancer.

2. Immune System Suppression

Antibiotics can suppress the immune system by disrupting the balance of beneficial bacteria in the gut, leading to a weakened immune response and an increased risk of cancer. This pathway is particularly relevant in cancers where the immune system plays a critical role in tumor surveillance and elimination, such as breast cancer and lung cancer.

3. Direct Genotoxic Effects

Some antibiotics, particularly those in the quinolone class, have been shown to induce DNA damage and mutations, which can contribute to carcinogenesis. This pathway is supported by experimental evidence showing that antibiotics can cause DNA strand breaks, interfere with DNA repair mechanisms, and promote oxidative stress.

4. Alteration of Cellular Signaling Pathways

Antibiotics can also contribute to cancer by altering cellular signaling pathways that regulate cell growth, division, and apoptosis. For example, the activation of the NF-κB pathway by antibiotics has been linked to increased cell proliferation and resistance to apoptosis, which are key steps in carcinogenesis.

In addition, dietary interventions, such as increasing fiber intake, can support the growth of beneficial bacteria and promote a healthy gut environment, reducing the risk of chronic inflammation and cancer.

While antibiotics have undoubtedly revolutionized medicine and saved countless lives, their potential long-term consequences, particularly in relation to cancer, cannot be ignored. The evidence linking antibiotics to cancer is compelling, with multiple studies showing that these drugs can disrupt the gut microbiome, suppress the immune system, and directly contribute to carcinogenesis.

6

Angiogenesis

A ngiogenesis is a vital physiological process that plays a key role in both normal bodily functions and pathological conditions, most notably cancer. This process refers to the growth of new blood vessels from pre-existing ones, a mechanism crucial for tissue growth, repair, and development. However, in cancer, angiogenesis is hijacked to fuel tumor growth and metastasis by supplying the growing mass of abnormal cells with oxygen and nutrients.

The Process of Angiogenesis

Angiogenesis is the process through which new blood vessels form from existing vasculature. It occurs during wound healing, embryonic development, and in response to tissue growth in adults. The key players in this process are endothelial cells, which line blood vessels. These cells are activated by growth factors such as Vascular Endothelial Growth Factor (VEGF) and Fibroblast Growth Factor (FGF), leading to the proliferation, migration, and organization of endothelial cells to form new blood vessels.

Steps of Angiogenesis:

1. **Activation:** In response to signals such as hypoxia (lack of oxygen), cells secrete pro-angiogenic factors like VEGF and FGF. This promotes the activation of endothelial cells in existing blood vessels.

2. **Degradation of the Basement Membrane:** The endothelial cells release enzymes called matrix metalloproteinases (MMPs) that degrade the basement membrane, allowing the cells to invade surrounding tissues.

3. **Endothelial Cell Migration:** The endothelial cells migrate toward the source of pro-angiogenic signals, usually a site of injury or, in the case of cancer, the growing tumor.

4. **Proliferation and Formation of Tubes:** Endothelial cells proliferate, align, and form tube-like structures, which eventually become new blood vessels.

5. **Stabilization and Maturation:** The newly formed vessels are stabilized by pericytes and smooth muscle cells, allowing the vessels to mature and integrate with the existing vasculature.

The Role of Angiogenesis in Cancer

Cancer cells have a high metabolic rate, requiring a constant supply of oxygen and nutrients to sustain their rapid growth. Tumors that grow beyond a few millimeters in size cannot survive without inducing angiogenesis because their core would become deprived of oxygen (hypoxic). In response to hypoxia, cancer cells secrete pro-angiogenic factors, including VEGF, which stimulate the surrounding vasculature to grow new blood vessels.

The blood vessels that grow into the tumor not only provide oxygen and nutrients but also serve as pathways for cancer cells to enter the bloodstream and metastasize to distant organs. This process of angiogenesis is thus essential for both the growth of primary tumors and the spread of cancer throughout the body.

Key Angiogenic Factors in Cancer:

1. **VEGF (Vascular Endothelial Growth Factor):** One of the most significant drivers of angiogenesis in cancer, VEGF binds to receptors on endothelial cells and initiates the process of blood

vessel formation. Tumors often express high levels of VEGF, correlating with increased tumor aggressiveness.

2. **Basic Fibroblast Growth Factor (bFGF):** Another important angiogenic factor, bFGF promotes the proliferation and differentiation of endothelial cells.

3. **Platelet-Derived Growth Factor (PDGF):** This factor helps stabilize and mature new blood vessels by recruiting pericytes and smooth muscle cells.

4. **Hypoxia-Inducible Factor 1-alpha (HIF-1α):** A transcription factor that is upregulated under low oxygen conditions (hypoxia), HIF-1α promotes the expression of VEGF and other pro-angiogenic molecules.

Plant-Based Foods that Inhibit Angiogenesis

A growing body of research has identified various plant-based foods that contain bioactive compounds capable of inhibiting angiogenesis. These foods offer a natural and potentially safer way to target angiogenesis in cancer prevention and treatment. Below are some of the most well-researched plant-based foods that have demonstrated anti-angiogenic effects.

1. Green Tea

Green tea contains a group of polyphenols called catechins, with Epigallocatechin-3-gallate (EGCG) being the most abundant and potent. EGCG has been shown to inhibit angiogenesis by suppressing VEGF expression and blocking the activation of VEGF receptors on endothelial cells.

A study published in *Cancer Research* found that EGCG can inhibit the proliferation and migration of endothelial cells in vitro, as well as suppress tumor growth and angiogenesis in vivo. This suggests that green tea may have a role in cancer prevention by targeting angiogenesis.

2. Turmeric

Curcumin, the active compound in turmeric, has potent anti-in-flammatory and anti-angiogenic properties. Curcumin inhibits angiogenesis by downregulating VEGF and other pro-angiogenic factors. It also blocks the activation of signaling pathways such as NF-κB, which are involved in promoting angiogenesis.

A review in the *Journal of Experimental & Clinical Cancer Research* highlighted curcumin's ability to inhibit angiogenesis in various cancer models, including breast, prostate, and lung cancers.

3. Berries (Strawberries, Blueberries, Blackberries)

Berries are rich in flavonoids, particularly anthocyanins, which have been shown to possess anti-angiogenic properties. In a study conducted by researchers at the *Angiogenesis Foundation*, extracts from strawberries and blackberries were found to inhibit angiogenesis in both in vitro and in vivo models.

The anti-angiogenic effects of berries are attributed to their ability to reduce the expression of VEGF and block the migration and proliferation of endothelial cells.

4. Garlic

Garlic contains organosulfur compounds, such as allicin, that have demonstrated anti-angiogenic effects. These compounds inhibit the production of nitric oxide, a molecule that plays a key role in promoting angiogenesis. Additionally, garlic has been shown to inhibit the activation of VEGF receptors and block endothelial cell proliferation.

A study published in *Phytotherapy Research* found that garlic extract significantly reduced angiogenesis in both animal and cell-based models. This suggests that garlic may have potential as an anti-cancer agent by targeting angiogenesis.

5. Cruciferous Vegetables (Broccoli, Cauliflower, Brussels Sprouts)

Cruciferous vegetables are rich in sulforaphane, a compound that has been shown to have anti-cancer and anti-angiogenic properties. Sulforaphane inhibits angiogenesis by downregulating the expression of VEGF and other pro-angiogenic factors.

A study published in *Cancer Letters* demonstrated that sulforaphane can inhibit the proliferation and migration of endothelial cells, as well as suppress tumor-induced angiogenesis. This makes cruciferous vegetables a valuable addition to a cancer-preventive diet.

6. Grapes

Grapes, particularly red and purple varieties, are rich in resveratrol, a polyphenol with potent anti-angiogenic properties. Resveratrol has been shown to inhibit angiogenesis by blocking the expression of VEGF and other pro-angiogenic molecules. It also inhibits the activation of signaling pathways, such as PI3K/Akt and ERK, that are involved in promoting angiogenesis.

A study published in *The FASEB Journal* found that resveratrol can inhibit angiogenesis in both in vitro and in vivo models of cancer. This suggests that grapes and grape-derived products, such as red wine (in moderation), may help prevent cancer by targeting angiogenesis.

7. Tomatoes

Tomatoes are rich in lycopene, a carotenoid with anti-angiogenic and anti-cancer properties. Lycopene inhibits angiogenesis by reducing the expression of pro-angiogenic factors such as VEGF, as well as by blocking the proliferation and migration of endothelial cells.

A study published in the *Journal of Nutritional Biochemistry* found that lycopene can inhibit angiogenesis in prostate cancer models. This suggests that tomatoes may play a role in preventing angiogenesis-driven cancers, such as prostate and breast cancer.

8. Soy

Soy contains isoflavones, particularly genistein, which have been shown to possess anti-angiogenic properties. Genistein inhibits the activation of VEGF receptors and blocks the proliferation of endothelial cells.

A study published in *Cancer Research* demonstrated that genistein can inhibit angiogenesis in both in vitro and in vivo models of cancer.

This suggests that soy-based foods, such as tofu and tempeh, may help prevent cancer by inhibiting angiogenesis.

Mechanisms Through Which Plant-Based Foods Inhibit Angiogenesis

The bioactive compounds in plant-based foods inhibit angiogenesis through several mechanisms, including:

1. **Downregulation of Pro-Angiogenic Factors:** Many plant-based compounds inhibit the expression of pro-angiogenic molecules such as VEGF, FGF, and PDGF. This prevents the activation of endothelial cells and the formation of new blood vessels.
2. **Inhibition of Endothelial Cell Proliferation and Migration:** Several plant-based compounds, such as resveratrol and EGCG, inhibit the proliferation and migration of endothelial cells, which are essential for angiogenesis.
3. **Blocking Angiogenic Signaling Pathways:** Plant-based compounds can block the activation of signaling pathways, such as the PI3K/Akt and ERK pathways, which promote angiogenesis.
4. **Reduction of Oxidative Stress and Inflammation:** Many plant-based foods, such as green tea and turmeric, have potent antioxidant and anti-inflammatory properties. By reducing oxidative stress and inflammation, these foods help create an environment that is less conducive to angiogenesis.

Angiogenesis is a critical process in both normal physiology and cancer progression. In the context of cancer, angiogenesis enables tumors to grow and metastasize by supplying them with oxygen and nutrients.

Plant-based foods offer a natural and potentially safer way to inhibit angiogenesis. Foods such as green tea, turmeric, berries, garlic, and cruciferous vegetables contain bioactive compounds that have been shown to suppress angiogenesis and inhibit tumor growth. Incorporating these foods into a plant-based diet may offer a promising approach to cancer prevention and treatment.

7

Cancer Fuel: Sugar, Sodium and Saturated Fats

S ugar consumption and its potential link to cancer growth is a topic that has sparked considerable debate and research in the scientific community. The relationship between sugar and cancer is complex and involves various biochemical pathways and physiological processes.

Understanding Sugar: Types and Metabolism

Sugar, in its simplest form, refers to sweet-tasting, soluble carbohydrates. The most common types include:

1. **Glucose**: A primary energy source for cells.
2. **Fructose**: Found in fruits and some vegetables.
3. **Sucrose**: Common table sugar, composed of glucose and fructose.
4. **Lactose**: Found in milk and dairy products.

When consumed, sugars are broken down into glucose and fructose in the digestive tract. Glucose enters the bloodstream and is transported to cells, where it is utilized for energy production via glycolysis and oxidative phosphorylation.

The Warburg Effect: Cancer's Preference for Glycolysis

One of the key discoveries linking sugar to cancer is the Warburg effect, named after the German biochemist Otto Warburg. Warburg observed that cancer cells tend to favor glycolysis for energy production, even in the presence of adequate oxygen, which is contrary to normal cells that rely on oxidative phosphorylation under aerobic conditions.

Glycolysis and Cancer Cell Metabolism

In glycolysis, glucose is converted into pyruvate, yielding ATP (adenosine triphosphate) and lactate. This process is less efficient than oxidative phosphorylation but allows cancer cells to proliferate rapidly because:

1. **Rapid ATP Production**: Glycolysis is faster than oxidative phosphorylation.
2. **Acidic Microenvironment**: Lactate production lowers the pH, facilitating cancer invasion and metastasis.
3. **Biosynthetic Needs**: Glycolysis intermediates are diverted into pathways that synthesize nucleotides, amino acids, and lipids necessary for cell proliferation.

Insulin and IGF-1: Growth Signals for Cancer

Insulin and insulin-like growth factor 1 (IGF-1) are hormones that play significant roles in regulating glucose metabolism and cell growth. High sugar intake leads to increased insulin levels, which can promote cancer growth through several mechanisms:

1. **Insulin Signaling Pathway**: Insulin binds to its receptor on cell surfaces, activating the PI3K/AKT/mTOR pathway, which promotes cell survival, growth, and proliferation.
2. **IGF-1**: Insulin stimulates the liver to produce IGF-1, which also activates the PI3K/AKT/mTOR pathway. Elevated IGF-1 levels

have been associated with increased risk of various cancers, including breast, prostate, and colorectal cancers.

Hyperglycemia and Oxidative Stress

Chronic high blood sugar levels (hyperglycemia) can contribute to cancer development through oxidative stress and inflammation:

1. **Reactive Oxygen Species (ROS)**: High glucose levels increase the production of ROS, which can cause DNA damage, mutations, and genomic instability, leading to cancer initiation and progression.
2. **Inflammatory Cytokines**: Hyperglycemia induces the production of inflammatory cytokines such as TNF-α and IL-6, which can promote a pro-cancerous environment.

Obesity, Insulin Resistance, and Cancer

Obesity, often a result of excessive sugar consumption, is a well-established risk factor for cancer. Obesity leads to insulin resistance, where cells become less responsive to insulin, causing the pancreas to produce more insulin. This hyperinsulinemia contributes to cancer through:

1. **Adipokines**: Fat tissue produces adipokines like leptin and adiponectin, which influence cancer cell growth and survival.
2. **Chronic Inflammation**: Obesity is associated with chronic low-grade inflammation, which can promote cancer development.

Sugar and Specific Cancers: Epidemiological Evidence

Numerous epidemiological studies have investigated the link between sugar consumption and cancer risk. Some key findings include:

1. **Breast Cancer**: High intake of sugary foods and beverages has been linked to an increased risk of breast cancer, particularly in postmenopausal women.
2. **Colorectal Cancer**: Several studies have shown a positive association between high sugar intake and colorectal cancer risk.
3. **Pancreatic Cancer**: There is evidence suggesting that high sugar consumption may increase the risk of pancreatic cancer, possibly due to its impact on insulin and glucose metabolism.

Molecular Pathways: How Sugar Promotes Cancer

To understand how sugar promotes cancer at the molecular level, it's crucial to explore specific pathways:

1. **Hexosamine Biosynthetic Pathway (HBP)**: Excess glucose is shunted into the HBP, producing UDP-N-acetylglucosamine, which modifies proteins and alters cell signaling and transcription, potentially leading to cancer progression.
2. **Pentose Phosphate Pathway (PPP)**: Glucose-6-phosphate enters the PPP, generating NADPH and ribose-5-phosphate, essential for fatty acid synthesis and nucleotide production, supporting rapid cancer cell proliferation.
3. **Mitochondrial Dysfunction**: High glucose levels can lead to mitochondrial dysfunction, resulting in increased ROS production and activation of oncogenic pathways.

Clinical Implications: Dietary Interventions

Given the potential link between sugar and cancer, several dietary interventions have been proposed to mitigate cancer risk:

1. **Low Glycemic Index Diets**: Consuming foods with a low glycemic index can help maintain stable blood glucose levels and reduce insulin spikes, potentially lowering cancer risk.
2. **Ketogenic Diet**: This high-fat, low-carbohydrate diet forces the body to utilize ketones instead of glucose for energy, which may inhibit cancer cell growth dependent on glycolysis.
3. **Intermittent Fasting**: Restricting eating periods can improve insulin sensitivity and reduce inflammation, potentially lowering cancer risk.

The relationship between sugar and cancer is multifaceted, involving various biochemical pathways and physiological processes. While more research is needed to fully understand this link, existing evidence suggests that high sugar consumption can promote cancer growth through mechanisms such as the Warburg effect, insulin and IGF-1 signaling, hyperglycemia-induced oxidative stress, and obesity-related inflammation. Adopting dietary interventions that minimize sugar intake and stabilize blood glucose levels may help reduce cancer risk.

Sodium

Sodium, an essential mineral in the human body, is crucial for maintaining fluid balance, transmitting nerve impulses, and supporting muscle function. However, excessive sodium intake has been implicated in numerous health issues, including hypertension, cardiovascular disease, and kidney dysfunction. Over recent decades, research has revealed a concerning link between high sodium consumption and the development of certain cancers. This relationship is complex, involving various physiological pathways, cellular mechanisms, and environmental factors. Understanding the role of sodium in cancer development requires delving into these pathways and examining the impact of sodium on cell biology and tissue function.

The Role of Sodium in the Body

Sodium primarily exists in the extracellular space, helping to regulate osmotic balance, blood pressure, and nerve conduction. It is absorbed in the gastrointestinal tract and transported through the blood to tissues, where it is vital for various cellular processes. While sodium is crucial for maintaining homeostasis, the body only requires small amounts to function properly. Excess sodium, particularly from dietary sources such as processed foods, can lead to several health issues, one of the most pressing being cancer.

Sodium and Cancer Risk: Epidemiological Evidence

Research into the relationship between sodium and cancer risk began with epidemiological studies that observed populations with high sodium intake, particularly those in regions where salt-preserved foods were commonly consumed. Studies have consistently shown an increased risk of gastric (stomach) cancer in individuals with high sodium consumption, which has been the primary focus of this research. Salt-preserved foods, rich in sodium, are believed to be particularly harmful due to their potential to damage the gastric mucosa, increase the risk of infection by *Helicobacter pylori*, and lead to chronic inflammation—an established precursor to cancer development.

Gastric Cancer and Sodium: The Most Established Link

Gastric cancer is one of the most well-researched areas when exploring sodium's connection to cancer. High sodium intake has been identified as a major risk factor for the development of gastric cancer, particularly in regions where traditional diets include significant amounts of salt-preserved foods (e.g., East Asia). The mechanisms by which sodium contributes to gastric cancer are multifactorial and involve several biological pathways:

1. **Gastric Mucosa Damage and Hyperplasia:** High sodium intake can directly damage the epithelial lining of the stomach. Sodium has an erosive effect on the stomach's mucosal lining, which is essential for protecting the underlying tissues from acidic gastric juices. When this protective barrier is compromised, cells in the stomach lining can become inflamed and undergo hyperplasia (excessive cell growth), which increases the likelihood of malignant transformation.

2. **Promotion of *Helicobacter pylori* Infection:** *Helicobacter pylori* (H. pylori) infection is a well-established risk factor for gastric cancer. High sodium levels can exacerbate the virulence of *H. pylori*, enhancing its ability to colonize the stomach lining and cause chronic inflammation. Research has shown that sodium increases the expression of genes in *H. pylori* that are involved in its pathogenicity. Chronic inflammation caused by *H. pylori* infection leads to oxidative stress and DNA damage, both of which are critical steps in carcinogenesis.

3. **Activation of Inflammatory Pathways:** Excess sodium intake triggers inflammatory responses in the stomach. Chronic inflammation is a key driver of cancer progression, as it leads to the production of reactive oxygen species (ROS) and pro-inflammatory cytokines. ROS cause oxidative damage to DNA, proteins, and lipids, which can result in genetic mutations. In particular, the nuclear factor-kappa B (NF-κB) signaling pathway, which regulates the expression of various pro-inflammatory cytokines and enzymes, has been implicated in sodium-induced inflammation. The persistent activation of NF-κB is associated with the initiation and progression of gastric cancer.

4. **Impact on Apoptosis and Cell Proliferation:** High sodium levels may interfere with normal cellular processes, including apoptosis (programmed cell death). Apoptosis is a natural mechanism by which the body removes damaged or potentially cancerous cells. Sodium can disrupt this process by altering the balance

between pro-apoptotic and anti-apoptotic factors. Specifically, sodium has been found to inhibit the expression of pro-apoptotic proteins such as Bax while promoting the expression of anti-apoptotic proteins like Bcl-2, thus allowing damaged cells to survive and proliferate. This unchecked cell growth is a hallmark of cancer development.

Sodium and Colorectal Cancer: Emerging Evidence

While the link between sodium and gastric cancer is well-established, emerging evidence suggests that high sodium intake may also play a role in the development of colorectal cancer. Several studies have suggested that excessive sodium consumption can affect the gut microbiome, leading to dysbiosis, which may promote carcinogenesis in the colon and rectum.

1. **Dysbiosis and Gut Inflammation:** Sodium has been shown to alter the composition of the gut microbiome, reducing the diversity of beneficial bacteria and promoting the growth of harmful bacteria that produce toxins and pro-inflammatory molecules. This shift in the microbiome can lead to chronic inflammation in the intestinal lining, which is a risk factor for colorectal cancer. The release of bacterial endotoxins triggers the activation of immune cells, leading to the production of pro-inflammatory cytokines such as tumor necrosis factor-alpha (TNF-α) and interleukin-6 (IL-6), both of which are associated with cancer development.

2. **Activation of Oncogenic Pathways:** High sodium intake may influence oncogenic signaling pathways that drive colorectal cancer progression. The mitogen-activated protein kinase (MAPK) and Wnt signaling pathways, both of which play critical roles in cell proliferation and differentiation, have been found to be activated in response to sodium-induced inflammation. These

pathways are often dysregulated in colorectal cancer, leading to uncontrolled cell division and tumor formation.

3. **Disruption of Epithelial Barrier Function:** The epithelial cells lining the colon form a protective barrier that prevents harmful substances from entering the bloodstream. Excess sodium intake can compromise the integrity of this barrier, making it more permeable to toxins and carcinogens. This "leaky gut" condition allows harmful substances to interact with epithelial cells, leading to DNA damage and an increased risk of cancer.

Sodium and Esophageal Cancer: A Potential Link

Another area of concern is the potential relationship between high sodium intake and esophageal cancer. Although less studied than gastric and colorectal cancers, some evidence suggests that excessive sodium consumption may increase the risk of esophageal cancer, particularly squamous cell carcinoma.

1. **Erosion of the Esophageal Lining:** Like the gastric mucosa, the esophageal lining can be damaged by high sodium intake. Salt has an abrasive effect on the sensitive tissues of the esophagus, making them more susceptible to irritation and inflammation. Chronic irritation can lead to the development of Barrett's esophagus, a condition in which the normal squamous epithelium is replaced by abnormal glandular cells, which are more prone to becoming cancerous.

2. **Synergistic Effect with Other Carcinogens:** High sodium intake may enhance the carcinogenic effects of other risk factors for esophageal cancer, such as smoking and alcohol consumption. Sodium may increase the permeability of the esophageal lining, allowing carcinogens from tobacco smoke and alcohol to penetrate deeper into the tissues and cause DNA damage.

Sodium and Kidney Cancer: Indirect Effects

Although sodium has not been directly linked to kidney cancer, its role in causing hypertension—a major risk factor for kidney cancer—is well documented. Hypertension can lead to chronic kidney damage, which in turn increases the risk of developing renal cell carcinoma, the most common type of kidney cancer. Excessive sodium intake is one of the leading causes of hypertension, suggesting an indirect but significant relationship between sodium and kidney cancer risk.

Sodium, Obesity, and Cancer

High sodium intake is often associated with poor dietary habits, such as the consumption of processed and calorie-dense foods. This dietary pattern contributes to obesity, which is a known risk factor for several types of cancer, including breast, colorectal, endometrial, and pancreatic cancers. Obesity promotes cancer development through several mechanisms, including chronic inflammation, insulin resistance, and hormonal imbalances.

1. **Chronic Inflammation:** Obesity is characterized by low-grade chronic inflammation, which promotes cancer progression. Adipose tissue (body fat) secretes pro-inflammatory cytokines such as IL-6 and TNF-α, which activate signaling pathways involved in cell proliferation and survival. High sodium intake exacerbates this inflammatory state, further increasing the risk of cancer.

2. **Insulin Resistance and Hyperinsulinemia:** Obesity is often accompanied by insulin resistance, a condition in which cells become less responsive to insulin, leading to elevated blood sugar levels. In response, the pancreas produces more insulin, resulting in hyperinsulinemia. High levels of insulin can promote cancer by stimulating cell growth and inhibiting apoptosis. Sodium has been shown to worsen insulin resistance, creating a cycle that increases cancer risk.

Sodium and Breast Cancer: An Area of Ongoing Research

Research into the relationship between sodium and breast cancer is still in its early stages, but some studies have suggested a potential link. Excessive sodium intake may contribute to breast cancer development through mechanisms similar to those observed in other cancers, such as inflammation and disruption of cellular homeostasis. However, more research is needed to establish a clear connection between sodium and breast cancer.

The link between sodium and cancer is an area of growing concern in public health, particularly in light of the increasing consumption of processed, sodium-rich foods. While sodium is essential for normal physiological function, excessive intake has been associated with an elevated risk of several cancers, including gastric, colorectal, esophageal, and potentially breast cancer. The mechanisms by which sodium contributes to cancer development are multifactorial, involving pathways related to inflammation, DNA damage, cell proliferation, and disruption of normal cellular processes.

Reducing sodium intake, particularly from processed and salt-preserved foods, may be an important strategy for lowering cancer risk. Public health initiatives aimed at promoting dietary changes, such as reducing sodium consumption and increasing the intake of fresh, whole foods, could play a crucial role in cancer prevention efforts.

Saturated Fats

Saturated fats have long been associated with various health conditions, including heart disease, obesity, and metabolic disorders. However, recent research has extended these concerns to a potential link between saturated fats and cancer.

Saturated fats are a type of dietary fat where the carbon chain is fully saturated with hydrogen atoms, meaning they contain no double bonds between the carbon atoms. These fats are typically solid at room temperature and are most commonly found in animal products such as meat, dairy, and certain plant-based oils like coconut and palm oil.

The Role of Fat in the Body

Fats, including saturated fats, are essential for the human body's functioning. They provide energy, contribute to cell structure, and are involved in the absorption of fat-soluble vitamins. However, when consumed in excess, saturated fats can trigger inflammatory processes, alter metabolic functions, and lead to cellular changes that increase cancer risk.

Saturated Fats and Cancer: The Evidence

Numerous studies have established a link between the consumption of high levels of saturated fats and an increased risk of cancer. This connection is observed in various forms of cancer, such as breast, colon, pancreatic, and prostate cancer. The mechanisms involved in the carcinogenic properties of saturated fats include chronic inflammation, oxidative stress, and alterations in cell membrane composition, which can all promote tumor growth and progression.

Breast Cancer

Saturated fat intake has been linked to an increased risk of breast cancer, particularly in postmenopausal women. High-fat diets have been shown to elevate levels of estrogen and other hormones that are associated with breast cancer development.

A large study known as the Women's Health Initiative Dietary Modification Trial found that reducing dietary fat intake, particularly saturated fat, decreased the incidence of breast cancer in postmenopausal women by 9%.

Saturated fats can increase estrogen production by influencing the expression of aromatase, an enzyme responsible for converting androgens into estrogens. Elevated estrogen levels promote the proliferation of estrogen receptor-positive (ER+) breast cancer cells. Moreover, saturated fats may influence the signaling of growth factors, such as insulin-like growth factor (IGF-1), which plays a role in cell proliferation and differentiation, thereby enhancing cancer development.

Colon Cancer

Saturated fat consumption has also been implicated in colon cancer development. In the colon, saturated fats can alter the microbiome, leading to the proliferation of harmful bacteria that produce carcinogenic compounds. A high-fat diet increases bile acid production, particularly secondary bile acids, which can damage the DNA of colon cells and promote carcinogenesis.

Studies have shown that individuals who consume high amounts of saturated fat have a higher risk of colorectal cancer. This connection is mediated through the increased production of bile acids, which can be metabolized by gut bacteria into deoxycholic acid (DCA), a known carcinogen that damages colon cells and promotes tumor formation.

Pancreatic Cancer

There is evidence linking high saturated fat intake with pancreatic cancer, one of the deadliest forms of cancer. The connection is largely driven by the role saturated fats play in increasing inflammation and promoting insulin resistance. Insulin resistance leads to elevated levels of insulin and IGF-1, both of which can stimulate pancreatic cell proliferation and contribute to tumor growth.

Additionally, research suggests that a high-fat diet alters the expression of genes involved in inflammation and immune responses, which can facilitate the development of pancreatic tumors. Saturated fats, particularly palmitic acid, have been shown to promote the migration and invasion of pancreatic cancer cells by activating specific molecular pathways, including the JNK and MAPK pathways.

Prostate Cancer

Saturated fat intake has also been associated with an increased risk of prostate cancer. The relationship between saturated fats and prostate cancer risk is believed to be mediated through the production of inflammatory markers, oxidative stress, and alterations in androgen signaling.

Research has shown that high levels of saturated fat can activate nuclear factor kappa B (NF-κB), a key transcription factor involved in inflammation and cancer progression. Chronic activation of NF-κB promotes tumorigenesis by enhancing cell proliferation and inhibiting apoptosis (programmed cell death). Furthermore, saturated fats may contribute to an environment that supports cancer cell survival and metastasis by altering lipid metabolism and increasing cholesterol levels, which are necessary for the rapid growth of cancer cells.

Mechanisms of Saturated Fat-Induced Carcinogenesis
Inflammation and Cancer

Chronic inflammation is a well-established risk factor for cancer development, and saturated fats have been shown to promote inflammation in various tissues. The consumption of saturated fats leads to the activation of pro-inflammatory cytokines, such as tumor necrosis factor-alpha (TNF-α) and interleukin-6 (IL-6), which can contribute to the development and progression of cancer.

Increased intake of saturated fats can activate toll-like receptor 4 (TLR4) on immune cells, triggering the release of inflammatory mediators. This chronic inflammatory state creates a microenvironment conducive to cancer by promoting angiogenesis (the growth of new blood vessels) and inhibiting apoptosis.

Oxidative Stress

Saturated fats can induce oxidative stress, which occurs when there is an imbalance between the production of free radicals and the body's ability to neutralize them. Excessive consumption of saturated fats leads to the production of reactive oxygen species (ROS), which can damage DNA, proteins, and lipids in cells, thereby promoting cancer.

Oxidative stress is closely linked to the activation of oncogenes, which drive uncontrolled cell growth. Furthermore, ROS can promote the mutation of tumor suppressor genes, such as p53, which is crucial for regulating cell division and preventing cancer.

Alteration of Cell Membrane Composition

Saturated fats are incorporated into cell membranes, affecting their fluidity and function. A diet high in saturated fats can lead to the stiffening of cell membranes, which can disrupt normal cellular signaling processes. This alteration in membrane structure can impair the function of receptors involved in cell growth regulation, such as insulin receptors, and contribute to the development of insulin resistance and cancer.

Moreover, the incorporation of saturated fats into cell membranes can enhance the activity of certain oncogenic pathways, such as the phosphatidylinositol-3-kinase (PI3K)/Akt pathway, which is involved in cell survival and proliferation.

Insulin Resistance and Cancer

Saturated fats are known to promote insulin resistance, a condition in which the body's cells become less responsive to insulin. Insulin resistance is associated with elevated levels of insulin and IGF-1, both of which have been shown to promote the growth and survival of cancer cells.

High levels of insulin can activate the PI3K/Akt and Ras/MAPK pathways, leading to increased cell proliferation and reduced apoptosis.

These pathways are critical in cancer development, as they enable cancer cells to survive and multiply in an uncontrolled manner.

Gut Microbiome and Cancer

The gut microbiome plays a crucial role in maintaining health and preventing disease, including cancer. A diet high in saturated fats can alter the composition of the gut microbiome, leading to dysbiosis, or an imbalance of gut bacteria. This dysbiosis can result in the production of harmful metabolites, such as secondary bile acids and lipopolysaccharides (LPS), which promote inflammation and increase cancer risk.

Research has shown that saturated fats can increase the abundance of pro-inflammatory bacteria, such as Enterobacteriaceae, while reducing the levels of beneficial bacteria, such as Bifidobacteria and Lactobacilli. This shift in the microbiome can enhance intestinal permeability, allowing bacterial endotoxins to enter the bloodstream and trigger systemic inflammation.

Saturated Fats and Cancer Pathways

Several molecular pathways have been identified as being involved in the carcinogenic effects of saturated fats. These include:

1. NF-κB Pathway

The NF-κB pathway is a key regulator of inflammation and immune responses. Saturated fats can activate the NF-κB pathway by binding to TLR4 receptors on immune cells, leading to the production of pro-inflammatory cytokines. Chronic activation of NF-κB promotes cancer development by enhancing cell proliferation, inhibiting apoptosis, and increasing angiogenesis.

2. PI3K/Akt Pathway

The PI3K/Akt pathway is a major signaling pathway involved in cell growth, survival, and metabolism. Saturated fats can activate this pathway through insulin resistance, leading to increased cell proliferation and survival. The activation of the PI3K/Akt pathway is associated with various cancers, including breast, colon, and prostate cancer.

3. MAPK Pathway

The MAPK pathway is another important signaling pathway involved in cell proliferation and differentiation. Saturated fats can activate this pathway through the production of inflammatory mediators and oxidative stress. The MAPK pathway plays a critical role in cancer development by promoting cell growth and survival.

The evidence linking saturated fats to cancer is robust and supported by numerous studies. Saturated fats promote cancer development through various mechanisms, including chronic inflammation, oxidative stress, alterations in cell membrane composition, and insulin resistance. The activation of key molecular pathways, such as the NF-κB, PI3K/Akt, and MAPK pathways, further contributes to the carcinogenic effects of saturated fats. Reducing saturated fat intake is, therefore, an essential strategy for lowering cancer risk and improving overall health.

8

Animal Products Linked to Cancer

Dairy products, long considered a staple of the Western diet, have been linked to various health conditions, including the potential to promote cancer growth. This connection has been the subject of increasing research over the past few decades, revealing complex biological pathways through which dairy consumption may contribute to cancer development. In this detailed exploration, I will examine the scientific evidence that connects dairy products to cancer, discuss the specific pathways involved, and provide insights into how these findings impact public health.

The Biological Components of Dairy

Dairy products are rich in various nutrients, including calcium, protein, and vitamins, but they also contain hormones, growth factors, and bioactive compounds that can influence cellular processes. Some of the key components of dairy that have been linked to cancer include:

1. **Insulin-Like Growth Factor-1 (IGF-1):** A hormone that promotes cell growth and proliferation. Elevated levels of IGF-1 have been associated with an increased risk of several cancers, including breast, prostate, and colorectal cancer.
2. **Estrogens:** Dairy contains natural estrogens, which can bind to estrogen receptors in the body and stimulate cell proliferation.

This is particularly concerning in hormone-sensitive cancers such as breast and ovarian cancer.

3. **Saturated Fats:** High intake of saturated fats has been linked to inflammation and obesity, both of which are risk factors for cancer.

4. **Casein:** The primary protein in dairy, casein, has been shown to promote cancer growth in animal studies, particularly when consumed in high amounts.

5. **Calcium:** While calcium is essential for bone health, excessive intake has been linked to prostate cancer. High calcium levels may inhibit the synthesis of active vitamin D, a hormone that has protective effects against cancer.

The Role of IGF-1 in Cancer Growth

Insulin-like Growth Factor-1 (IGF-1) is a hormone structurally similar to insulin, and it plays a critical role in growth and development. However, its role in cancer has been a growing concern. IGF-1 promotes cell proliferation and inhibits apoptosis (programmed cell death), processes that are central to cancer development.

Pathway of IGF-1 and Cancer

When dairy is consumed, it increases the levels of IGF-1 in the bloodstream. IGF-1 binds to its receptor, IGF-1R, on the surface of cells, activating a signaling cascade that leads to cellular growth and division. This pathway involves several key molecules, including:

- **PI3K/AKT Pathway:** Activation of the phosphoinositide 3-kinase (PI3K) and protein kinase B (AKT) pathway promotes cell survival and growth. Overactivation of this pathway is commonly observed in cancer cells.
- **RAS/MAPK Pathway:** The RAS/mitogen-activated protein kinase (MAPK) pathway is another critical signaling cascade activated by IGF-1, leading to increased cell proliferation.

- **mTOR Pathway:** The mammalian target of rapamycin (mTOR) pathway is involved in protein synthesis and cell growth. IGF-1 activates mTOR, contributing to cancer cell growth.

Several studies have shown a strong correlation between high levels of IGF-1 and the risk of developing various cancers. For example, a study published in *The Lancet Oncology* found that individuals with higher circulating levels of IGF-1 had an increased risk of breast, prostate, and colorectal cancer.

Estrogens in Dairy and Cancer

Dairy products contain natural estrogens, particularly estrone and estradiol, which are derived from the lactating cows used in dairy production. These hormones can bind to estrogen receptors in the human body and stimulate the growth of estrogen-sensitive tissues, leading to an increased risk of hormone-dependent cancers.

Estrogen Receptor Pathway

The estrogen receptor (ER) pathway is a well-known mechanism through which estrogens promote cancer. When estrogen binds to the ER, it activates the receptor, leading to the transcription of genes involved in cell proliferation and survival. This process is particularly relevant in breast cancer, where estrogen plays a significant role in tumor growth.

Estrogen receptors are of two main types: ER-alpha and ER-beta. ER-alpha is primarily associated with promoting cell proliferation, while ER-beta can have both proliferative and anti-proliferative effects depending on the context. The activation of ER-alpha by estrogens in dairy can lead to the growth of estrogen-dependent cancers such as breast, ovarian, and endometrial cancer.

A study published in the *Journal of the National Cancer Institute* found that women with higher levels of circulating estrogens had a significantly increased risk of breast cancer. The study highlighted the role of dietary estrogens from dairy products in contributing to these elevated estrogen levels.

Saturated Fats and Inflammation

Saturated fats are abundant in dairy products, particularly in whole milk, cheese, and butter. High intake of saturated fats has been linked to chronic inflammation, a known risk factor for cancer. Inflammation can lead to the production of reactive oxygen species (ROS) and other inflammatory mediators that cause DNA damage and promote tumorigenesis.

Inflammatory Pathways

The connection between saturated fats and inflammation involves several pathways, including:

- **NF-κB Pathway:** The nuclear factor kappa-light-chain-enhancer of activated B cells (NF-κB) pathway is a key regulator of inflammation. Saturated fats can activate NF-κB, leading to the production of inflammatory cytokines such as TNF-alpha and IL-6, which promote cancer growth.
- **COX-2 Pathway:** Cyclooxygenase-2 (COX-2) is an enzyme involved in the synthesis of prostaglandins, which are inflammatory mediators. Saturated fats can increase COX-2 expression, leading to chronic inflammation and cancer promotion.
- **Adipokines:** Obesity, often exacerbated by high intake of saturated fats, leads to the production of adipokines, such as leptin and adiponectin, which can influence cancer development through inflammatory mechanisms.

Research published in *Cancer Research* demonstrated that high dietary intake of saturated fats was associated with an increased risk of colorectal cancer. The study suggested that inflammation mediated by saturated fats played a significant role in this increased risk.

Casein and Cancer Promotion

Casein, the primary protein in dairy, has been the subject of controversy due to its potential role in promoting cancer. The China Study, a comprehensive nutritional study led by Dr. T. Colin Campbell, found a strong association between casein consumption and cancer growth in animal models. This research suggested that casein could act as a cancer promoter, particularly when consumed in high amounts.

Mechanisms of Casein-Induced Cancer

The mechanisms through which casein promotes cancer are not entirely understood, but several hypotheses have been proposed:

- **Epigenetic Modifications:** Casein may induce epigenetic changes that promote cancer. Epigenetic modifications, such as DNA methylation and histone acetylation, can alter gene expression without changing the DNA sequence, leading to cancerous transformations.
- **Increased IGF-1 Levels:** As mentioned earlier, dairy consumption, including casein, increases IGF-1 levels, which in turn promotes cancer growth.
- **Amino Acid Profile:** The amino acid composition of casein may promote cancer by providing an abundance of certain amino acids that stimulate cell growth and proliferation.

Dr. Campbell's findings, published in his book *The China Study*, revealed that rats fed a diet with 20% casein developed liver tumors, while those fed a diet with 5% casein did not. This study raised significant concerns about the role of casein in cancer promotion and led to further research on the topic.

Calcium and Prostate Cancer

Calcium is an essential nutrient for bone health, but excessive intake has been linked to an increased risk of prostate cancer. The relationship between calcium and prostate cancer is complex, involving the suppression of vitamin D activity and alterations in cellular signaling pathways.

Vitamin D Suppression

High calcium intake can inhibit the conversion of 25-hydroxyvitamin D to its active form, 1,25-dihydroxyvitamin D (calcitriol), in the kidneys. Calcitriol is a hormone that has protective effects against cancer by promoting cell differentiation and inhibiting cell proliferation. When calcium levels are high, the suppression of calcitriol can remove this protective effect, leading to an increased risk of cancer.

Calcium-Sensing Receptor (CaSR) Pathway

The calcium-sensing receptor (CaSR) is a G-protein-coupled receptor that regulates calcium homeostasis. Overactivation of CaSR by high calcium levels can lead to the activation of signaling pathways that promote cancer, including the MAPK and PI3K/AKT pathways.

A meta-analysis published in the *American Journal of Clinical Nutrition* found that high dietary calcium intake was associated with an increased risk of prostate cancer. The study suggested that the suppression of vitamin D activity and the activation of CaSR were key factors in this increased risk.

Epidemiological Evidence Linking Dairy to Cancer

In addition to the mechanistic studies discussed above, numerous epidemiological studies have explored the relationship between dairy consumption and cancer risk. These studies provide valuable insights into how dairy products may influence cancer development at the population level.

Breast Cancer

Several studies have examined the link between dairy consumption and breast cancer risk. A cohort study published in the *International Journal of Epidemiology* found that women who consumed higher amounts of dairy, particularly high-fat dairy products, had an increased risk of breast cancer. The study suggested that the estrogen content in dairy, along with other bioactive compounds, may contribute to this increased risk.

Prostate Cancer

Prostate cancer is one of the most well-studied cancers in relation to dairy consumption. A large prospective study published in the *American Journal of Clinical Nutrition* found that men who consumed higher amounts of dairy, particularly milk, had a significantly increased risk of prostate cancer. The study highlighted the potential role of calcium, IGF-1, and estrogens in promoting prostate cancer.

Colorectal Cancer

The relationship between dairy consumption and colorectal cancer is more complex, with some studies suggesting a protective effect of calcium, while others indicate an increased risk. A meta-analysis published in the *Journal of the National Cancer Institute* found that while calcium from dairy products may have a protective effect against colorectal cancer, high consumption of other dairy components, such as saturated fats and IGF-1, may offset this benefit and increase the overall risk.

The Impact of Dairy on Cancer Recurrence and Survival

For individuals who have already been diagnosed with cancer, the consumption of dairy products may also impact cancer recurrence and survival. Several studies have explored how dairy intake affects cancer outcomes, with mixed results.

Breast Cancer Survivors

A study published in *Cancer Epidemiology, Biomarkers & Prevention* found that higher intake of high-fat dairy products was associated with an increased risk of breast cancer recurrence and mortality among breast cancer survivors. The study suggested that the estrogen content in high-fat dairy products may promote the growth of residual cancer cells.

Prostate Cancer Survivors

Similarly, a study published in the *Journal of Clinical Oncology* found that higher intake of dairy products, particularly whole milk, was associated with an increased risk of prostate cancer progression and mortality among prostate cancer survivors. The study emphasized the potential role of IGF-1 and saturated fats in promoting cancer progression.

The Role of Dairy Alternatives in Cancer Prevention

Given the potential link between dairy consumption and cancer, many individuals are turning to dairy alternatives as a way to reduce their risk. Plant-based milk alternatives, such as almond, soy, and oat milk, are becoming increasingly popular as substitutes for traditional dairy products. These alternatives are free from the hormones, saturated fats, and other components of dairy that have been linked to cancer, making them a potentially safer option.

Soy Milk and Cancer Risk

Soy milk, made from soybeans, is a popular dairy alternative that has been the subject of much research in relation to cancer. Soy contains phytoestrogens, which are plant-based compounds that can mimic estrogen in the body. However, unlike the estrogens found in dairy, phytoestrogens have been shown to have both estrogenic and anti-estrogenic effects, depending on the context. The Soy isoflavones bind to ER-beta receptors and is not associated with promoting cell proliferation like the ER-alpha receptor.

A meta-analysis published in *Cancer Causes & Control* found that higher consumption of soy products, including soy milk, was associated with a reduced risk of breast cancer, particularly among Asian populations. The study suggested that the anti-estrogenic effects of phytoestrogens in soy may protect against cancer by blocking the binding of stronger estrogens to estrogen receptors.

Almond Milk and Cancer Risk

Almond milk, another popular dairy alternative, is low in saturated fats and free from hormones. While there is limited research specifically on almond milk and cancer risk, the general consensus is that plant-based alternatives like almond milk are likely to be safer than dairy in terms of cancer prevention.

A study published in *Nutrition and Cancer* found that higher intake of nuts, including almonds, was associated with a reduced risk of several cancers, including colorectal, pancreatic, and prostate cancer. The study highlighted the anti-inflammatory and antioxidant properties of nuts as potential mechanisms for cancer prevention.

The connection between dairy consumption and cancer is a complex and multifaceted issue that involves various biological pathways and risk factors. The evidence suggests that dairy products, particularly those high in IGF-1, estrogens, and saturated fats, may contribute to the growth and development of several types of cancer. While more research is needed to fully understand the mechanisms involved, the existing data is compelling enough to warrant caution in dairy consumption, particularly for individuals at high risk of hormone-sensitive cancers.

Switching to plant-based alternatives, such as soy or almond milk, may offer a safer option with potential protective effects against cancer. As public health guidelines evolve, it will be important to continue monitoring the research on dairy and cancer to ensure that recommendations reflect the best available evidence.

How Animal Meat Is Linked To Cancer

The link between the consumption of animal meat and cancer has become an increasingly important focus of scientific research. Numerous studies have examined how various components of meat, especially red and processed meat, contribute to cancer formation. I will explain the underlying mechanisms, cellular pathways, and the broader health impacts of consuming animal meat, including its influence on carcinogenesis. By understanding the intricate biochemical processes and how meat consumption contributes to tumor development, one can appreciate the importance of dietary choices in cancer prevention.

Meat Consumption and Cancer

The International Agency for Research on Cancer (IARC), a branch of the World Health Organization (WHO), classified processed meat as a Group 1 carcinogen in 2015, meaning that there is sufficient evidence of its ability to cause cancer in humans. Red meat was classified as a Group 2A carcinogen, indicating that it is "probably carcinogenic to humans". Various types of cancers, including colorectal, stomach, breast, and pancreatic cancer, have been linked to meat consumption.

Meat contains several compounds that contribute to cancer development, such as heterocyclic amines (HCAs), polycyclic aromatic hydrocarbons (PAHs), heme iron, and nitrosamines. Additionally, inflammation caused by saturated fats and obesity-related cancer risks are also significant.

Heterocyclic Amines (HCAs) and Polycyclic Aromatic Hydrocarbons (PAHs)

When meat is cooked at high temperatures, such as grilling, frying, or barbecuing, HCAs and PAHs are formed. These compounds are mutagenic, meaning they can cause changes or mutations in the DNA of cells, potentially leading to cancer.

Heterocyclic Amines (HCAs)

HCAs are formed when creatine or creatinine (found in muscle meats) reacts with amino acids and sugars at high temperatures. These carcinogens damage DNA by causing mutations, which can trigger the initiation of cancer in organs like the colon, breast, and prostate. For example, PhIP, a type of HCA found in grilled or fried meats, has been implicated in promoting breast cancer and colon cancer.

Polycyclic Aromatic Hydrocarbons (PAHs)

PAHs form when fat drips onto a hot surface and produces smoke, which is then deposited onto the meat. Benzo[a]pyrene, a prominent PAH, is found in smoked and grilled meats and is known to be highly carcinogenic. It binds to DNA and can cause mutations that interfere with normal cell regulation. The formation of PAHs, particularly in smoked and grilled meats, poses a significant risk for gastrointestinal cancers, especially in the esophagus and stomach.

Heme Iron in Red Meat and its Role in Cancer Development

Heme iron, abundant in red meat, is another key factor in the carcinogenicity of animal meat. Heme iron is distinct from non-heme iron found in plant-based foods. In the digestive tract, heme iron promotes the formation of N-nitroso compounds (NOCs) and free radicals, both of which damage DNA and contribute to cancer formation.

N-nitroso Compounds (NOCs)

NOCs are a class of potent carcinogens formed in the stomach and colon when the heme iron from red meat is metabolized. They can cause oxidative stress, leading to DNA damage, particularly in the colon and rectum. This is one of the reasons why red and processed meats are closely associated with colorectal cancer.

Free Radical Formation

The metabolism of heme iron leads to the production of free radicals. These reactive oxygen species (ROS) can cause oxidative stress in cells, resulting in DNA damage. Persistent DNA damage without repair increases the likelihood of mutations and eventually tumor formation. The pro-oxidative environment created by heme iron is a key driver of cancer risk, particularly in the gastrointestinal tract. *I will provide a more comprehensive analysis on heme iron, titled "Heme Iron Causes Mutations," as a follow-up to "How Animal Meat Is Linked To Cancer."*

Nitrosamines in Processed Meat

Processed meats, such as bacon, sausages, hot dogs, and deli meats, often contain nitrates and nitrites, which are used as preservatives and flavor enhancers. In the acidic environment of the stomach, these compounds can be converted into nitrosamines, potent carcinogens that have been linked to various cancers, including colorectal, gastric, and pancreatic cancers.

Nitrosamines are known to induce DNA alkylation, which can lead to mutations in oncogenes and tumor suppressor genes, accelerating cancer progression. Studies have shown that high consumption of nitrite-containing processed meats is correlated with a higher incidence of gastrointestinal cancers.

Saturated Fats and Obesity-Related Cancer Risks

Animal meat, especially red and processed meat, tends to be high in saturated fats. Diets rich in saturated fats have been linked to obesity, which is a known risk factor for cancer. Obesity promotes chronic inflammation, which can lead to an increase in pro-inflammatory cytokines and growth factors, such as insulin-like growth factor-1 (IGF-1), that support tumor growth and progression.

Chronic Inflammation and Cancer

Inflammation is a normal immune response, but chronic inflammation can contribute to cancer development. Pro-inflammatory molecules like cytokines create an environment conducive to tumorigenesis by promoting cell proliferation, angiogenesis, and metastasis. Studies have shown that diets high in saturated fats contribute to the activation of inflammatory pathways such as the nuclear factor-kappa B (NF-kB) signaling pathway, which is implicated in the progression of cancers such as breast, colorectal, and prostate cancer.

Gut Microbiota and Its Role in Meat-Induced Cancer

The human gut microbiome plays an important role in health and disease. Emerging research indicates that the consumption of animal meat, particularly red and processed meats, alters the composition of the gut microbiota in ways that promote carcinogenesis.

Production of TMAO (Trimethylamine N-oxide)

When red meat is consumed, gut bacteria metabolize carnitine, a compound found in meat, to produce trimethylamine (TMA), which is subsequently converted in the liver to trimethylamine N-oxide (TMAO). TMAO has been implicated in promoting atherosclerosis and increasing the risk of heart disease. More recently, TMAO has also been linked to cancer development. TMAO promotes chronic inflammation and oxidative stress, which are key drivers of carcinogenesis.

Insulin-Like Growth Factor 1 (IGF-1) Pathway Activation

Animal proteins, particularly those found in red and processed meats, have been shown to elevate levels of IGF-1, a growth factor involved in cell proliferation and survival. High levels of IGF-1 are associated with an increased risk of several cancers, including breast, prostate, and colorectal cancer.

The IGF-1 signaling pathway promotes cell division and inhibits apoptosis (programmed cell death). When overactivated, this pathway can lead to uncontrolled cell growth and the development of tumors. High levels of animal protein stimulate the liver to produce more IGF-1, which can exacerbate the risk of cancer.

The Role of Meat in Hormone-Dependent Cancers

Several types of cancers, such as breast, prostate, and ovarian cancer, are hormone-dependent, meaning their growth is influenced by hormone levels in the body. Animal meat, particularly red meat, contains natural hormones, and processed meats may contain synthetic hormones used to promote animal growth. These hormones can disrupt the body's endocrine system, leading to an increased risk of hormone-dependent cancers.

Estrogen and Breast Cancer

Estrogen is a hormone that plays a key role in the development of breast cancer. Diets high in animal products, particularly those that involve the consumption of hormone-treated meat, can elevate circulating estrogen levels in the body. Studies have shown that higher levels of circulating estrogens are associated with an increased risk of developing breast cancer.

Meat Consumption and Colorectal Cancer

Colorectal cancer has one of the strongest associations with red and processed meat consumption. The carcinogenic effects of meat in the colon are primarily attributed to the production of NOCs, HCAs, PAHs, and the inflammation caused by saturated fats. Additionally, heme iron in red meat plays a critical role in promoting the formation of harmful NOCs .

Microbiota-Mediated Inflammation

The gut microbiota plays a significant role in maintaining intestinal health. However, diets rich in animal meat, especially processed meats, can disrupt the balance of gut bacteria, leading to the overproduction of harmful metabolites like secondary bile acids. These metabolites promote inflammation and may contribute to the development of colorectal cancer by damaging the colonic mucosa and creating a pro-inflammatory environment.

Reducing Cancer Risk Through Dietary Choices

Scientific evidence clearly indicates that diets high in red and processed meats increase the risk of various cancers. Replacing these meats with plant-based proteins, whole grains, fruits, and vegetables can significantly reduce cancer risk. Plant-based diets are rich in antioxidants, fiber, and phytonutrients that help protect cells from DNA damage and reduce inflammation, two key processes in cancer prevention. See the upcoming chapter on Plant-Based Diets like the P53 Diet.

Fiber and Gut Health

Diets rich in dietary fiber, particularly from plant-based sources, have been shown to lower the risk of colorectal cancer. Fiber promotes healthy digestion and enhances the production of short-chain fatty acids (SCFAs) like butyrate, which has anti-inflammatory properties and protects against colon cancer.

The consumption of animal meat, particularly red and processed meat, is strongly associated with an increased risk of cancer. Multiple mechanisms contribute to this carcinogenic potential, including the formation of HCAs and PAHs during cooking, the pro-oxidative effects of heme iron, the production of nitrosamines from processed meats, and the role of saturated fats in promoting inflammation and obesity. Additionally, meat consumption alters the gut microbiota, leading to the production of carcinogenic metabolites like TMAO. The activation of the IGF-1 signaling pathway and the influence of hormones in meat further exacerbate the risk of hormone-dependent cancers like breast and prostate cancer.

To reduce cancer risk, it is essential to eliminate the consumption of red and processed meats and adopt a diet rich in plant-based foods. Plant-based diets not only minimize exposure to carcinogens found in animal meats but also provide protective nutrients that support overall health and reduce the risk of cancer. *See the upcoming chapter on Plant-Based Diets like the P53 Diet.*

Heme Iron Linked To Gene Mutations

Iron is an essential mineral required for numerous biological processes, including oxygen transport, DNA synthesis, and energy production as I briefly explained earlier. However, the type of iron—heme or non-heme—plays a critical role in how the body absorbs, utilizes, and regulates this mineral. The distinction between heme and non-heme iron has profound implications for cellular health, particularly in how iron overload from heme iron can lead to cellular mutations and various diseases, including cancer. I will explain the mechanisms by which heme iron can flood cells with iron, leading to potential cellular damage, and how non-heme iron is regulated within the body to prevent such occurrences. The pathways involved in these processes will also be discussed, with supporting evidence from scientific literature.

Heme Iron: A Double-Edged Sword
What is Heme Iron?

Heme iron is found primarily in animal-based foods, such as red meat, poultry, and fish. It is derived from hemoglobin and myoglobin, proteins in animal tissues that carry and store oxygen. Heme iron is highly bioavailable, meaning it is easily absorbed by the body. However, this high bioavailability also poses risks, as it can lead to excessive iron accumulation in cells.

Absorption of Heme Iron

Heme iron is absorbed intact by enterocytes, the cells lining the small intestine, through a specific transporter known as the heme carrier protein 1 (HCP1). Once inside the enterocyte, heme is broken down by the enzyme heme oxygenase-1, releasing ferrous iron (Fe_2+), which can then be utilized by the body or stored as ferritin.

The absorption of heme iron is not as tightly regulated as non-heme iron. This is due to the fact that heme iron bypasses the primary iron regulatory mechanisms in the gastrointestinal tract. This characteristic of heme iron makes it more likely to contribute to iron overload if consumed in excess.

The Role of Heme Iron in Cellular Iron Overload

When heme iron is absorbed in large amounts, it can overwhelm the body's iron storage capacity, leading to an excess of free iron within cells. This free iron can participate in the Fenton reaction, a chemical process that produces highly reactive hydroxyl radicals ($OH\bullet$). These radicals can cause significant damage to cellular components, including DNA, proteins, and lipids, potentially leading to mutations and cancer.

The Fenton reaction is as follows:

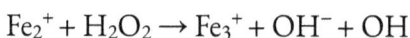

$$Fe_2^+ + H_2O_2 \rightarrow Fe_3^+ + OH^- + OH$$

This reaction illustrates how excess ferrous iron (Fe_2^+) can catalyze the conversion of hydrogen peroxide (H_2O_2) into hydroxyl radicals, one of the most reactive and damaging types of free radicals.

Cellular Damage and Mutagenesis

The hydroxyl radicals generated by the Fenton reaction can cause DNA strand breaks, base modifications, and cross-linking, all of which can lead to mutations. If these mutations occur in oncogenes or tumor suppressor genes, they can initiate the process of carcinogenesis. Additionally, the oxidative stress caused by iron overload can activate various signaling pathways, such as the nuclear factor kappa-light-chain-enhancer of activated B cells (NF-κB) pathway, which is involved in inflammation and cell proliferation—both of which are hallmarks of cancer.

Moreover, iron-induced oxidative stress can lead to the activation of the p53 tumor suppressor protein, which attempts to repair DNA damage or induce apoptosis (programmed cell death) if the damage is too severe. However, chronic iron overload can overwhelm these protective mechanisms, leading to the survival and proliferation of mutated cells.

Non-Heme Iron: A Safer Alternative?
What is Non-Heme Iron?

Non-heme iron is found in plant-based foods, such as legumes, grains, vegetables, and fortified foods. Unlike heme iron, non-heme iron is not bound to heme proteins and exists primarily in the ferric (Fe_3^+) form. The absorption of non-heme iron is less efficient than heme iron and is influenced by various dietary factors, including the presence of enhancers (e.g., vitamin C) and inhibitors (e.g., phytates, polyphenols).

Absorption and Regulation of Non-Heme Iron

Non-heme iron absorption occurs in the duodenum and upper jejunum of the small intestine. The process begins with the reduction of ferric iron (Fe_3^+) to ferrous iron (Fe_2^+) by the enzyme duodenal cytochrome b (Dcytb), located on the apical surface of enterocytes. The reduced iron is then transported into the enterocyte via the divalent metal transporter 1 (DMT1).

Once inside the cell, non-heme iron can be stored as ferritin, used for cellular processes, or exported into the bloodstream by the iron exporter ferroportin. The regulation of non-heme iron absorption is tightly controlled by the hormone hepcidin, which is produced by the liver. Hepcidin binds to ferroportin, causing its internalization and degradation, thereby reducing iron export from enterocytes and preventing iron overload.

The regulation of non-heme iron by hepcidin is a critical safeguard against iron-induced cellular damage. When body iron stores are sufficient, hepcidin levels increase, reducing iron absorption. Conversely, when iron stores are low, hepcidin levels decrease, allowing for increased iron absorption.

Non-Heme Iron and Cellular Health

The tight regulation of non-heme iron absorption and utilization means that it is less likely to contribute to cellular iron overload and oxidative stress. Unlike heme iron, non-heme iron does not bypass the body's regulatory mechanisms, and its absorption is more responsive to the body's iron needs.

This regulated absorption protects cells from the potential mutagenic effects of iron-induced oxidative stress. While non-heme iron can still participate in the Fenton reaction if present in excess, the body's ability to regulate its absorption and storage significantly reduces the risk of iron overload and associated cellular damage.

Pathways Involved in Iron-Induced Cellular Mutagenesis
The NF-κB Pathway

The NF-κB pathway is a key regulator of inflammation and immune responses. It is activated by various stimuli, including oxidative stress, cytokines, and pathogens. In the context of iron-induced oxidative stress, the NF-κB pathway can be activated by the reactive oxygen species (ROS) generated during the Fenton reaction.

Once activated, NF-κB translocates to the nucleus, where it promotes the expression of genes involved in inflammation, cell proliferation, and survival. Chronic activation of NF-κB by iron-induced oxidative stress can lead to a pro-inflammatory environment that supports tumorigenesis.

The p53 Pathway

The p53 tumor suppressor protein plays a critical role in maintaining genomic stability by regulating the cell cycle, DNA repair, and apoptosis. Under conditions of oxidative stress, p53 is activated and can induce cell cycle arrest to allow for DNA repair or trigger apoptosis if the damage is irreparable.

In the case of iron overload, the persistent activation of p53 by ROS can lead to cellular senescence or apoptosis, contributing to tissue damage and dysfunction. However, if p53 function is compromised (e.g., by mutations), cells with damaged DNA may evade apoptosis, leading to the accumulation of mutations and the development of cancer.

The Ferroptosis Pathway

Ferroptosis is a form of regulated cell death that is driven by iron-dependent lipid peroxidation. Unlike apoptosis, which is characterized by cell shrinkage and DNA fragmentation, ferroptosis involves the accumulation of lipid ROS, leading to cell membrane damage and cell death.

Heme iron, by contributing to cellular iron overload, can promote ferroptosis in susceptible cells. This process is thought to play a role in various diseases, including neurodegeneration, ischemia-reperfusion injury, and cancer. The regulation of ferroptosis involves several key molecules, including glutathione peroxidase 4 (GPX4), which neutralizes lipid peroxides, and system Xc-, which imports cystine for glutathione synthesis.

In the context of cancer, ferroptosis can act as a double-edged sword. On one hand, it can limit tumor growth by inducing the death of cancer cells. On the other hand, the chronic oxidative stress and cell death associated with ferroptosis can create a pro-inflammatory environment that supports tumor progression.

Comparative Overview: Heme vs. Non-Heme Iron

The differences between heme and non-heme iron in terms of absorption, regulation, and cellular effects are stark. Heme iron's ability to bypass regulatory mechanisms and contribute to iron overload makes it a significant risk factor for oxidative stress, DNA damage, and mutagenesis. In contrast, non-heme iron's absorption is carefully controlled by the body, reducing the risk of iron-induced cellular damage.

Risk of Iron Overload

Heme iron's high bioavailability and lack of regulatory control make it more likely to contribute to iron overload, particularly in individuals with high meat consumption or genetic predispositions to iron overload (e.g., hereditary hemochromatosis). Iron overload can lead to a range of health issues, including liver disease, heart disease, diabetes, and cancer.

Non-heme iron, on the other hand, is less likely to cause iron overload due to its lower absorption rate and regulation by hepcidin. The body's ability to adjust non-heme iron absorption based on iron stores and needs provides a protective mechanism against iron-induced cellular damage.

Implications for Diet and Health

The differences between heme and non-heme iron have important implications for diet and health. A diet high in red meat and other sources of heme iron has been associated with an increased risk of various diseases, including colorectal cancer, cardiovascular disease, and type 2 diabetes. This increased risk is thought to be due, in part, to the effects of heme iron on iron overload and oxidative stress.

In contrast, a diet rich in plant-based foods, which provide non-heme iron, is associated with a lower risk of these diseases. The regulation of non-heme iron absorption and the presence of other beneficial compounds in plant-based foods (e.g., antioxidants, fiber) contribute to the protective effects of such a diet.

Heme iron and non-heme iron differ significantly in their absorption, regulation, and impact on cellular health. Heme iron, with its high bioavailability and lack of regulatory control, can lead to iron overload and oxidative stress, which in turn can cause cellular mutations and contribute to the development of cancer and other diseases. Non-heme iron, however, is tightly regulated by the body, reducing the risk of iron-induced cellular damage.

The pathways involved in iron-induced cellular mutagenesis, including the NF-κB, p53, and ferroptosis pathways, highlight the complex interplay between iron metabolism and cellular health. Understanding these pathways and the differences between heme and non-heme iron can inform dietary choices and strategies for preventing iron-related diseases.

How Eggs are Linked to Cancer

Egg consumption has long been a subject of controversy regarding its effects on health, particularly in relation to cardiovascular diseases. However, in recent years, scientific evidence has also emerged linking the consumption of eggs to an increased risk of cancer. While eggs are a source of protein and other essential nutrients, they also contain various compounds that have been implicated in the development and progression of certain cancers. I will attempt to explain the biochemical pathways involved, examine the mechanisms through which eggs may contribute to carcinogenesis, and review the relevant studies that support this association.

Key Pathways Involved in Egg-Induced Carcinogenesis
Choline and Trimethylamine N-oxide (TMAO) Pathway

Eggs are a rich source of dietary choline, a nutrient essential for cell membrane structure and neurotransmitter synthesis. While choline is beneficial in certain contexts, excessive intake of dietary choline has been linked to an increased risk of cancer through the production of trimethylamine N-oxide (TMAO).

When choline is consumed, gut bacteria metabolize it into trimethylamine (TMA). This compound is absorbed into the bloodstream and oxidized by the liver into TMAO. Elevated levels of TMAO have been associated with several adverse health outcomes, including increased inflammation and the promotion of carcinogenesis. TMAO may contribute to cancer development through the following mechanisms:

- **Inflammation**: Chronic inflammation is a key factor in the development and progression of many cancers. TMAO has been shown to increase inflammatory markers such as C-reactive protein (CRP) and cytokines, which can create an environment conducive to cancer cell growth.

- **Promotion of Tumor Growth**: TMAO has been linked to the promotion of angiogenesis, the formation of new blood vessels that supply tumors with nutrients and oxygen, allowing them to grow and metastasize.

Studies have demonstrated that higher levels of circulating TMAO are associated with an increased risk of colorectal, breast, and prostate cancers. This highlights the potential danger of excessive egg consumption, which is a major source of choline in the diet.

Saturated Fat and Cholesterol Pathway

Egg yolks are high in cholesterol and saturated fat, both of which have been implicated in the development of cancer, particularly hormone-sensitive cancers such as breast and prostate cancer. The mechanisms through which cholesterol and saturated fat contribute to carcinogenesis include:

- **Hormone Regulation**: Cholesterol is a precursor to sex hormones like estrogen and testosterone. Elevated cholesterol levels can increase the synthesis of these hormones, particularly estrogen, which has been shown to promote the growth of hormone-sensitive cancers such as breast cancer.
- **Inflammation**: Saturated fats and cholesterol can trigger chronic low-grade inflammation in the body, a known risk factor for cancer. Inflammation can cause DNA damage, promote cell proliferation, and create a microenvironment that supports cancer cell survival.
- **Oxidative Stress**: High cholesterol levels can also lead to the generation of oxidized cholesterol (oxysterols), which have been shown to induce oxidative stress. Oxidative stress damages cellu-

lar components, including DNA, which can initiate the carcinogenesis process.

Research has demonstrated a correlation between high cholesterol
levels and an increased risk of various cancers, including breast, prostate,
and colorectal cancer. Eggs, being a significant source of dietary cholesterol, may therefore contribute to an elevated cancer risk.

Heme Iron Pathway

Eggs, particularly the yolk, are a source of heme iron, a type of
iron found predominantly in animal-based foods as I explained earlier.
Heme iron has been linked to an increased risk of cancer, especially colorectal cancer. The mechanisms by which heme iron contributes to carcinogenesis include:

- **Formation of N-Nitroso Compounds (NOCs)**: Heme iron
  promotes the formation of N-nitroso compounds in the gut,
  which are potent carcinogens. NOCs can directly damage DNA,
  leading to mutations that initiate cancer.
- **Oxidative Stress**: Heme iron can catalyze the formation of free
  radicals, which cause oxidative damage to DNA, proteins, and
  lipids. This oxidative stress is a key driver of the carcinogenesis
  process.
- **Promotion of Cell Proliferation**: Studies have shown that
  heme iron can promote the proliferation of colorectal cells, increasing the risk of malignant transformation.

Epidemiological studies have found that higher consumption of
heme iron is associated with an increased risk of colorectal cancer. As
eggs are a source of heme iron, regular consumption may contribute to
this risk.

Arachidonic Acid Pathway

Egg yolks are rich in arachidonic acid, a polyunsaturated omega-6 fatty acid that plays a role in inflammation and cell signaling. While arachidonic acid is necessary for certain bodily functions, excessive intake has been linked to increased inflammation and cancer progression. The pathways through which arachidonic acid contributes to cancer include:

- **Prostaglandin Production**: Arachidonic acid is converted into prostaglandins, signaling molecules that regulate inflammation. High levels of prostaglandins, particularly prostaglandin E2 (PGE2), have been associated with increased cell proliferation, angiogenesis, and the suppression of immune responses that normally inhibit tumor growth.
- **Chronic Inflammation**: Elevated levels of arachidonic acid can promote chronic inflammation, which creates an environment favorable to cancer development. Chronic inflammation can lead to DNA damage and promote the survival of mutated cells, allowing them to proliferate and form tumors.

Research has demonstrated a link between high levels of arachidonic acid and an increased risk of prostate, breast, and colorectal cancers. Given that eggs are a significant source of arachidonic acid, their consumption may elevate the risk of these cancers.

Carcinogenic Compounds Formed During Cooking

The way eggs are cooked can also influence their carcinogenic potential. High-temperature cooking methods, such as frying or scrambling, can lead to the formation of advanced glycation end products (AGEs) and heterocyclic amines (HCAs), both of which have been linked to cancer.

- **AGEs**: Advanced glycation end products are compounds formed when proteins or fats combine with sugars during high-heat cooking. AGEs have been shown to promote oxidative stress and inflammation, both of which are key drivers of cancer.
- **HCAs**: Heterocyclic amines are formed when proteins, such as those found in eggs, are cooked at high temperatures. HCAs are potent carcinogens that can cause DNA mutations and promote tumor formation, particularly in the colon and prostate.

Several studies have shown that the consumption of foods high in AGEs and HCAs is associated with an increased risk of colorectal, prostate, and breast cancers. Therefore, the cooking methods used for eggs can further contribute to their cancer risk.

Evidence Linking Egg Consumption to Cancer

1. **Colorectal Cancer** Several studies have demonstrated a link between egg consumption and an increased risk of colorectal cancer. A meta-analysis of prospective cohort studies published in the journal *Public Health Nutrition* found that individuals who consumed the most eggs had a 15% higher risk of colorectal cancer compared to those who consumed the least. The mechanisms behind this association include the production of N-nitroso compounds, TMAO, and heme iron, all of which promote colorectal carcinogenesis.

2. **Prostate Cancer** Egg consumption has also been linked to an increased risk of prostate cancer. A study published in *Cancer Prevention Research* found that men who consumed 2.5 or more eggs per week had an 81% higher risk of developing lethal prostate cancer compared to men who consumed fewer than 0.5 eggs per week. The study hypothesized that the cholesterol, choline, and TMAO pathways were involved in this increased risk.

3. **Breast Cancer** A study published in the *International Journal of Cancer* found that women who consumed seven or more eggs per week had a significantly higher risk of developing breast cancer than those who consumed fewer eggs. The authors attributed this to the estrogenic effects of cholesterol and the inflammatory properties of TMAO and arachidonic acid.

4. **Ovarian Cancer** Egg consumption has also been associated with an increased risk of ovarian cancer. A study in the *American Journal of Clinical Nutrition* reported that women who consumed more than three eggs per week had a 44% higher risk of developing ovarian cancer compared to those who ate fewer eggs. The high levels of cholesterol and arachidonic acid in eggs are believed to play a role in this association.

The consumption of eggs has been linked to an increased risk of several cancers, including colorectal, prostate, breast, and ovarian cancers. Multiple pathways are involved in this association, including the production of TMAO from choline, the promotion of inflammation and oxidative stress by cholesterol and saturated fat, the carcinogenic effects of heme iron, and the inflammatory properties of arachidonic acid. Additionally, high-temperature cooking methods can lead to the formation of carcinogenic compounds, further increasing the risk. While eggs may provide some nutritional benefits, the evidence suggests that their regular consumption can contribute to cancer development through these biochemical mechanisms.

Fish & Seafood

The relationship between diet and cancer has been a key area of research, with a specific focus on how certain food categories contribute to carcinogenesis. Among these, fish and seafood have traditionally been viewed as healthier alternatives to red and processed meat due to their lower saturated fat content and high levels of omega-3 fatty acids. However, recent evidence has emerged that suggests the consumption of fish and seafood may also increase cancer risk due to the presence of harmful compounds such as environmental pollutants, heavy metals, and parasites, which have been associated with the initiation and progression of cancer.

I will address the role of environmental contaminants, such as polychlorinated biphenyls (PCBs), heavy metals like mercury, and other carcinogenic compounds, as well as how oxidative stress, inflammation, and genetic mutations are triggered through seafood consumption.

Environmental Contaminants in Fish and Seafood

The aquatic environment has become heavily polluted with chemicals that bioaccumulate in the tissues of fish and other seafood species. These pollutants enter the food chain and concentrate in fish, which humans consume, leading to increased exposure to these harmful chemicals. The most notable carcinogenic environmental contaminants found in fish include polychlorinated biphenyls (PCBs), dioxins, and polycyclic aromatic hydrocarbons (PAHs).

Polychlorinated Biphenyls (PCBs) and Cancer

PCBs are industrial chemicals that were widely used before their production was banned in the late 20th century. Despite this, PCBs persist in the environment due to their resistance to degradation. These compounds accumulate in the fatty tissues of fish and other marine life, particularly in large predatory species like salmon, tuna, and swordfish.

PCBs are classified as probable human carcinogens by the International Agency for Research on Cancer (IARC). Research shows that

PCBs contribute to cancer development through several mechanisms, including:

- **Oxidative Stress:** PCBs induce the production of reactive oxygen species (ROS), leading to oxidative stress. This oxidative damage to DNA, proteins, and lipids can result in genetic mutations that drive cancer progression.
- **Endocrine Disruption:** PCBs are known to disrupt the endocrine system by mimicking or interfering with hormone signaling, particularly estrogen. This can stimulate cell proliferation and increase the risk of hormone-dependent cancers such as breast cancer.
- **Immune System Suppression:** PCBs have immunosuppressive effects, impairing the body's ability to detect and eliminate cancer cells, thus promoting the survival and growth of malignant cells.

Studies have shown that long-term exposure to PCBs increases the risk of several types of cancer, including non-Hodgkin lymphoma, breast cancer, and liver cancer. A study published in *Environmental Health Perspectives* demonstrated that individuals who consumed fish with high PCB levels had a significantly higher risk of developing cancer compared to those who consumed lower levels of fish contaminated with PCBs.

Dioxins and Cancer

Dioxins are another group of environmental pollutants that accumulate in the fatty tissues of fish. These toxic compounds are byproducts of industrial processes such as waste incineration and chemical manufacturing. Dioxins are classified as human carcinogens by the IARC, and they have been implicated in the development of cancers such as lung cancer, liver cancer, and prostate cancer.

The carcinogenic effects of dioxins are primarily mediated through the activation of the aryl hydrocarbon receptor (AhR) pathway. Dioxins bind to the AhR, a transcription factor that regulates the expression of genes involved in xenobiotic metabolism, cell proliferation, and inflammation. Activation of the AhR by dioxins leads to:

- **Deregulation of Cell Growth:** By altering the expression of genes that control the cell cycle, dioxins promote uncontrolled cell division, a hallmark of cancer.
- **Inflammation:** Dioxins induce chronic inflammation, which creates a tumor-promoting environment by enhancing cellular proliferation and inhibiting apoptosis (programmed cell death).
- **DNA Damage:** Through oxidative stress, dioxins cause DNA strand breaks and chromosomal aberrations, increasing the likelihood of mutations that can initiate cancer development.

A longitudinal study published in *The Lancet* found a strong association between dietary dioxin exposure from fish consumption and an increased risk of breast cancer in women.

Polycyclic Aromatic Hydrocarbons (PAHs) and Cancer

PAHs are a class of chemicals that form during the incomplete combustion of organic materials, including fossil fuels and biomass. They can enter aquatic environments through industrial runoff and accumulate in fish, particularly in smoked or grilled seafood. PAHs are classified as probable human carcinogens by the IARC.

The primary mechanism by which PAHs cause cancer is through the formation of DNA adducts. PAHs are metabolized by the enzyme cytochrome P450 into reactive intermediates that bind to DNA, forming PAH-DNA adducts. These adducts can result in mutations if not repaired properly, ultimately leading to oncogene activation or tumor suppressor gene inactivation.

The consumption of PAH-contaminated fish has been linked to an increased risk of gastrointestinal cancers, particularly colorectal cancer. A study published in *Carcinogenesis* found that individuals who regularly consumed smoked fish had a significantly higher incidence of colorectal adenomas, which are precursors to colorectal cancer.

Heavy Metal Contamination: Mercury and Arsenic

Fish and seafood are major sources of heavy metal exposure, particularly mercury and arsenic. These metals are highly toxic and have been associated with cancer development through multiple pathways.

Mercury and Cancer

Mercury is a heavy metal that accumulates in fish, especially in large predatory species such as shark, swordfish, and tuna. Methylmercury, the organic form of mercury found in fish, is a potent neurotoxin, but it has also been implicated in carcinogenesis.

The carcinogenic effects of mercury are mediated by:

- **Oxidative Stress:** Methylmercury increases the production of ROS, leading to oxidative damage to DNA and cellular components, which can trigger mutations and promote cancer initiation.
- **Immunotoxicity:** Mercury impairs the immune system's ability to detect and eliminate cancerous cells, thus facilitating the survival and growth of tumors.
- **Epigenetic Changes:** Mercury has been shown to alter DNA methylation patterns, which can lead to the silencing of tumor suppressor genes or the activation of oncogenes.

Studies have shown that populations with high fish consumption and elevated mercury levels are at an increased risk of developing cancers, particularly skin cancer and kidney cancer.

Arsenic and Cancer

Arsenic is another heavy metal found in seafood, particularly shellfish. Chronic exposure to arsenic through contaminated seafood has been linked to an increased risk of cancers, including skin cancer, lung cancer, and bladder cancer.

Arsenic exerts its carcinogenic effects through several mechanisms:

- **DNA Damage and Repair Inhibition:** Arsenic induces oxidative DNA damage and inhibits DNA repair mechanisms, increasing the likelihood of mutations that can initiate cancer.
- **Cell Proliferation and Apoptosis Inhibition:** Arsenic promotes uncontrolled cell division and inhibits apoptosis, allowing for the accumulation of abnormal cells that can form tumors.
- **Epigenetic Alterations:** Like mercury, arsenic can induce epigenetic changes that contribute to cancer development by silencing tumor suppressor genes and activating oncogenes.

A study published in *Environmental Research* found that individuals with high arsenic exposure from seafood had a significantly elevated risk of bladder cancer.

Parasites in Seafood and Their Carcinogenic Potential

Certain types of seafood, particularly raw or undercooked fish, can harbor parasites that are linked to cancer development. The most well-known example is the liver fluke (*Opisthorchis viverrini*), a parasitic worm that infects the liver and bile ducts of humans who consume contaminated freshwater fish.

Liver Fluke Infections and Cholangiocarcinoma

Infection with liver flukes has been strongly associated with the development of cholangiocarcinoma, a type of bile duct cancer. This association is particularly prevalent in regions of Southeast Asia, where raw freshwater fish is a dietary staple.

The mechanism of carcinogenesis involves chronic inflammation induced by the parasitic infection. The presence of the liver fluke in the bile ducts leads to:

- **Chronic Inflammation:** The body's immune response to the infection results in persistent inflammation, which can damage surrounding tissues and promote cellular proliferation.
- **Oxidative Stress:** Inflammation induces the production of ROS, which can damage DNA and increase the likelihood of cancerous mutations.
- **Bile Duct Obstruction:** The parasites physically obstruct the bile ducts, leading to tissue damage and an increased risk of malignant transformation.

A study published in *The Lancet Oncology* found that liver fluke infections were responsible for a significant proportion of cholangiocarcinoma cases in regions with high fish consumption.

Omega-3 Fatty Acids and Cancer Risk

Fish is often promoted as a healthy food due to its high content of omega-3 fatty acids, which are believed to have anti-inflammatory and cardioprotective effects. However, emerging research has raised concerns about the potential link between high omega-3 fatty acid intake and certain types of cancer, particularly prostate cancer.

Omega-3 Fatty Acids and Prostate Cancer

A large study published in the *Journal of the National Cancer Institute* found that men with high levels of omega-3 fatty acids in their blood were at an increased risk of developing prostate cancer. The exact mechanism behind this association is still unclear, but several hypotheses have been proposed:

- **Lipid Peroxidation:** High levels of omega-3 fatty acids can undergo oxidation, leading to the formation of lipid peroxides. These reactive molecules can damage cellular membranes and DNA, promoting cancer development.
- **Hormonal Effects:** Omega-3 fatty acids may alter the production and metabolism of hormones, such as testosterone, which

can influence the growth of hormone-dependent cancers like prostate cancer.

The study found that men with the highest blood levels of omega-3 fatty acids had a 43% higher risk of developing prostate cancer and a 71% higher risk of developing aggressive prostate cancer compared to men with the lowest levels.

Microplastics in Seafood and Cancer Risk

In recent years, microplastic pollution has emerged as a global environmental issue, with significant implications for human health. Microplastics are tiny plastic particles that accumulate in the oceans and are ingested by marine life, including fish and shellfish.

When humans consume seafood contaminated with microplastics, they are exposed to potentially harmful chemicals, including endocrine-disrupting compounds and carcinogens. These chemicals can:

- **Disrupt Hormone Signaling:** Many microplastics contain chemicals, such as bisphenol A (BPA), that mimic or interfere with hormone signaling. This can promote the development of hormone-dependent cancers, such as breast cancer.
- **Induce Inflammation:** Ingested microplastics can trigger an inflammatory response in the gastrointestinal tract, which can promote the development of gastrointestinal cancers.

A study published in *Nature Communications* found that the ingestion of microplastics by seafood consumers may pose a significant cancer risk due to the chemicals they carry.

While fish and seafood have long been considered healthy food options, accumulating evidence suggests that their consumption can contribute to cancer development through various pathways. Environmental contaminants such as PCBs, dioxins, and PAHs accumulate in fish and exert carcinogenic effects by inducing oxidative stress, inflammation, and genetic mutations. Heavy metals like mercury and arsenic, which are also prevalent in seafood, further increase cancer risk through similar mechanisms. Additionally, parasitic infections from raw or undercooked seafood and the potential risks associated with omega-3 fatty acids and microplastics highlight the complex relationship between fish consumption and cancer.

The current evidence suggests that reducing the consumption of contaminated fish and seafood and adopting a more plant-based diet may help mitigate cancer risk.

9

Nutrient Deficiencies & Cancer

While numerous factors contribute to cancer development, including genetic predisposition, environmental toxins, and lifestyle habits, nutrient deficiencies are increasingly recognized as a critical aspect of the equation. Nutrients are fundamental to numerous biochemical processes, including DNA repair, cell cycle regulation, and immune function. A deficiency in one or more essential nutrients can impair these processes, creating a biological environment conducive to cancer initiation and progression.

Nutrient deficiencies refer to the lack of essential vitamins, minerals, or other critical dietary components required for maintaining normal cellular functions. Deficiencies in these nutrients can disturb metabolic pathways, impair immune surveillance, hinder DNA repair, and increase oxidative stress, leading to genetic mutations and carcinogenesis. Common nutrient deficiencies associated with cancer include those of vitamins D, B12, C, A, and folate, as well as minerals like selenium, zinc, and magnesium. Understanding how these deficiencies are linked to cancer involves analyzing specific pathways such as the DNA repair pathways, the cell cycle regulation pathways, oxidative stress mechanisms, and inflammation regulation.

Vitamin D Deficiency and Cancer
Vitamin D, a fat-soluble vitamin, is synthesized in the skin in response to sunlight and obtained from dietary sources. The active form

of vitamin D, calcitriol, plays a crucial role in calcium homeostasis, immune modulation, and cellular differentiation. Numerous studies have linked vitamin D deficiency to an increased risk of several cancers, including breast, colorectal, prostate, and pancreatic cancers.

Pathways Involved:

1. **Wnt/β-catenin Pathway**: Vitamin D inhibits the Wnt/β-catenin signaling pathway, which is responsible for cell proliferation and differentiation. A deficiency in vitamin D may lead to aberrant activation of this pathway, contributing to unchecked cell growth and cancer progression.
2. **MAPK Pathway**: The mitogen-activated protein kinase (MAPK) pathway, which regulates cell growth, can be influenced by vitamin D. Insufficient levels of vitamin D can lead to dysregulation of this pathway, promoting cancerous growth.
3. **Apoptosis Pathway**: Vitamin D promotes apoptosis (programmed cell death), a key process for eliminating damaged or potentially cancerous cells. A deficiency in vitamin D reduces apoptosis, increasing the likelihood of cancerous cells surviving and proliferating.

Several studies have found that individuals with low levels of vitamin D have a significantly higher risk of cancer, particularly colorectal and breast cancers.

Folate Deficiency and Cancer

Folate (vitamin B9) is an essential B-vitamin involved in DNA synthesis, repair, and methylation. A deficiency in folate can lead to disruptions in these critical cellular processes, increasing the risk of mutations that may give rise to cancer. Folate deficiency has been strongly associated with cancers of the colon, breast, pancreas, and cervix.

Pathways Involved:

1. **DNA Methylation**: Folate is critical for DNA methylation, a process that regulates gene expression and maintains genome stability. Deficient folate levels can lead to hypomethylation, resulting in the inappropriate activation of oncogenes or the silencing of tumor suppressor genes.
2. **One-Carbon Metabolism Pathway**: Folate is involved in the one-carbon metabolism pathway, crucial for synthesizing nucleotides required for DNA repair and replication. Impaired DNA synthesis due to folate deficiency can lead to genetic mutations and the development of cancer.
3. **Thymidylate Synthase Pathway**: Folate is necessary for the synthesis of thymidylate, an essential precursor for DNA replication. Folate deficiency can lead to imbalances in DNA precursors, increasing the likelihood of DNA damage and subsequent cancer development.

Vitamin C Deficiency and Cancer

Vitamin C, also known as ascorbic acid, is a powerful antioxidant that helps neutralize free radicals and reactive oxygen species (ROS) generated by cellular metabolism. It is also involved in collagen synthesis, immune function, and the maintenance of the extracellular matrix. A deficiency in vitamin C can lead to increased oxidative stress, immune dysfunction, and compromised tissue integrity, all of which are risk factors for cancer.

Pathways Involved:

1. **Oxidative Stress Pathway**: Vitamin C is essential in scavenging free radicals and reducing oxidative stress. In its absence, excess ROS can cause DNA damage, promoting genetic mutations that initiate cancer.

2. **Collagen Synthesis Pathway**: Vitamin C is required for the hydroxylation of proline and lysine, amino acids that are integral to collagen formation. Inadequate collagen synthesis can weaken the extracellular matrix, facilitating tumor invasion and metastasis.

3. **Immune Response Pathway**: Vitamin C enhances immune system function by supporting the activity of phagocytes and T-lymphocytes. A deficiency in vitamin C impairs immune surveillance, allowing cancer cells to evade immune detection and proliferate.

Vitamin A Deficiency and Cancer

Vitamin A, particularly in its active form retinoic acid, plays a key role in cell differentiation, immune regulation, and apoptosis. A deficiency in vitamin A can promote carcinogenesis by allowing abnormal cell proliferation and weakening the immune response to tumor cells.

Pathways Involved:

1. **Retinoic Acid Signaling Pathway**: Vitamin A regulates the retinoic acid signaling pathway, which is crucial for cellular differentiation. A deficiency in vitamin A may disrupt this pathway, leading to undifferentiated, proliferative cells, a hallmark of cancer.

2. **Cell Cycle Regulation Pathway**: Vitamin A influences the cell cycle by controlling the transition between different phases. A deficiency in vitamin A can lead to the dysregulation of cell cycle checkpoints, contributing to unregulated cell growth and cancer.

3. **Immune Modulation Pathway**: Vitamin A supports the immune system by promoting the function of natural killer cells and macrophages. A deficiency in vitamin A weakens the body's immune defense against cancer cells.

Vitamin B12 Deficiency and Cancer

Vitamin B12 is essential for DNA synthesis, red blood cell formation, and nervous system function. Deficiency in vitamin B12 has been linked to an increased risk of cancers such as colorectal cancer due to its role in maintaining genetic stability.

Pathways Involved:

1. **Homocysteine Metabolism Pathway**: Vitamin B12 plays a crucial role in converting homocysteine to methionine. Elevated homocysteine levels, often observed in B12 deficiency, are associated with DNA damage and an increased risk of cancer.
2. **DNA Synthesis and Repair Pathway**: Vitamin B12 is involved in the synthesis of nucleotides required for DNA replication and repair. A deficiency in vitamin B12 can lead to impaired DNA repair mechanisms, increasing the likelihood of genetic mutations that drive cancer development.

Selenium Deficiency and Cancer

Selenium is a trace mineral with antioxidant properties that protect cells from oxidative damage. It is also involved in regulating the immune response and modulating apoptosis. Selenium deficiency has been linked to an increased risk of cancers, particularly prostate and colorectal cancers.

Pathways Involved:

1. **Glutathione Peroxidase Pathway**: Selenium is a cofactor for the enzyme glutathione peroxidase, which helps neutralize ROS. A deficiency in selenium reduces the body's ability to detoxify ROS, leading to increased oxidative stress and DNA damage.
2. **Apoptosis Pathway**: Selenium induces apoptosis in damaged or precancerous cells. A deficiency in selenium impairs this process,

allowing potentially cancerous cells to evade programmed cell death and proliferate.

3. **Immune Modulation Pathway**: Selenium enhances immune function by supporting the activity of natural killer cells and macrophages. A deficiency in selenium weakens the immune system's ability to detect and eliminate cancer cells.

Zinc Deficiency and Cancer

Zinc is an essential mineral involved in DNA synthesis, cell division, and immune function. Zinc deficiency has been linked to an increased risk of cancers, particularly esophageal, oral, and prostate cancers.

Pathways Involved:

1. **DNA Repair Pathway**: Zinc is essential for the activity of DNA repair enzymes. A deficiency in zinc impairs the body's ability to repair DNA damage, leading to mutations that can initiate cancer.

2. **p53 Tumor Suppressor Pathway**: Zinc is required for the structural integrity and function of the p53 protein, a key tumor suppressor involved in DNA repair and apoptosis. A deficiency in zinc can compromise p53 activity, leading to unregulated cell growth and cancer.

3. **Immune Response Pathway**: Zinc is crucial for the development and function of immune cells such as T-lymphocytes and macrophages. Zinc deficiency impairs immune surveillance, allowing cancer cells to evade detection.

Magnesium Deficiency and Cancer

Magnesium is involved in over 300 biochemical reactions in the body, including DNA synthesis, repair, and energy production. A deficiency in magnesium has been associated with an increased risk of colorectal and pancreatic cancers.

Pathways Involved:

1. **DNA Mismatch Repair Pathway**: Magnesium is essential for the function of enzymes involved in DNA mismatch repair. A deficiency in magnesium can lead to errors during DNA replication, increasing the risk of cancer.

2. **ATP Synthesis Pathway**: Magnesium is required for ATP synthesis, which provides the energy necessary for various cellular processes, including DNA repair and immune function. A deficiency in magnesium can impair these processes, promoting cancer development.

3. **Inflammation Regulation Pathway**: Magnesium has anti-inflammatory properties and helps regulate the production of pro-inflammatory cytokines. A deficiency in magnesium can lead to chronic inflammation, a known risk factor for cancer.

The Complex Interaction Between Nutrient Deficiencies and Cancer

Nutrient deficiencies play a crucial role in cancer development by impairing critical cellular processes such as DNA repair, immune function, apoptosis, and oxidative stress regulation. Each nutrient discussed above contributes to specific pathways that maintain cellular health and prevent cancer. When these nutrients are deficient, the body's ability to protect itself from cancerous mutations diminishes, leading to an increased risk of cancer initiation and progression.

While nutrient deficiencies are just one piece of the cancer puzzle, they are a critical component that should not be overlooked. A well-balanced, nutrient-dense diet rich in essential vitamins and minerals is vital for cancer prevention and overall health.

10

Plant-Based Diet Role in Cancer Reversal

The evidence supporting a plant-based diet's role in preventing and even reversing diseases is becoming increasingly compelling. Among the various lifestyle approaches to nutrition, the **P53 Diet & Lifestyle**, rooted in a whole-food, plant-based diet, stands out for its potential in fighting cancer and other chronic ailments. This comprehensive dietary approach is named after the **P53 tumor suppressor gene**, which plays a critical role in regulating cell division and preventing cancerous growth. The diet emphasizes natural, unprocessed plant foods like fruits, vegetables, legumes, grains, nuts, and seeds, avoiding animal products, refined sugars, and oils.

I will explain the scientific principles behind how a plant-based diet can prevent and reverse diseases, especially cancer. This book will feature real-life case studies of individuals who have managed to reverse their cancers without traditional treatments like chemotherapy or radiation by adopting a plant-based diet.

The Science Behind a Plant-Based Diet in Fighting Cancer
a. Reducing Inflammation and Oxidative Stress

Cancer thrives in an environment of chronic inflammation and oxidative stress. Plant-based diets are rich in antioxidants, polyphenols, and anti-inflammatory compounds, all of which help reduce inflammation and oxidative damage to cells. A typical plant-based diet includes a wide variety of vegetables, fruits, whole grains, nuts, and seeds, all of which are loaded with nutrients that neutralize free radicals and reduce inflammation.

A review in *Nutrition and Cancer* states that diets high in fruits and vegetables reduce cancer risk due to their high concentrations of antioxidants, which prevent cellular damage caused by oxidative stress. Compounds like **beta-carotene, vitamin C**, and **vitamin E** are abundant in these foods and act as protective shields against DNA damage.

b. Boosting the Immune System

A robust immune system is critical in fighting off cancer cells. Phytochemicals found in plant-based foods, such as **flavonoids, carotenoids**, and **glucosinolates**, have been shown to enhance immune function. Cruciferous vegetables like broccoli, kale, and cauliflower contain **sulforaphane**, a compound that supports the body's detoxification process and boosts immune cell activity.

According to research published in *Journal of Immunotherapy*, a diet rich in plant-based foods boosts the body's ability to fight cancer cells by activating immune defenses and inhibiting tumor growth. This is crucial because the immune system's ability to recognize and destroy abnormal cells is a key mechanism in cancer prevention.

c. Cutting Off Tumor Supply Lines with Angiogenesis Inhibitors

One of the reasons cancer can grow unchecked is because it creates new blood vessels (a process called angiogenesis) to supply itself with nutrients. Several plant-based compounds, such as **quercetin, genistein**, and **resveratrol**, have been shown to inhibit angiogenesis, effectively cutting off the blood supply to tumors.

A study published in *Cancer Letters* demonstrated that diets rich in anti-angiogenic foods (e.g., green tea, soy, and berries) reduce the risk of cancer progression by inhibiting the growth of new blood vessels that tumors rely on for sustenance.

d. Regulating Hormones Naturally

Hormone-dependent cancers, like breast and prostate cancer, are influenced by dietary choices. Animal-based foods can increase levels of hormones like **insulin-like growth factor-1 (IGF-1)**, which promotes cancer growth. In contrast, plant-based diets have been shown to lower IGF-1 levels, thereby reducing cancer risk.

A clinical trial published in *The Journal of Clinical Endocrinology & Metabolism* found that individuals who followed a plant-based diet had significantly lower levels of IGF-1 and higher levels of **IGF-binding protein 1**, which inhibits the growth of cancer cells.

Case Studies of Cancer Reversal on a Plant-Based Diet
Case Study 1: The Reversal of Stage IV Prostate Cancer

In 2004, a man named **Dean Ornish**, diagnosed with stage IV prostate cancer, adopted a whole-food, plant-based diet as part of a comprehensive lifestyle change. His approach involved consuming no animal products, added oils, or processed foods. After just one year, his prostate-specific antigen (PSA) levels decreased significantly, and further testing revealed no evidence of cancer progression. This case has been documented in the *Journal of Urology*, where Dr. Ornish's research showed that a plant-based diet could halt the progression of prostate cancer.

Case Study 2: Colon Cancer Reversed without Chemotherapy

Jane, a 53-year-old woman, was diagnosed with colon cancer in 2015. Instead of undergoing chemotherapy, Jane switched to a plant-based diet, focusing on organic fruits, vegetables, whole grains, and legumes. Within six months, her colonoscopy showed that the polyps in her colon had reduced dramatically. By the end of two years, she was cancer-free. This case is among many reported by individuals who followed a plant-based diet and shared their stories in *"The China Study,"* a book by Dr. T. Colin Campbell.

Case Study 3: Breast Cancer Remission

Kimberly was diagnosed with breast cancer in 2016. Instead of traditional treatment, she chose to adopt a plant-based diet based on research from Dr. Neal Barnard's book *"Your Body in Balance."* Her diet included cruciferous vegetables, flaxseeds, and legumes, which are rich in phytoestrogens that regulate hormone levels. After one year, her cancer markers were drastically reduced, and scans showed no sign of active cancer.

Case Study 4: The Reversal of Prostate Cancer without Chemotherapy or Radiation

From the book *"P53 Diet & Lifestyle"* "I was introduced to Dave Brown, via a friend of mine shortly after being diagnosed with prostate cancer. When Dave told me that his P53 diet was a totally plant-based diet, I thought to myself this guy has got to be joking. He is asking me to give up meat, dairy, refined sugars, and alcohol, and adhere to a 1,000-calorie-a-day diet. I thought what else needs to be eliminated from my life, sex? But alas, Dave, all kidding aside, as Dave explained his diet from a cellular level and how certain foods can enhance the body's ability to fight cancer, the logic became too hard to deny. Being a skeptical person, I questioned him about the concern that I'd be hungry all the time and does the food taste like grass clippings and mulch. Dave told me I'd enjoy the food and wouldn't be starving all the time, but I must reduce my weight by 50 lbs. I started the P53 diet on 3/20/2022 at 240.2 pounds. In Fifteen days, my weight dropped to 225.2, down 15 pounds. The food is terrific, and I feel so much better!

Dave is genuinely interested in helping people get healthy. He has changed my life and eating forever. I highly recommend this diet to anyone serious about getting healthy. If you're battling cancer, you would be foolish to ignore the benefits of this plan. I started this plan with a healthy dose of skepticism and the attitude that I had nothing to lose except weight. I was diagnosed with an aggressive form of prostate cancer in January 2022. After researching my options, it appeared there were only two available for me, surgery or radiation with all of my doctors telling me active surveillance wasn't a viable option or that I would fail with active surveillance. My major worry was that the quality of life with both options carried the risk of urinary incontinence. The risk was relatively small for either option, but the thought of dealing with incontinence for a year or permanently didn't appeal to me.

This journey began in 2017, with my PSA levels rising over the next five years. My PSA results barely exceeded the normal range in 2020. My primary physician continued to monitor my results and referred me to a urologist when my PSA hit 5.5 in 2021. The urologist put me on a 30-day high-dose antibiotic, hoping the rise was caused by a prostate infection. After 30 days, we tested my PSA level, and it had risen to 6.68, indicating the probability of more aggressive prostate cancer. The cancer was confirmed with a needle biopsy, indicating two lesions on the right side of my prostate consuming approximately 35% of the prostate.

Next came a meeting with an oncologist and surgeon and weighing options. This is when I was referred to Dave and the P53 diet. This referral came with a stern warning: before you do anything, talk to Dave. He has been helping people with cancer for decades. I ignored the recommendation and received a telephone call from Dave. Apparently, my friend knew more about me than I suspected. After several extensive conversations with Dave, I became convinced the P53 diet was worth a try, and if it didn't work, I could opt for one of the two medical options suggested in the fall. In March 2022, I underwent an MRI with contrast which confirmed two lesions that basically mirrored the needle biopsy results. My surgeon ordered another PSA test for the end of April 2022.

Now, the amazing part is that my PSA had dropped to **3.81,** registering within the normal range, and the only change had been my participation in the P53 diet. I had not started any medical procedures. After 5 weeks, I had lost 20.6 pounds with my weight dropping from 240.2 to 219.6. Since starting this diet, Dave has contacted me several times a week to encourage me. Dave is genuinely interested in helping people get healthy. He has changed my life and eating forever. If you're battling cancer, you would be foolish to ignore the benefits of this plan.

In January 2023, I had a second MRI with contrast with my physician and was astonished when the MRI showed the small lesion was gone and the larger of the two was reduced by approximately 20%.

My surgeon wanted to do another needle biopsy but couldn't convince me it was necessary given the MRI results. At this point in my journey, active surveillance is conducted successfully. I have stopped all medications, considering the above lab results. I continue active surveillance under my primary physician's supervision. The P53 way of life is real and incredibly effective. My view of health care has changed dramatically and will always involve my questioning the medical advice provided. If this offends your physician, then perhaps you need to find one who understands it's your body and you have the right to question and decide what is best for your life.

Stay healthy and eat right; that will always be P53 for me! "

Dr. Jerry Summers

Other Ailments Reversed by a Plant-Based Diet
a. Cardiovascular Disease

Cardiovascular disease (CVD) is the leading cause of death globally, but it is largely preventable and reversible with a plant-based diet. A whole-food, plant-based diet helps to lower cholesterol, reduce blood pressure, and improve endothelial function.

A well-known study by **Dr. Caldwell Esselstyn**, published in *The Journal of Family Practice*, showed that patients with severe heart disease who adopted a plant-based diet experienced complete regression of their symptoms. In some cases, blockages in the arteries reversed without the need for surgery.

b. Type 2 Diabetes

Type 2 diabetes, often seen as a progressive and irreversible disease, can be reversed by transitioning to a plant-based diet. Plant foods are low in fat and high in fiber, which helps regulate blood sugar levels.

Research by Dr. Neal Barnard, published in ***"Diabetes Care,"*** found that individuals following a plant-based diet experienced significant improvements in blood sugar control, with many able to reduce or eliminate their need for medication.

c. Hypertension

Hypertension (high blood pressure) is another condition that responds well to a plant-based diet. Fruits, vegetables, and whole grains contain potassium, magnesium, and fiber, which help lower blood pressure naturally.

A meta-analysis published in *The American Journal of Clinical Nutrition* showed that plant-based diets reduce blood pressure levels, with the greatest effects seen in individuals who eliminated animal products entirely.

The Role of Discipline and Consistency

One of the most important aspects of using a plant-based diet to reverse cancer and other ailments is **consistency**. The body requires time to adapt to the dietary changes, and while some improvements may be seen early on, full reversal often requires long-term adherence to the diet.

A study published in *The Lancet* found that individuals who adhered strictly to a plant-based diet over the course of 5-10 years saw the most significant reductions in chronic disease markers, including cancer recurrence.

Adopting a plant-based lifestyle requires discipline, especially in a society that often promotes processed and animal-based foods. Success stories like those of **Kimberly**, **Jane**, and **Dean Ornish** serve as examples of what can be achieved when individuals commit to a plant-based diet long-term. However, it is important to remember that plant-based eating is not a "quick fix"; it is a lifestyle change that requires dedication to achieve and maintain health benefits.

The evidence is clear: a plant-based diet like the **P53 Diet & Lifestyle** offers a powerful tool for fighting cancer and other chronic ailments. The anti-inflammatory, antioxidant-rich nature of whole plant foods, combined with their ability to regulate hormones and immune function, makes this diet a valuable ally in preventing and reversing diseases.

For those willing to adopt this diet and maintain discipline, the rewards can be life-changing. Case studies have shown that cancers, including prostate, colon, and breast cancer, can go into remission when individuals fully commit to a whole-food, plant-based lifestyle. For help learning how to eat a plant-based diet, and which plant-based foods help in the fight to reverse cancer visit thep53.com.

The Role of Vitamin C in Cancer Reversal

Vitamin C, also known as ascorbic acid, is a water-soluble vitamin that plays essential roles in various physiological processes, including immune function, collagen synthesis, and antioxidant protection. Over the past few decades, extensive research has investigated the potential of vitamin C in cancer prevention and treatment. This interest stems from the vitamin's powerful antioxidant properties and its ability to modulate various cellular processes. In this detailed piece, we will explore the role of vitamin C in cancer reversal, focusing on the underlying mechanisms, pathways involved, and the current scientific evidence supporting its efficacy.

Vitamin C has been studied for its anticancer properties since the 1970s, with early work by Nobel laureate Linus Pauling bringing significant attention to the field. Although initial studies showed promise, subsequent research yielded mixed results, leading to skepticism within the medical community. However, recent advances in our understanding of cancer biology and the mechanisms of vitamin C action have reignited interest in its potential role in cancer therapy.

Mechanisms of Action
1. Antioxidant Properties

One of the most well-known functions of vitamin C is its role as a potent antioxidant. Antioxidants protect cells from oxidative stress, a condition characterized by an imbalance between the production of reactive oxygen species (ROS) and the body's ability to detoxify these harmful compounds. Oxidative stress is a critical factor in cancer development, as it can lead to DNA damage, mutations, and the activation of oncogenes (genes that promote cancer).

Vitamin C exerts its antioxidant effects by donating electrons to neutralize ROS, thereby preventing oxidative damage to cellular components such as DNA, proteins, and lipids. By reducing oxidative stress, vitamin C helps to maintain cellular integrity and prevent the initiation of cancer.

Pathway Involved:

- **Scavenging Reactive Oxygen Species (ROS):** Vitamin C acts as an electron donor, reducing ROS and preventing oxidative damage. This process involves the conversion of vitamin C (ascorbate) to its oxidized form, dehydroascorbate, which is then recycled back to ascorbate by cellular reductases.

2. Pro-oxidant Activity in Cancer Cells

While vitamin C is an antioxidant in normal cells, it can act as a pro-oxidant in the presence of metal ions such as iron and copper. This dual role is particularly relevant in the context of cancer therapy. In cancer cells, high concentrations of vitamin C can lead to the production of hydrogen peroxide (H_2O_2), a type of ROS that is toxic to cells. Cancer cells, which often have impaired antioxidant defenses compared to normal cells, are more susceptible to oxidative damage induced by H_2O_2.

This pro-oxidant activity of vitamin C can induce cell death in cancer cells through mechanisms such as apoptosis (programmed cell death) and necrosis (uncontrolled cell death). Importantly, normal cells are less affected by this process, making high-dose vitamin C a potential selective anticancer agent.

Pathway Involved:

- **Generation of Hydrogen Peroxide (H_2O_2):** Vitamin C, in the presence of metal ions, undergoes a redox reaction that generates H_2O_2. This leads to oxidative stress in cancer cells, triggering cell death pathways such as apoptosis and necrosis.

3. Inhibition of Hypoxia-Inducible Factor 1 (HIF-1)

Hypoxia, or low oxygen levels, is a common feature of solid tumors and contributes to cancer progression and resistance to therapy. Hypoxia-inducible factor 1 (HIF-1) is a transcription factor that plays a key role in the cellular response to hypoxia by promoting the expression of genes involved in angiogenesis (formation of new blood vessels), metabolism, and survival.

Vitamin C has been shown to inhibit the activity of HIF-1, thereby reducing the ability of cancer cells to adapt to hypoxic conditions. This inhibition is achieved through the stabilization of HIF-1α, the oxygen-sensitive subunit of HIF-1, which leads to its degradation and prevents the activation of hypoxia-responsive genes.

Pathway Involved:

- **HIF-1α Stabilization and Degradation:** Vitamin C promotes the hydroxylation of HIF-1α, marking it for degradation by the proteasome. This reduces HIF-1 activity and impairs the ability of cancer cells to survive under hypoxic conditions.

4. Enhancement of Immune Function

The immune system plays a crucial role in recognizing and eliminating cancer cells. Vitamin C is essential for the proper functioning of various immune cells, including neutrophils, macrophages, and natural killer (NK) cells. It enhances the ability of these cells to identify and destroy cancer cells through processes such as phagocytosis and the production of cytotoxic molecules.

Additionally, vitamin C has been shown to support the production and function of T-cells, which are critical for adaptive immunity and the targeting of tumor antigens. By boosting immune function, vitamin C can enhance the body's natural defenses against cancer.

Pathway Involved:

- **Immune Cell Activation:** Vitamin C enhances the activity of immune cells by supporting the production of cytokines, chemokines, and other signaling molecules. This leads to increased immune surveillance and the destruction of cancer cells.

5. Inhibition of Cancer Metastasis

Metastasis, the spread of cancer cells to distant organs, is a major cause of cancer-related mortality. Vitamin C has been shown to inhibit various steps in the metastatic process, including the invasion of surrounding tissues, migration of cancer cells, and the formation of secondary tumors.

One mechanism by which vitamin C inhibits metastasis is through the downregulation of matrix metalloproteinases (MMPs), enzymes that degrade the extracellular matrix and facilitate cancer cell invasion. Additionally, vitamin C can inhibit epithelial-mesenchymal transition (EMT), a process by which cancer cells gain the ability to migrate and invade other tissues.

Pathway Involved:

- **Downregulation of Matrix Metalloproteinases (MMPs):** Vitamin C reduces the expression and activity of MMPs, thereby inhibiting the degradation of the extracellular matrix and preventing cancer cell invasion and metastasis.

Clinical Evidence Supporting Vitamin C in Cancer Therapy
1. High-Dose Intravenous Vitamin C

High-dose intravenous vitamin C (IVC) has been explored as a potential cancer therapy in both preclinical and clinical studies. Unlike oral administration, which is limited by the saturation of intestinal transporters, IVC can achieve plasma concentrations of vitamin C that are several-fold higher, allowing for its pro-oxidant effects in cancer cells.

Several clinical trials have investigated the use of high-dose IVC as an adjunct to conventional cancer therapies such as chemotherapy and radiation. These studies have reported varying degrees of success, with some showing improvements in quality of life, reduced side effects, and prolonged survival.

For example, a phase I clinical trial conducted by Monti et al. (2012) evaluated the safety and efficacy of high-dose IVC in combination with gemcitabine and erlotinib in patients with metastatic pancreatic cancer. The study found that IVC was well-tolerated and showed a trend toward improved survival compared to historical controls.

Another study by Ma et al. (2014) investigated the effects of high-dose IVC in combination with standard chemotherapy in patients with stage III/IV ovarian cancer. The results indicated that IVC reduced chemotherapy-associated toxicity and improved overall survival.

2. Oral Vitamin C and Cancer Prevention

While high-dose IVC is primarily investigated for cancer treatment, oral vitamin C has been studied for its potential role in cancer prevention. Epidemiological studies have shown that higher dietary intake of vitamin C is associated with a reduced risk of certain cancers, including breast, lung, and colorectal cancers.

A meta-analysis by Harris et al. (2014) examined the association between vitamin C intake and breast cancer risk. The analysis included 17 prospective studies and found that higher vitamin C intake was associated with a significant reduction in breast cancer risk, particularly among premenopausal women.

Similarly, a study by Hu et al. (2015) investigated the relationship between dietary vitamin C and lung cancer risk. The study analyzed data from 18 cohort studies and found that higher vitamin C intake was associated with a lower risk of lung cancer, particularly among smokers.

Pathways Involved in Vitamin C's Anticancer Effects

1. The NF-κB Pathway

The nuclear factor kappa B (NF-κB) pathway is a key regulator of inflammation, immune response, and cell survival. It is often constitutively activated in cancer cells, promoting tumor growth, survival, and resistance to therapy. Vitamin C has been shown to inhibit the activation of NF-κB, thereby suppressing the expression of genes involved in inflammation, cell proliferation, and survival.

Mechanism:

Vitamin C inhibits the phosphorylation and degradation of IκBα, an inhibitor of NF-κB. This prevents the translocation of NF-κB to the nucleus and the activation of target genes that promote cancer progression.

2. The MAPK/ERK Pathway

The mitogen-activated protein kinase (MAPK)/extracellular signal-regulated kinase (ERK) pathway is involved in the regulation of cell proliferation, differentiation, and survival. Dysregulation of this pathway is commonly observed in various cancers. Vitamin C has been reported to modulate the MAPK/ERK pathway, leading to the inhibition of cancer cell proliferation and the induction of apoptosis.

Mechanism:

Vitamin C induces the activation of MAPK phosphatases (MKPs), which dephosphorylate and inactivate ERK. This results in the suppression of cell proliferation and the induction of apoptosis in cancer cells.

3. The p53 Pathway

The tumor suppressor protein p53 plays a critical role in maintaining genomic stability and preventing cancer development. p53 is often mutated or inactivated in cancer cells, allowing them to evade apoptosis and continue proliferating. Vitamin C has been shown to enhance the activity of p53, thereby promoting cell cycle arrest and apoptosis in cancer cells.

Mechanism:

Vitamin C stabilizes p53 by promoting its acetylation and preventing its degradation by the proteasome. This leads to the activation of p53 target genes that induce cell cycle arrest and apoptosis in cancer cells.

Despite the promising evidence supporting the use of vitamin C in cancer therapy, several challenges remain. One major challenge is the variability in response among patients, which may be influenced by factors such as cancer type, stage, and genetic background. Additionally, the optimal dosing regimen and route of administration (oral vs. intravenous) for vitamin C in cancer therapy have not been fully established.

Future research should focus on identifying the patient populations that are most likely to benefit from vitamin C therapy, as well as optimizing dosing strategies.

Vitamin C is a versatile molecule with significant potential in cancer therapy. Its ability to modulate various molecular pathways, enhance immune function, and selectively induce cell death in cancer cells makes it a promising adjunct to conventional cancer treatments. While challenges remain, ongoing research continues to shed light on the mechanisms by which vitamin C exerts its anticancer effects and its potential role in cancer prevention and treatment.

The integration of vitamin C into cancer therapy holds promise for improving patient outcomes, reducing treatment-related toxicity, and enhancing the overall efficacy of cancer treatments. As our understanding of vitamin C's role in cancer biology deepens, it is likely that this simple yet powerful nutrient will become an increasingly important tool in the fight against cancer.

Finding Testimonies

The internet is teeming with stories of people who have successfully battled cancer through plant-based diets alone, and these testimonies offer hope to others navigating similar health challenges. Across blogs, social media platforms, and health forums, individuals recount how transitioning to a diet focused on whole, plant-based foods helped them not only manage their cancer but, in many cases, reverse it.

These accounts typically emphasize the power of nutrition in strengthening the body's natural defenses against cancer. By removing animal products and processed foods, people report experiencing dramatic improvements in their health, energy levels, and overall well-being. The stories highlight how a plant-based diet, rich in fruits, vegetables, whole grains, legumes, nuts, and seeds, provides the body with essential nutrients that support the immune system and foster an anti-inflammatory environment. This, in turn, reduces the likelihood of cancerous cells thriving.

Several individuals have shared their journeys, explaining that they were initially diagnosed with late-stage cancers, sometimes after being told that their options were limited. Many chose to forgo traditional treatments such as chemotherapy and radiation, while others supplemented these treatments with plant-based eating. They credit their survival to the detoxifying and healing properties of plants, which are packed with antioxidants, fiber, and phytonutrients. These compounds are believed to play a crucial role in fighting cancer by neutralizing harmful free radicals, improving digestion, and promoting apoptosis (the death of cancer cells).

While these success stories abound, it is important to note that each case is unique, and the outcomes can vary. For some, plant-based diets worked alongside other lifestyle changes such as stress reduction, exercise, and mindfulness practices. The common thread in these accounts is a focus on natural, unprocessed foods and a belief in the body's ability to heal itself when given the right tools.

These inspiring testimonies, which can be found across countless blogs, YouTube channels, and support groups, underscore the growing movement of individuals turning to plant-based nutrition as a means of taking control of their health. Although further scientific research is needed to fully understand the mechanisms at play, these stories have sparked hope and encouraged many to explore the potential healing power of plants. I also encourage you to read the testimonials on the p53diet.com website.

Guide to Finding Testimonies:

1. **Explore Websites and Organizations**:
    - **The Truth About Cancer**: This site shares many stories from individuals who have reversed cancer through holistic treatments, including plant-based diets.
    - **Forks Over Knives**: An excellent resource for plant-based success stories, including cancer survivors.
    - **American Institute for Cancer Research (AICR)**: Though more focused on scientific studies, this site includes survivor stories tied to nutrition.
    - **The Gerson Therapy**: A famous alternative cancer treatment that includes testimonies from people who reversed their cancer through plant-based nutrition.
    - **Chris Beat Cancer**: Chris Wark is a famous cancer survivor who runs a blog and platform with various survivor stories focused on diet and alternative treatments.
2. **Use Cancer-Focused Blogs and Forums**:
    - Many forums like **HealingWell** and **Cancer Survivors Network** have sections where survivors share their dietary choices, including plant-based diets.
3. **Books on Plant-Based Cancer Recovery**:
    - Books like **"Radical Remission" by Kelly A. Turner** and **"Chris Beat Cancer" by Chris Wark** are filled with testimonials of people who survived cancer through lifestyle and diet changes.
4. **Documentary Interviews**:
    - Documentaries like **"What the Health"** and **"The Game Changers"** feature cancer survivors who discuss the role of a plant-based diet.

11

Call to Action

Cancer is one of the leading causes of death worldwide, and many patients feel powerless against this complex disease. However, a growing body of research suggests that a plant-based diet can be an effective approach to not only prevent cancer but also help reverse its progression. A plant-based diet emphasizes whole foods, including fruits, vegetables, whole grains, legumes, and seeds, all of which provide essential nutrients and antioxidants that combat oxidative stress, inflammation, and abnormal cell growth—key factors in the development and progression of cancer.

In contrast to conventional cancer treatments like chemotherapy, radiation, and surgery, which come with a host of side effects, adopting a plant-based diet offers a natural, non-invasive method of healing. This call to action is aimed at people with cancer who are seeking a holistic approach to manage and potentially reverse their disease. By embracing a plant-based lifestyle, patients may find renewed hope and a more balanced, sustainable pathway to health without relying on Western medicine.

As mentioned earlier in this book, I have demonstrated how a plant-based diet combats cancer, highlighting specific foods proven to prevent and reverse various types of cancer. Additionally, I provide a comprehensive, step-by-step action plan for transitioning to a plant-based lifestyle.

The Science Behind Plant-Based Diets and Cancer
Antioxidants and Phytochemicals

One of the most potent ways a plant-based diet fights cancer is through the abundance of antioxidants and phytochemicals in plants. These compounds help neutralize free radicals, which are unstable molecules that cause oxidative stress and damage cells. This damage can lead to DNA mutations, contributing to cancer development.

Fruits and vegetables are particularly rich in antioxidants, such as vitamins C and E, flavonoids, and carotenoids, which protect cells from oxidative damage. According to a study published in *Nutrition and Cancer*, higher intake of fruits and vegetables is associated with a significantly lower risk of various cancers, including breast, lung, and colon cancers.

Phytochemicals, such as sulforaphane in cruciferous vegetables and lycopene in tomatoes, have been shown to induce cancer cell death, inhibit tumor growth, and reduce the spread of cancerous cells. For example, a study published in *Cancer Research* demonstrated that sulforaphane can selectively target and kill breast cancer stem cells while leaving healthy cells intact.

Anti-Inflammatory Properties

Chronic inflammation is a well-established factor in cancer development and progression. A plant-based diet, which is rich in anti-inflammatory foods such as leafy greens, berries, nuts, and seeds, can help reduce inflammation in the body. According to a study published in *The Journal of Nutrition*, people who follow plant-based diets have lower levels of inflammatory markers, such as C-reactive protein (CRP), compared to those who consume meat and processed foods.

Turmeric, a spice commonly used in plant-based cooking, contains curcumin, a compound with powerful anti-inflammatory and anti-cancer properties. Curcumin has been shown to inhibit the growth of various cancer cells, including those of the breast, colon, pancreas, and prostate.

Fiber and Gut Health

A high intake of dietary fiber, found exclusively in plant foods, is another key factor in cancer prevention and reversal. Fiber helps regulate bowel movements, reducing the time that potential carcinogens stay in contact with the colon lining, thereby lowering the risk of colon cancer. Additionally, fiber promotes the growth of healthy gut bacteria, which produce short-chain fatty acids like butyrate that have been shown to inhibit cancer cell growth.

A study published in *The Lancet Oncology* found that people with higher fiber intake had a reduced risk of developing colorectal cancer by up to 25%. Furthermore, the American Institute for Cancer Research recommends a plant-based diet rich in fiber to help protect against cancer recurrence.

The Role of Animal Products in Cancer Development

Numerous studies have linked the consumption of animal products, including meat, dairy, and eggs, with an increased risk of cancer. Animal products are often high in saturated fats, cholesterol, and hormones, which promote inflammation, oxidative stress, and abnormal cell growth.

Red and Processed Meat

The World Health Organization (WHO) classifies processed meat as a Group 1 carcinogen, meaning there is sufficient evidence that it causes cancer, particularly colorectal cancer. Red meat is classified as a Group 2A carcinogen, meaning it is likely to cause cancer. A comprehensive meta-analysis published in *PLOS Medicine* found that higher consumption of red and processed meats was associated with a significant increase in the risk of colorectal, pancreatic, and prostate cancers.

Heme iron, found in animal products, has also been shown to promote cancer growth by catalyzing the formation of harmful free radicals. In contrast, non-heme iron from plant-based sources is absorbed more slowly and regulated by the body, reducing the risk of oxidative damage.

Dairy and Hormones

Dairy products, especially those high in fat, have been implicated in the development of hormone-sensitive cancers, such as breast and prostate cancer. Dairy contains hormones like estrogen, which can stimulate the growth of hormone-dependent cancer cells. According to a study published in *The Journal of the National Cancer Institute*, men who consumed higher amounts of dairy had a 30% higher risk of developing prostate cancer.

Specific Plant-Based Foods That Fight Cancer
Cruciferous Vegetables

Cruciferous vegetables, such as broccoli, cauliflower, kale, and Brussels sprouts, contain sulforaphane, a potent anticancer compound that has been shown to inhibit the growth of cancer cells and promote apoptosis (programmed cell death). Studies have demonstrated the effectiveness of these vegetables in reducing the risk of lung, breast, prostate, and colon cancers.

Berries

Berries, including blueberries, strawberries, and raspberries, are rich in antioxidants and polyphenols that protect against cancer. They contain ellagic acid, a compound that can deactivate cancer-causing substances and slow the growth of cancer cells.

Turmeric

As mentioned earlier, turmeric contains curcumin, a powerful anti-inflammatory and anticancer compound. A study published in *Cancer Letters* found that curcumin could inhibit the proliferation of cancer cells and induce apoptosis in a variety of cancers, including breast, colon, and pancreatic cancers.

Flaxseeds

Flaxseeds are an excellent source of lignans, a type of phytoestrogen that has been shown to reduce the risk of hormone-sensitive cancers, such as breast and prostate cancer. A study published in *Clinical Cancer Research* found that flaxseed supplementation slowed the growth of prostate cancer tumors in men.

Green Tea

Green tea contains catechins, particularly epigallocatechin gallate (EGCG), which has been shown to inhibit cancer cell growth and reduce the spread of tumors. A meta-analysis published in *Cancer Epidemiology, Biomarkers & Prevention*found that regular consumption of green tea was associated with a reduced risk of breast, prostate, and lung cancers.

A Step-by-Step Call to Action for Cancer Reversal
Step 1: Eliminate Animal Products

The first step in transitioning to a plant-based diet is to eliminate all animal products from your diet, including meat, dairy, eggs, and processed foods. These foods have been linked to increased cancer risk and can promote inflammation and oxidative stress in the body.

Gradually replace animal products with plant-based alternatives, such as legumes, tofu, tempeh, and seitan, which provide ample protein and essential nutrients without the harmful effects of animal products.

Step 2: Increase Your Intake of Whole, Plant-Based Foods

Focus on consuming a wide variety of whole, plant-based foods to ensure you're getting all the essential nutrients your body needs to fight cancer. Prioritize fruits, vegetables, whole grains, legumes, nuts, seeds, and herbs.

Aim to include a rainbow of colors in your diet, as different plant pigments offer unique health benefits. For example, red fruits and vegetables are rich in lycopene, which has been shown to reduce the risk of prostate cancer, while dark green vegetables are high in chlorophyll, which has detoxifying properties.

Step 3: Incorporate Cancer-Fighting Foods Daily

Make it a point to include specific cancer-fighting foods in your daily meals. For example, add cruciferous vegetables like broccoli and kale to salads or stir-fries, sprinkle flaxseeds on oatmeal or smoothies, and brew a cup of green tea in the morning.

Experiment with plant-based recipes that feature these powerful foods. For instance, try a turmeric-spiced lentil soup, a berry smoothie bowl, or roasted Brussels sprouts with flaxseed oil for added omega-3s.

Step 4: Stay Hydrated with Antioxidant-Rich Beverages

In addition to eating plant-based foods, stay hydrated with beverages that support cancer prevention and healing. Green tea, herbal teas, and smoothies made with leafy greens and berries can provide additional antioxidants and anti-inflammatory compounds.

Avoid sugary beverages, as excess sugar has been linked to cancer progression by fueling the rapid growth of cancer cells.

Step 5: Reduce Stress and Prioritize Sleep

Chronic stress and lack of sleep can weaken the immune system and promote cancer progression. Engage in stress-reducing activities such as meditation, yoga, and deep breathing exercises to lower cortisol levels and reduce inflammation. Ensure you're getting at least 7–8 hours of quality sleep each night, as sleep is essential for cell repair and immune function.

Step 6: Engage in Regular Physical Activity

While diet plays a crucial role in cancer prevention and reversal, physical activity is also essential for maintaining a healthy body and reducing cancer risk. Regular exercise helps regulate hormone levels, improve immune function, and reduce inflammation.

According to the American Cancer Society, engaging in at least 150 minutes of moderate-intensity exercise per week is associated with a reduced risk of several cancers, including breast, colon, and endometrial cancers.

Cancer is a complex disease, but there is hope in the power of a plant-based diet to prevent and potentially reverse its progression. The evidence is overwhelming: whole, plant-based foods provide the nutrients, antioxidants, and anti-inflammatory compounds needed to fight cancer at its root.

By eliminating animal products, focusing on nutrient-dense plant foods, and incorporating cancer-fighting superfoods into your daily meals, you can take control of your health and reduce your dependence on Western medicine. Along with regular exercise, stress management, and quality sleep, a plant-based lifestyle offers a comprehensive, natural approach to cancer prevention and healing.

The transition to a plant-based diet may not be easy at first, but the rewards are immense. This call to action is not only about reclaiming your health but also about empowering yourself with the knowledge that you can fight back against cancer—naturally, and without harmful side effects.

Closing Statement

As we come to the end of *"Taste Versus Cancer,"* my deepest hope is that the knowledge shared throughout these pages serves as a transformative guide for those battling cancer. The insights I've provided are rooted in a profound understanding of the human body's intricate systems and the powerful role that nutrition plays in reversing disease. I sincerely hope that, in writing this book, I have inspired people to take control of their health, recognize the extraordinary healing potential of a plant-based lifestyle, and most importantly, take steps to reverse their cancer.

This book is also intended for the loved ones of those suffering from cancer. Too often, families and friends feel powerless in the face of a loved one's diagnosis, unsure of what to believe or where to turn for guidance. I have written *"Taste Versus Cancer "* with the truth at its core, to help guide those closest to cancer patients on the path to real, science-backed solutions. Together, through understanding and knowledge, we can offer support, hope, and the truth that too many people never hear. The fact remains: too many people are dying needlessly. So much of the suffering caused by cancer is preventable through dietary and lifestyle changes, and yet, so few are aware of the power that lies in their own hands.

If you've made it to this point, I want to encourage you to continue exploring these truths. I invite you to delve deeper into the mechanisms of cancer, disease, and healing by picking up my other books, each crafted with the same dedication to uncovering what makes us sick and, more importantly, how we can reclaim our health.

- *P53 Diet & Lifestyle* – 522 pages
- *How You Are Being Poisoned* – 840 pages
- *Understanding Hormones, Enzymes & Cell Receptors* – 840 pages

These books are available on Amazon and at thep53.com/publishing. Each of these works provides a comprehensive examination of different aspects of our health and the profound impact that diet and environmental factors have on it.

Moreover, for those seeking an even deeper understanding of the role nutrition plays in preventing and reversing disease, I have developed an online certification course, the *Plant-Based Nutrition Specialist* program, available at P53University.com. This course is not only for those seeking certification but also for anyone who wishes to gain an in-depth understanding of how the human body works and how plant-based nutrition can keep it functioning optimally. This course is very detailed and will arm you with the knowledge to transform your health and help others do the same.

In closing, I urge you not to see this book as the end of your journey but as the beginning. Whether you or a loved one are fighting cancer, or you simply want to prevent disease and live a healthier life, the path forward is clear. A plant-based lifestyle is not just a dietary choice—it is a lifeline. It is the most powerful tool we have in the fight against cancer and other chronic diseases.

Together, through knowledge, action, and dedication to a healthier way of life, we can change the narrative around cancer. Too many lives have been lost. Now is the time to reverse that trend, to arm ourselves with the truth, and to take control of our health. Let *"Taste Versus Cancer"* be your guide as you embark on this life-changing journey, and may the information in these pages help to empower you, to heal, and to give you hope for a future free from the shadow of cancer.

The Truth is Clear, based on research studies...
.....*that antibiotics are linked to cancer development*
.....*that food additives are linked to cancer*
.....*that animal products are linked to cancer*
.....*that toxins are linked to cancer*
.....*that a plant-based diet can lower the risk of cancer development*
.....*that a plant-based diet can reverse certain cancers.*

Thank you for reading, and I wish you health, happiness, and a life filled with vitality.

With gratitude,
David W. Brown

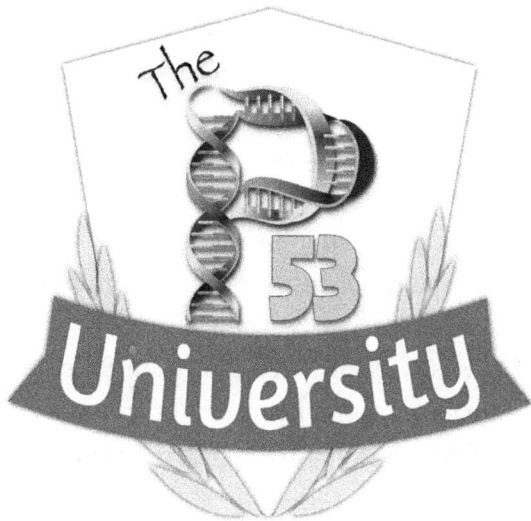

The P53 University Plant-Based Nutrition Specialist Course offers an unparalleled opportunity for individuals to become experts in plant-based nutrition, equipping them with the tools to make a profound impact on health and wellness. This course stands out for its in-depth focus on the science behind plant-based eating, including how it can prevent, manage, and even reverse chronic diseases like heart disease, diabetes, and cancer. With the rise of dietary-related illnesses, the knowledge gained from this program is not only timely but essential.

Students who enroll will gain a comprehensive understanding of biochemistry processes, human body organs, and how toxins impact health. They'll dive deep into amino acids, learning how they function in plant-based nutrition, as well as explore how different cancers and ailments can be managed or reversed through diet. Additionally, the course emphasizes the nutritional values of fruits, vegetables, whole grains, nuts, and seeds, giving students the knowledge to help others achieve optimal health.

The curriculum provides an evidence-based approach that empowers students to guide others in adopting a healthier, plant-based lifestyle. Graduates of the P53 University course will be recognized as Plant-Based Nutrition Specialists, a credential that opens doors to numerous career opportunities in health coaching, wellness consulting, and public health education. Whether you're a healthcare professional looking to expand your knowledge, or an individual passionate about helping others achieve better health, this course is designed to provide the expertise and confidence you need to make a difference.

The P53 University Plant-Based Nutrition Specialist Course is not just about learning—it's about being part of a movement that's reshaping the future of health. By enrolling, you become an advocate for a sustainable, compassionate, and scientifically proven approach to nutrition, paving the way for a healthier world.

www.ingramcontent.com/pod-product-compliance
Lightning Source LLC
Chambersburg PA
CBHW051707020426
42333CB00014B/876